Basic Medical Sciences For MRCP Part 1

For Churchill Livingstone

Publisher: Laurence Hunter
Project Editor: Janice Urquhart
Copy Editor: Teresa Brady
Design Direction: Erik Bigland
Project Controller: Frances Affleck

Basic Medical Sciences For MRCP Part 1

Philippa J. Easterbrook
MB BChir BSc (Hons) MRCP DTM & H, MPH
Professor of Infectious Diseases and HIV, Guy's, Kings and St Thomas' School of Medicine, Kings College Hospital, London; Formerly Senior Lecturer in Infectious Diseases, Imperial College School of Medicine, Chelsea and Westminster Hospital, London

SECOND EDITION

CHURCHILL LIVINGSTONE
EDINBURGH LONDON NEW YORK OXFORD PHILADELPHIA ST LOUIS
SYDNEY TORONTO 1999

CHURCHILL LIVINGSTONE
An imprint of Elsevier Limited

First published 1994
Second edition 1999
Reprinted 2001, 2002, 2004

ISBN 0 443 06156 4

British Library Cataloguing in Publication Data
A catalogue record for this book is available from the British Library.

Library of Congress Cataloging in Publication Data
A catalog record for this book is available from the Library of Congress.

Printed in China
B/04

Preface

An understanding of the scientific principles underlying disease pathogenesis provides the basis for a more rational approach to the management of clinical problems. Recognition of the importance of the basic sciences in medicine has led to a growing emphasis on such questions in both the MRCP Part 1 and 2 examinations. However, many doctors, once involved in clinical work rapidly forget the basic science information they learned for examinations in their pre-clinical years. This book was written as the result of a need for a concise revision guide of the core basic sciences, namely genetics, microbiology, immunology, anatomy, physiology, biochemistry, statistics and epidemiology. It is intended primarily for MRCP Part 1 candidates, although those studying for other postgraduate examinations, such as the US Medical Licensing Examination (MLE) and PLAB, may also find it useful. Information is presented in the form of lists, tables, flow diagrams and simple illustrations to provide a useful framework for revision of the important concepts and facts. A chapter on clinical pharmacology has also been included since many of the Part 1 multiple choice questions on this subject focus on drug-induced disease and drug interactions, which are not covered adequately by other MRCP exam tests. No book of this length covering such a wide area could hope to be comprehensive, and I have therefore concentrated on recurring examination themes and topical issues. When a particular topic is unfamiliar or a point needs further clarification, one of the basic science textbooks listed in the reference section should be consulted.

In this second edition the immunology and genetics chapters have been updated, and there is a new section on molecular medicine contributed by Dr Kevin Talbot. A series of new illustrations has also been added to the anatomy chapter.

I am grateful to many former colleagues at the John Radcliffe Hospital in Oxford, the Johns Hopkins University School of Medicine in Baltimore and at the Chelsea and Westminster Hospital who provided valuable criticism on the contents of each chapter.

I would appreciate any corrections, clarifications or suggestions for future editions.

London
1998

P.J.E.

Contents

Recommended Reference Books

GENETICS AND MOLECULAR MEDICINE

Connor J M, Ferguson-Smith M A 1997 Essential medical genetics, 5th edn. Blackwell Science

Rimoin D L, Connor J M, Pyeritz R E 1996 Emery and Rimoin's Principles and practice of medical genetics, 3rd edn. Churchill Livingstone

Trent R J A 1997 Molecular medicine: an introductory text, 2nd edn. Churchill Livingstone

MICROBIOLOGY

Brooks G F 1995 Medical microbiology, 20th edn. Appleton and Lange

Elliot T, Hastings M, Desselberger N 1997 Lecture notes on clinical microbiology, 3rd edn. Blackwell Science

Zuckerman A J 1995 Principles of practice of clinical virology, 3rd edn. Wiley

IMMUNOLOGY

Reeves G, Todd I 1996 Lecture notes on immunology, 3rd edn. Blackwell Science

Roitt I 1997 Essential immunology, 9th edn. Blackwell Science

Roitt I, Brostoff J, Male D 1996 Immunology, 4th edn. Mosby

ANATOMY

Ellis H 1997 Clinical anatomy, 9th edn. Blackwell Science

Sinnatamby C 1999 Last's anatomy: regional and applied, 10th edn. Churchill Livingstone

Moore K L 1992 Clinically orientated anatomy, 3rd edn. William and Wilkins

Snell R S 1995 Clinical anatomy for medical students, 5th edn. Little, Brown and Co

PHYSIOLOGY

Ganong W R 1997 Review of medical physiology, 18th edn. Appleton and Lange

Guyton A C, Hall J E 1996 Textbook of medical physiology, 9th edn. Saunders

BIOCHEMISTRY

Marshall W J 1995 Clinical chemistry, 3rd edn. Mosby

Murray R K 1996 Harper's biochemistry, 24th edn. Appleton and Lange
Stryer L 1995 Biochemistry, 4th edn. W H Freeman
Smith A F, Beckett G J, Walker S W, Rae P 1998 Lecture notes on clinical biochemistry, 6th edn. Blackwell Science

STATISTICS AND EPIDEMIOLOGY

Altman D G 1990 Practical statistics for medical research. Chapman and Hall
Barker D J P, Cooper C, Rose G 1998 Epidemiology in medical practice, 5th edn. Churchill Livingstone
Bland M 1995 Introduction to medical statistics, 2nd edn. Oxford University Press
Fletcher R H, Fletcher S W, Wagner E H 1996 Clinical epidemiology: the essentials, 3rd edn. Williams and Wilkins

CLINICAL PHARMACOLOGY

Davies D M 1991 Textbook of adverse drug reactions, 4th edn. Oxford University Press
Goodman L, Gilman A 1996 Pharmacological basis of therapeutics, 9th edn. Pergamon/McGraw
Laurence D R, Bennett P N, Brown M J 1997 Clinical pharmacology, 8th edn. Churchill Livingstone
Reid J L 1996 Lecture notes on clinical pharmacology, 5th edn. Blackwell Science

1. Genetics and molecular medicine

CHAPTER CONTENTS

GLOSSARY

Alleles: Alternative forms of a gene found at the same locus on a particular chromosome.

Amplification: (i) Treatment designed to increase the proportion of plasmid DNA relative to that of bacterial DNA.

(ii) Replication of a gene library in bulk. (See polymerase chain reaction page 16.)

Aneuploidy: A chromosome profile with fewer or greater than the normal diploid number: e.g. 45 (Turner's syndrome) or 47 (Down's syndrome) chromosomes.

Antisense technology: Use of synthetic nucleotide sequences, complementary to specific DNA or RNA sequences, to block expression of a gene.

Autosome: Any chromosome other than the sex chromosomes: i.e. 22 pairs in humans.

Barr body: All X chromosomes in excess of one per cell are inactivated so that only one is active (Lyon hypothesis), which is visible in interphase as a dark-staining Barr body: i.e. no Barr body in male or XO female.

cDNA: A single-stranded DNA complementary to an RNA, synthesized from it by the enzyme reverse transcriptase in vitro; often used as a probe in chromosome mapping.

Chimera: An individual composed of two populations of cells from different genotypes: e.g. blood group chimerism.

Chromatids: Equal halves of a chromosome following replication.

Chromosome mapping: The assigning of a gene or other DNA sequence to a particular position on a specific chromosome.

Clone: A cell line derived by mitosis from a single diploid cell.

Cloning: The isolation of a particular gene or DNA sequence. In recombinant technology, genes or DNA sequences are cloned by inserting them into a bacterium or other microorganism, which is then selected and propagated.

Concordant twins: Members of a pair of twins exhibiting the same trait. (See also discordant twins.)

Conserved sequence: A DNA sequence that has remained virtually unchanged throughout evolution. This is usually taken to imply that the sequence has an important function.

Deletion: A chromosomal aberration in which part of the chromosome is lost.

Diploid: The chromosome number of a somatic cell: i.e. 46 in humans.

Discordant twins: Only one twin has the trait. (See also concordant twins.)

Dizygotic twins: Twins produced by two separately fertilized

	ova: i.e. no more genetically similar than brothers and sisters (see also monozygotic twins).
DNA fingerprinting:	A pattern of DNA sequences, e.g. tandem repeat sequences, unique to an individual. This DNA profile can be detected in cells (e.g. blood or semen) and can be used in criminal cases and paternity suits.
Exon:	Portion of the DNA that codes for the final mRNA and is then translated into protein.
Expressivity:	Variation in the level of expression of a particular gene.
Gamete:	Haploid sperm or egg cell.
Gene:	A region of DNA that encodes a protein.
Gene therapy:	See p. 17.
Genome:	The complete set of genes of an organism and the intervening DNA sequences. The Human Genome Project is an international research programme aimed at mapping all the genes in the human genome.
Genotype:	The genetic constitution of an individual, usually at a particular locus.
Haploid:	The chromosome number of a normal gamete: i.e. 23 in humans.
Haplotype:	The particular combination of alleles in a defined region of a chromosome. Originally used to define the HLA type of an individual, it is now routinely used to describe any combination of alleles, such as those used in prenatal diagnosis by genetic linkage.
Heteroploidy:	Abnormal appearance of the karyotype due to alteration in the (i) number of chromosomes or (ii) their shape and form.
Homologous chromosomes:	The two matching members of a pair of chromosomes.
Hybridization:	The joining of the complementary sequences of DNA (or DNA and RNA) by base pairing.
Index case:	See **proband**.
In situ hybridization:	Use of a labelled probe to detect any complementary DNA or RNA sequence in a tissue section, cultured cell or cloned bacterial cell.
Intron:	Intervening sequence on DNA that does not appear in the final RNA transcript.
Karyotype:	The presentation of a cellular chromosome profile. Normal human karyotype is 44 autosomes and two sex chromosomes – XX female, XY male.
Library:	A collection of DNA clones representing

either all expressed genes – a cDNA library – or a whole genome – a genomic library.

Linkage disequilibrium: The association of two linked alleles more frequently than would be expected by chance.

Linkage map: A map of the relative positions of gene loci on a chromosome deduced from the frequency with which they are inherited together.

Locus: Site of a gene on a chromosome.

Meiosis: Sex cell division or reduction division. Formation of gametes with half the number of chromosomes (haploid) as the parent cell (diploid): i.e. 23.

Mitosis: Somatic cell division: Each daughter cell has the same complement of chromosomes as the parent: i.e. 46.

Monozygotic twins: Twins produced from a single fertilized ovum. (See also dizygotic twins.)

Mosaic: An individual with abnormal genotypic or phenotypic variation from cell to cell within the same tissue.

Non-dysjunction: The failure of two members of a chromosome to separate during cell division, so that both pass to the same daughter cell.

Northern blotting: See p. 12.

Oncogenes: Genes of either viral or mammalian origin that cause transformation of cells in culture. In normal cells, they are 'switched-off' or downregulated. They have copies in both viruses (v-onc) and mammalian cells (c-onc or protooncogenes) and have products that are essential to normal cell function or development. These include proteins (guanine-nucleotide binding proteins), cell surface receptors (epidermal growth factor receptor), and cellular growth factors (platelet-derived growth factor).

Penetrance: The proportion of individuals with a given genotype (usually a disease-causing mutation) manifesting a phenotype (usually a disease).

Phage: Virus that multiplies in bacteria.

Phenotype: The characteristics of an organism which result from an interaction between gene (the genotype) and environment.

Physical mapping: A linear map of the location of genes on a chromosome, as determined by the physical detection of overlaps between cloned DNA fragments rather than by linkage analysis.

Plasmid:	An autonomously replicating DNA element, separate from the chromosome. These units, which only occur in bacteria, can be used as vectors of small fragments of foreign DNA.
Pleiotropy:	The production of multiple effects by a single gene.
Polymerase chain reaction:	See p. 16.
Polymorphism:	The occurrence in one population of two or more genetically determined forms (alleles), all of which are too frequent to be ascribed to mutation: e.g. blood group systems, the HLA system and various forms of G6PDH deficiency.
Polyploidy:	Homologous chromosome numbers in more than two complete sets: i.e. three sets: triploid or 69 chromosomes, four sets: tetraploid or 92 chromosomes.
Primer (oligonucleotide primer):	A short DNA sequence used to initiate the synthesis of DNA, as in a polymerase chain reaction.
Proband or propositus:	The family member who first presents with a given trait.
Probe:	A specific DNA sequence, radioactively or fluorescently labelled, used with hybridization techniques to detect complementary sequences in a sample of genetic material.
Protooncogene:	See p. 29.
Reporter gene:	A gene whose product can be used as a genetic 'label'. For example, a gene for neomycin resistance incorporated into a plasmid before transfection allows the detection of successfully transfected cells.
Restriction endonuclease:	An enzyme that cleaves DNA at a specific site.
Restriction fragment length: polymorphism (RFLP):	See p. 12.
Reverse transcription:	DNA synthesis from RNA templates, catalysed by the enzyme reverse transcriptase. It is used to synthesize DNA for probes and occurs naturally in retroviruses.
Southern blotting:	See p. 13.
Splicing:	The removal of introns from messenger RNA and the joining together of adjacent exons.
Tandem repeat sequences:	Multiple copies of a short DNA sequence lying in a series along a chromosome; used in physical mapping, linkage mapping and also

in DNA fingerprinting because each person's pattern of tandem repeats is likely to be unique.

Tetraploid: See **polyploidy**.

Transfection: The transfer of new genetic material into cells.

Translocation: The transfer of genetic material from one chromosome to another non-homologous chromosome.

Transposition: Movement from one site in the genome to another.

Transposon: A segment of DNA that can move from one position in the genome to another.

Triploid: See polyploidy.

Trisomy: The presence of an extra chromosome, rather than the usual diploid set: i.e. 47 in humans.

Tumour suppressor gene (antioncogene): See p. 30.

Vector: A DNA molecule, usually derived from a virus or bacterial plasmid, which acts as a vehicle to introduce foreign DNA into host cells for cloning, and then to recover it.

Zygote: Fertilized egg.

NUCLEIC ACIDS

NUCLEIC ACID STRUCTURE

All nucleic acids are polynucleotides. A nucleotide consists of three components (Fig. 1.1):

1. a base
2. a pentose sugar
3. 1–3 phosphate groups.

There are two kinds of nucleic acids:
- deoxyribonucleic acid (DNA)
- ribonucleic acid (RNA).

DNA (Tables 1.1 and 1.2)

- Double-stranded, double helix. Found primarily in the chromosomes of the cell nucleus.
- Two polynucleotide chains are antiparallel (i.e. one chain runs in a 5′ to 3′ direction; the other runs 3′ to 5′) and held together by hydrogen bonds between the bases:
  adenine pairs only with thymidine (2 hydrogen bonds)
  guanine pairs only with cytosine (3 hydrogen bonds).

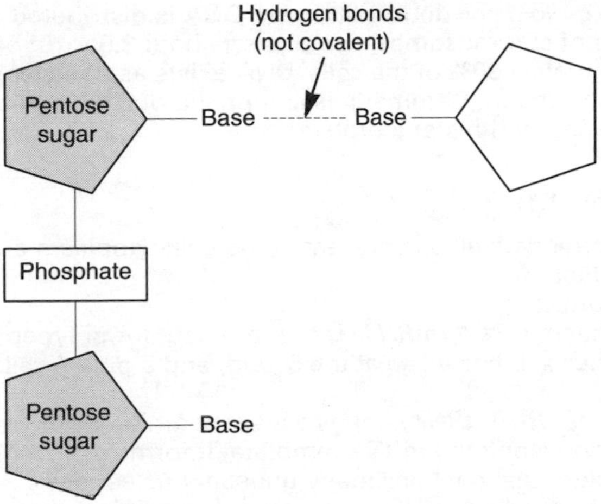

Fig. 1.1

Table 1.1 Proportions of different types of nuclear DNA

Type of DNA	*Percentage of total DNA*
Single copy	70
Repetitive DNA	30
Tandem repeats	(10)
Microsatellites	
Minisatellites	
Macrosatellites	
Interspersed repeats	(20)
Short interspersed repeats (SINES)	
Long interspersed repeats (LINES)	

Table 1.2 Structure of nucleic acids

Nucleic acid	*Sugar*	*Bases*		*Monomeric unit**
		Purines†	*Pyrimidines*	
DNA	2′ Deoxy-ribose	Adenine (A) Guanine (G)	Thymidine (T) Cytosine (C)	Deoxyribonucleotides, e.g. adenylic acid (AMP), thymidylic acid (TMP)
RNA	Ribose	Adenine (A) Guanine (G)	Uracil (U) Cytosine (C)	Ribonucleotides, e.g. adenylic acid (AMP), uridylic acid (UMP)

*If the sugar is not phosphorylated, the structure is called a nucleoside.
†Xanthine and hypoxanthine are also purines.

- In each *diploid cell* double-stranded DNA is distributed between 23 pairs of chromosomes, comprising about 3.5×10^9 base pairs.
- Approximately 90% of the cells' DNA exists as a nucleoprotein called chromatin. Chromatin is comprised of DNA and both histone and non-histone proteins.

RNA (Table 1.1)

- Single-stranded; 90% is present in the cell cytoplasm and 10% in the nucleolus.
- Three forms:
  1. *Messenger RNA (mRNA)* is the template for polypeptide synthesis. It has a cap at the 5′ end, and a poly A tail at the 3′ end.
  2. *Transfer RNA (tRNA)* brings activated amino acids into position along the mRNA template. It forms a cloverleaf structure that contains many unusual nucleotides.
  3. *Ribosomal RNA (rRNA)* is a component of ribosomes which functions as a non-specific site of polypeptide synthesis. In eukaryotic cells, there are four rRNA molecules of 18, 28, 5 and 5.8s.

PROTEIN SYNTHESIS (Fig. 1.2)

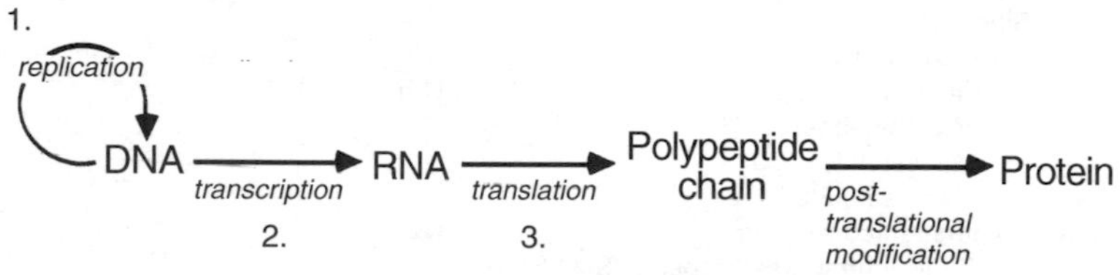

Fig. 1.2

1: DNA replication (Fig. 1.3)

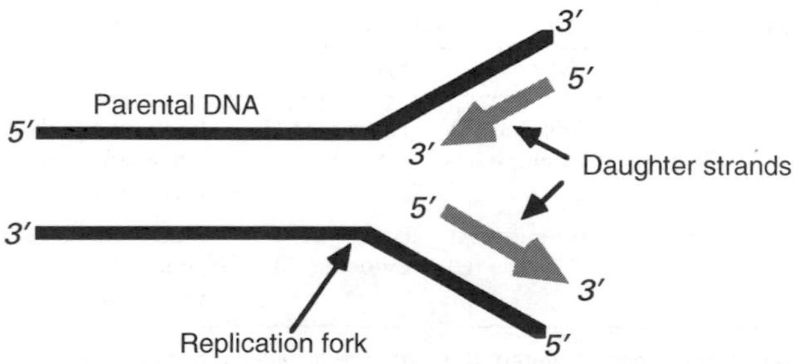

Fig. 1.3

- Replication is semi-conservative, i.e. each daughter molecule receives one strand from the parent DNA molecule.
- Unwinding proteins, DNA-directed RNA polymerase, DNA polymerase and ligase are also required.
- DNA polymerase synthesizes the new strand in a 5′ to 3′ direction.
- Discontinuous replication, i.e. one or both DNA strands may be synthesized in pieces known as Okazaki fragments, which are then linked together to yield a continuous DNA chain.

2: Transcription

- Synthesis of complete RNA molecules from DNA.
- Takes place in nucleus. One of the two DNA strands acts as a template for the formation of a mRNA molecule with a complementary base sequence.
- Transcription yields three types of RNA: mRNA, tRNA and rRNA.
- Fully conservative replication.
- Synthesis in 5′ → 3′ direction.
- DNA-dependent RNA polymerase is required (see Note).
- Processing: the RNA must be further modified to make it functionally active, e.g. introns cut out, exons spliced and in some cases polyadenylation before delivery of mRNA to the cytoplasm.

Note: Unlike DNA polymerase, RNA polymerase can initiate the synthesis of new strands. The RNA of an RNA virus is replicated by an RNA-dependent RNA polymerase. Oncogenic RNA viruses synthesize DNA from RNA, and insert the DNA into the chromosomes of animal cells. This reverse transcription is mediated by an RNA-directed DNA polymerase (*reverse transcriptase*).

3: Translation

- Protein synthesis according to the amino acid code in mRNA.
- Takes place in cytoplasm.
- Occurs on ribosomes when a tRNA molecule with three bases (anticodons) specific for a particular amino acid binds to the complementary mRNA codon.
- Four stages:
  1. Amino acid activation
  2. Initiation of polypeptide chain formation begins with the amino acid, methionine.
  3. Chain elongation
  4. Chain termination. Three codons, UAA, UGA and UAG, are signals for chain termination.

GENETIC CODE

- Each DNA strand codes for the synthesis of many polypeptides. A segment of DNA that codes for one polypeptide chain is called a gene.

- Genetic information is encoded by a sequence of bases in a non-overlapping code. Three bases (a *triplet*) specify one amino acid. There are 4^3, or 64 possible trinucleotide sequences of the four nucleotides in mRNA.
- The genetic code is degenerate: i.e. some aminoacids are coded for by more than one triplet codon. AUG is the codon for chain initiation and for the amino acid methionine.
- Coding sequences (*exons*) are interrupted by sequences of unknown function (*introns*).
- Single base or point mutations may involve base transitions, transversion, deletion or insertion.

CONTROL OF PROTEIN SYNTHESIS

In eukaryotes, this may occur by modification of DNA, or at the level of transcription and translation.

1. Regulation by induction-derepression.
2. Regulation by repression.

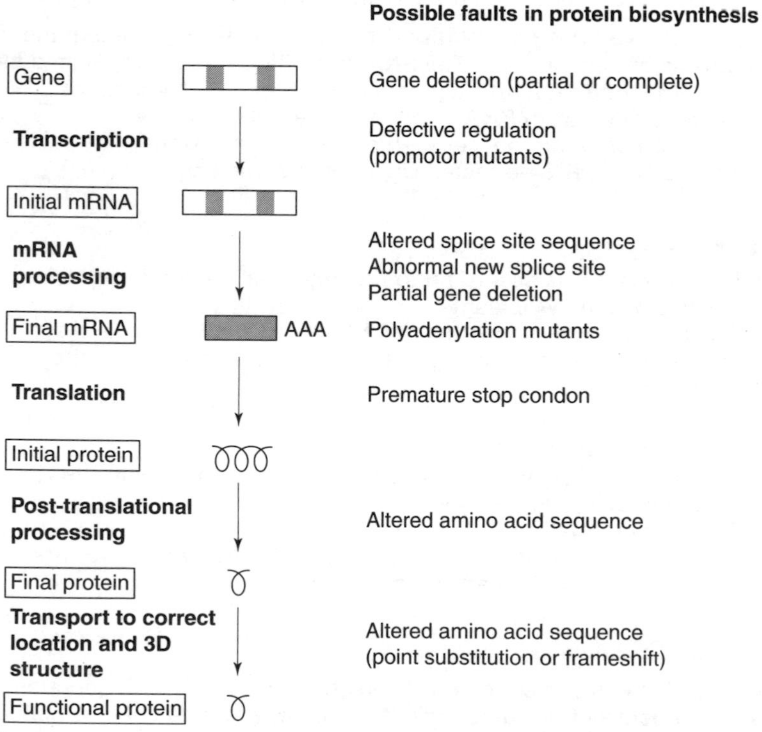

Fig. 1.4

Inhibitors of protein synthesis include rifampicin, streptomycin, tetracyline, chloramphenicol and erythromycin, pyrimidine analogues (5-fluorouracil, cytosine arabinoside, idoxuridine), and purine analogues (mercaptopurine, adenine arabinoside, thioguanine).

CELL CYCLE (See p. 368)

Replication of DNA occurs during the S phase of the cell cycle (i.e. DNA synthetic phase). This is preceded by G_1 (the first gap phase), when the cells prepare to duplicate their chromosomes. After the S phase, there is a second gap phase (G_2), during which cells prepare to divide. Cell division occurs during the mitotic (M) phase.

RECOMBINANT DNA TECHNOLOGY

BASIC TECHNIQUES OF GENE ANALYSIS

DNA can be extracted using standard techniques from any tissue containing nucleated cells, including blood and chorionic villus material.

1. DNA PROBE HYBRIDIZATION

A probe is a piece of single-stranded DNA which is used to detect homologous sequences in a sample of genomic DNA. If the probe is radiolabelled, its location after binding can be identified by exposure to X-ray film.
There are three main sources of gene probes:

1. complementary DNA (cDNA), i.e. DNA that is complementary to mRNA.
2. cloned cDNA.
3. DNA fragments prepared from genomic DNA.

2. GENE MAPPING

Restriction enzymes

- These are bacterial enzymes that recognize specific DNA sequences and cleave DNA at these sites. Each enzyme has its own recognition sequence and will cut genomic DNA into a series of fragments that can be analysed.
- The enzymes are named according to their organism of origin, e.g. Eco R1 is derived from *E. coli*.
- Because DNA is negatively charged, the DNA fragments can be ordered according to their size by electrophoresis in an agarose gel. It is possible to build up restriction enzyme maps of areas of the genome using different restriction enzymes that cleave DNA within or outside the gene of interest.

Preparation of and uses of a gene probe (Figs 1.5 and 1.6)

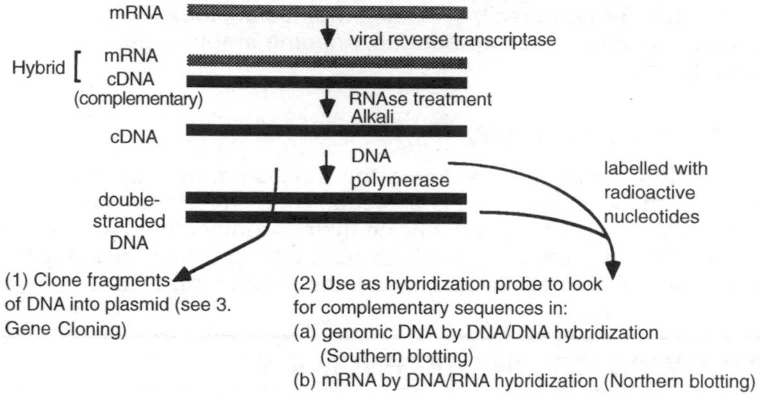

Fig. 1.5

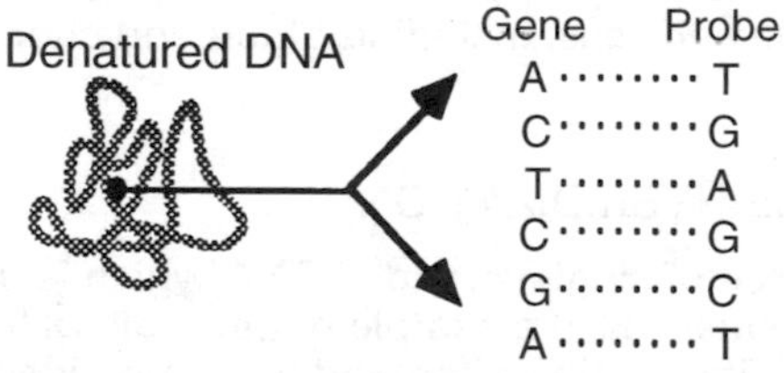

Fig. 1.6

Restriction fragment length polymorphisms (RFLP)

- Variations in non-coding DNA sequences are extremely frequent throughout the genome, and when they affect restriction enzyme cleavage sites, DNA fragments of different sizes will result. These variations are called restriction fragment length polymorphisms.
- If they occur in or near the gene of interest they provide potential linkage markers for following mutant genes through families.

Other markers

Other markers used in gene mapping include dinucleotide repeats (usually CA repeated many times, the number varying as a polymorphism can be detected by PCR); variable number tandem repeats (VNTRs; arrays or repetitive DNA sequences which vary in number and can be detected by blotting); and single nucleotide polymorphisms (variations in one base pair which are randomly scattered throughout the genome and provide a virtually limitless source of markers to explore the variation in the human genome).

Southern blot technique

- A method of transferring DNA fragments that have been size-fractionated by gel electrophoresis to a nylon membrane such that the relative positions of the DNA fragments are maintained. The DNA is then usually visualized on an autoradiograph following hybridization with a specific DNA or RNA probe.
- Useful for detection and size determination of specific restriction fragments in a DNA digest, e.g. detection of a sickle cell globin gene (Fig. 1.7).

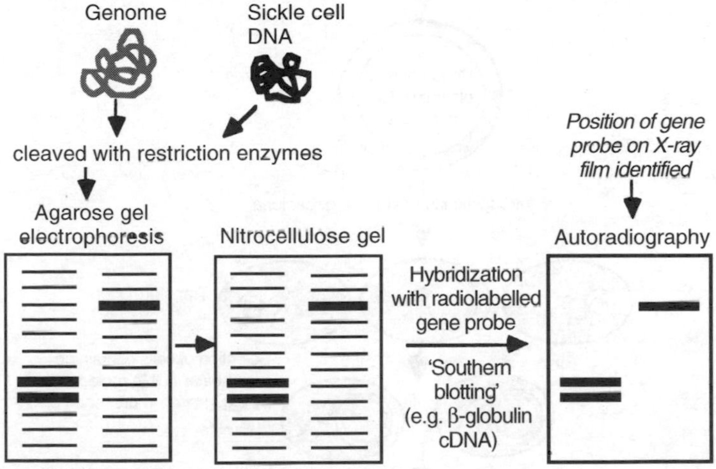

Fig. 1.7

3. GENE CLONING

- The insertion of foreign DNA into bacterial plasmids, bacteriophages or cosmids (see Note).
- Used in the preparation of gene libraries.

Note: *Plasmids*; Closed circular extrachromosomal DNA molecules which replicate autonomously in bacteria. *Bacteriophages*: Viruses that multiply in bacteria. *Cosmids*: Artificial vectors which are hybrids between a bacteriophage and a plasmid.

The cloning of DNA into a plasmid (Fig. 1.8)

Essential requirements

1. A method of specifically cutting and then religating DNA.
2. A source of carrier DNA (e.g. plasmid).

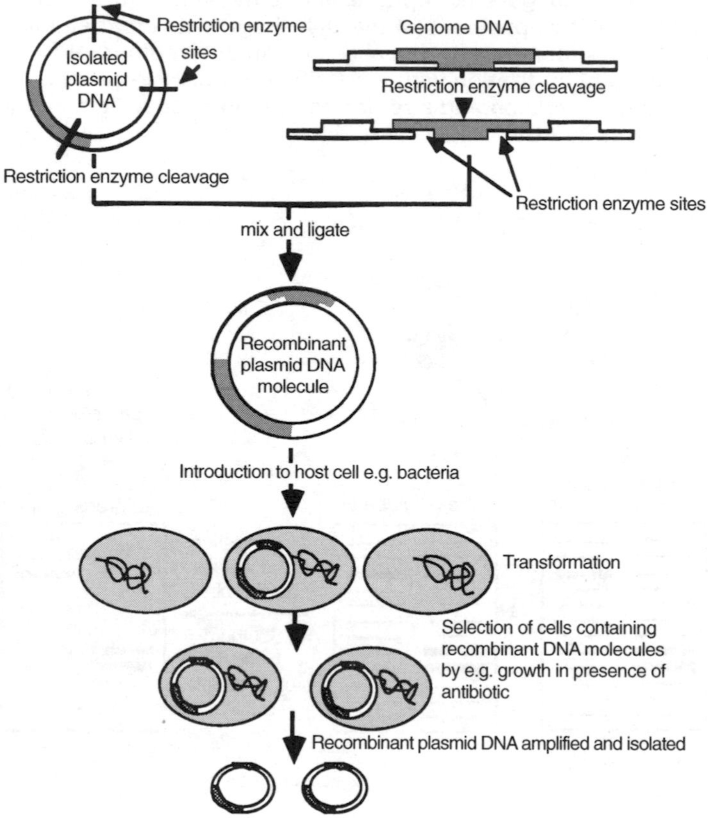

Fig. 1.8

3. A transfer method (e.g. conjugation).
4. A method of selecting the recombinant (e.g. antibiotic resistance).
5. A method of detecting the product of the cloned gene, e.g. enzyme-linked immunoabsorbent assay (ELISA).

Gene library

- A set of different bacterial and viral recombinants, each representing approximately one gene attached to a plasmid or bacteriophage.

- A particular colony containing a desired gene may be selected from a bacterial plate using a technique called colony hybridization.

4. GENE SEQUENCING

The identification and localization of new genes has been greatly enhanced by the development of methods for the large-scale sequencing of whole genomes in bacteria (e.g. *E. coli, H. pylori*), yeasts and nematodes (*C. elegans*). The Human Genome Project is a concerted effort to identify and sequence all human genes and to compare them with genes in the above organisms and others such as the fruitfly *Drosophila* and mouse.

Tools used

1. Expressed sequence tags (ESTs): short sequences of cDNA clones which are available on public databases. Currently about 50% of all human genes are represented and this figure will rapidly increase until all human coding sequence has been identified and can be characterized.
2. Sequence tagged sites (STSs): ESTs which have been assigned a map location by PCR (see below) of various genomic resources.
3. Bioinformatics: a variety of computational methods is now available for rapid comparison of raw sequence data, so that eventually the evolutionary relationship between all genes from bacteria to human will be understood.
4. Gene targeting: homologous genes in a variety of organisms can be simultaneously inactivated and the phenotype observed to give clues to the function of the gene product. A 'knockout mouse' is one in which a particular gene has been inactivated such that the animal will no longer produce the protein corresponding to that gene. This allows the modelling of particular human diseases in which a naturally occurring mouse mutant does not exist.
5. Transgenic analysis: the insertion of a foreign (usually human) gene into another organism, such as a mouse, to look at its effect on phenotype. Mutations can be systematically introduced to alter the protein function and the gene can be expressed under the control of tissue-specific promoters to look at function in particular cell types.

USES OF RECOMBINANT CLONED DNA

1. Isolation and sequencing of individual genes.
2. Preparation of probes for studying function of isolated genes, e.g. gene mapping using Southern blot technique.
3. As gene probes for rapid diagnosis of certain bacterial, viral and parasitic illnesses, in addition to diagnostic pathology, e.g. classification of lymphomas.

4. Pharmaceutical production of large quantities of proteins, such as human insulin, growth hormone, somatostatin, erythropoetin, interferon and hepatitis B vaccine.
5. Carrier detection, especially X-linked recessive disorders; presymptomatic diagnosis of autosomal dominant disorders and prenatal diagnosis of all categories of Mendelian disorders (see Note).
6. Potential correction of genetic defects in animals (i.e. gene therapy).

Note: Some diseases for which genetic prediction using DNA analysis is currently available are: haemophilia A and B; sickle cell disease; thalassaemia (alpha and beta); muscular dystrophy (Duchenne and Becker's); adult polycystic disease; phenylketonuria; cystic fibrosis; glucose-6-phosphate-dehydrogenase deficiency; and familial hypercholesterolaemia.

5. POLYMERASE CHAIN REACTION (PCR)

This is an amplification reaction in which a small amount of a DNA template is amplified to provide enough to perform analysis (prenatal diagnosis, detection of an infectious organism or the presence of a mutated oncogene).

The crucial feature of PCR is that to detect a given sequence of DNA it only needs to be present in one copy (i.e. one molecule of DNA). It is therefore an extremely sensitive technique.

Outline of the procedure (Fig. 1.9)

- A small sample of DNA is placed in a tube.
- Two oligonucleotides are added. These have sequences matching two sequences of the DNA that flank the region of interest.
- A thermostable DNA polymerase is added.
- The mixture is heated to just below 100°C and the DNA dissociates into two single strands (Fig. 1.9).
- The solution is allowed to cool and the single strands bind to the oligonucleotides, which are in excess.
- The oligonucleotide now acts as a primer for DNA polymerase and is extended to form a new double-stranded molecule.
- The cycle is repeated, with the amount of DNA doubling each time.

Application to molecular genetics

- Analysis of restriction fragment length polymorphisms.
- Analysis of messenger RNA.
- Amplification of fragments for identification by Southern blotting.
- Assessment of genetic polymorphism in linkage analysis.
- DNA sequencing.
- Site-directed mutagenesis.

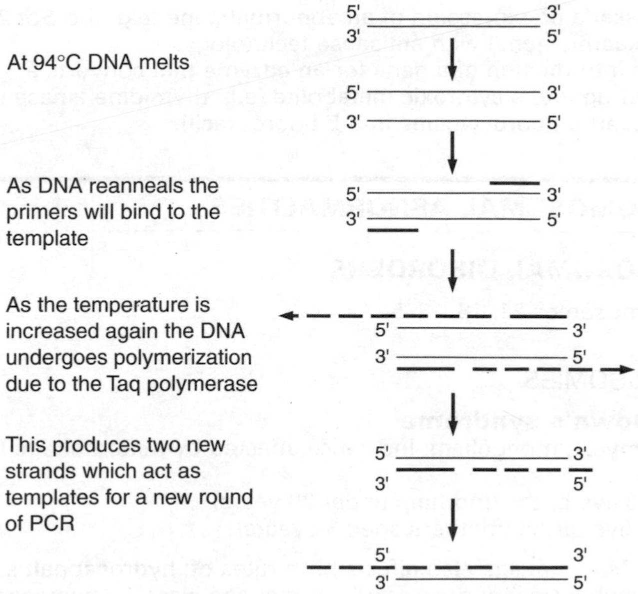
At 94°C DNA melts
As DNA reanneals the primers will bind to the template
As the temperature is increased again the DNA undergoes polymerization due to the Taq polymerase
This produces two new strands which act as templates for a new round of PCR
5'
3'

Fig. 1.9

Application to medicine

- Diagnosis of infections, e.g. mycobacteria, HIV, meningococcus, herpes simplex.
- Forensics (hair, blood, semen).
- Quantification of gene expression (where mRNA template is first reverse transcribed into a cDNA equivalent before amplification (RT-PCR)).
- Prenatal diagnosis from chorionic villus sampling, of known genetic mutations, e.g. cystic fibrosis, Duchenne muscular dystrophy.
- Detection of minimal residual tumour (e.g. *bcr-abl* in chronic myeloid leukaemia) and mutations in malignant tumours to assess prognosis.
- Investigation of evolution of pathogens, e.g. HIV, HCV.
- Tissue typing by PCR and detection of genetic variants, especially of MHC (major histocompatibility complex) class II alleles.

GENE THERAPY

This is the use of genetic intervention to treat disease. Techniques (still mostly experimental) include the following.

- Treatment of a genetic defect by insertion of a normal gene (e.g. in cystic fibrosis).

- Blockade of expression of an abnormal gene (e.g. the *BCL2* leukaemia gene) with antisense technology.
- The introduction of a gene for an enzyme that converts a prodrug into a cytotoxic metabolite (e.g. thymidine kinase to convert 5-fluorocytosine into 5-fluorouracil).

CHROMOSOMAL ABNORMALITIES

AUTOSOMAL DISORDERS

Chromosomes 21, 18, 13, 5.

1. TRISOMIES

(a) Down's syndrome

Trisomy 21, mongolism. Incidence affected by maternal age (see Note).
1:1200 live births (mothers under 30 years)
1:100 live births (mothers aged 39 years)

Note: Maternal age also affects birth rates of: hydrocephalus, anencephaly, achondroplasia (paternal age also); i.e. increased frequency with age.

Causes

- Non-dysjunction (94% of cases). Sporadic incidence related to maternal age.
- Mosaicism (2% of cases). Less marked physical or intellectual dysfunction.
- Translocation (4% of cases). Abnormalities in parents' chromosomes.

Clinical features

- Mental retardation, short stature, hypotonia and characteristic craniofacial abnormalities (flat occiput, oval face, epicanthic folds, Brushfield spots, macroglossia) simian palmar creases.
- Associated anomalies: e.g. congenital heart disease (atrial septal defect, patent ductus arteriosus and Fallot's tetralogy), tracheo-oesophageal fistulae, duodenal atresia, leukaemia and hypothyroidism.

(b) Edward's syndrome

Trisomy 18.

Clinical features

- Mental retardation, craniofacial abnormalities (prominent occiput, low-set ears, micronathia). 'Rocker bottom' foot deformity. Cardiac abnormalities.

(c) Patau's syndrome

Trisomy 13.

Clinical features

- Mental retardation, cleft palate and lip, polydactyly and microophthalmia.

2. DELETIONS

'Cri du chat' syndrome

Partial deletion of short arm of chromosome 5.

Clinical features

- Mental retardation, spasticity, high-pitched cry, craniofacial abnormalities (micronathia, low-set ears, epicanthic folds).

PHILADELPHIA CHROMOSOME

This is an *acquired* chromosomal abnormality present in 85% of cases of chronic myeloid leukaemia, due to the deletion of the long arm of chromosome 22 with translocation, usually on to chromosome 9. It persists during remission, and the prognosis is worse if absent. Also reported to occur in myelofibrosis and polycythaemia rubra vera.

SEX CHROMOSOME DISORDERS

Present in 25–30% of early abortions and 7% of deaths in first year of life.
Incidence 1:550 live births.

(a) Turner's syndrome

Karyotype 45 XO, i.e. no sex chromatin body.
Incidence 1:2000 live female births.

Causes

- Non-dysjunction of sex chromosomes.
- Mosaicism (XO/XX, XO/XY or XO/XXX).

Clinical features

- Phenotypically female, short stature, wide carrying angle, webbing of neck, short metacarpals (retarded bone age), sexual infantilism (lack of breast development with widely spaced nipples, scanty pubic and axillary hair).
- Primary amenorrhoea (occasional menstruation occurs in mosaicism), high gonadotrophin levels, low oestrogen level.
- Slight intellectual defect.
- Associated anomalies include coarctation of the aorta and renal abnormalities.

(b) Noonan's syndrome
Karyotype 45 XY.

Clinical features
- Similar features to Turner's syndrome but phenotypically male.
- Complete absence of testicles, cryptorchidism.
- Gonadal function may be normal.

(c) Testicular feminization syndrome
Karyotype 46 XY, i.e. one sex chromatin body.

Clinical features
- Inadequately virilized due to target organ failure.
- Phenotypically female, well developed breasts and female contours but lacking body hair with small, blind vaginas. No uterus or fallopian tubes. Gonads are testes, producing testosterone.

(d) Kleinfelter's syndrome
Karyotype 47 XXY, XXXYY or XXYY, i.e. one or two sex chromatin bodies.
Incidence: 1:400–600 male births.

Clinical features
- Tall, thin men with bilateral gynaecomastia and infertility due to hypogonadism (small, azoospermic testes).
- Increased incidence of mental subnormality.
- High urinary gonadotrophins with 17-ketosteroid content.

(e) 47 XYY
Incidence: 1:2000 live female births.

- Tall, aggressive males with increased tendency to psychiatric illness. More common in prison communities.

SINGLE-GENE ABNORMALITIES

Table 1.3 Proportions of genes in common among different relatives

Degree of relationship	*Examples*	*Proportion of genes in common*
First	Parents to child, sib to sib	1/2
Second	Uncles or aunts to nephews or nieces, grandparents to grandchildren	1/4
Third	First cousins, great-grandparents to great-grandchildren	1/8

AUTOSOMAL DOMINANT INHERITANCE

Approximately 1500 conditions described (generally 'structural-type' disorders), for example:

Achondroplasia
Adult polycystic kidney disease
Myotonic dystrophy
Facio-scapula-humeral muscular dystrophy
Ehlers–Danlos and Marfan's syndromes
Gardner's syndrome
Hereditary haemorrhagic telangiectasia
Familial hypercholesterolaemia
Hereditary spherocytosis
Huntington's chorea
Intestinal polyposis
Neurofibromatosis
Osteogenesis imperfecta
Tuberose sclerosis
Retinoblastoma
Hepatic porphyrias
Erythropoietic protoporphyria (See Note)
Charcot–Marie–Tooth syndrome

Note: An exception is congenital erythropoietic porphyria which has an autosomal recessive inheritance.

Summary

1. Both sexes are equally affected.
2. Heterozygotes are phenotypically affected, i.e. no carrier condition.
3. 50% of children are affected (Fig. 1.10).
4. Risk remains the same for each successive pregnancy.
5. Variable expressivity and penetrance.
6. Rare, and generally less severe than autosomal recessive.
7. High new mutation rate.

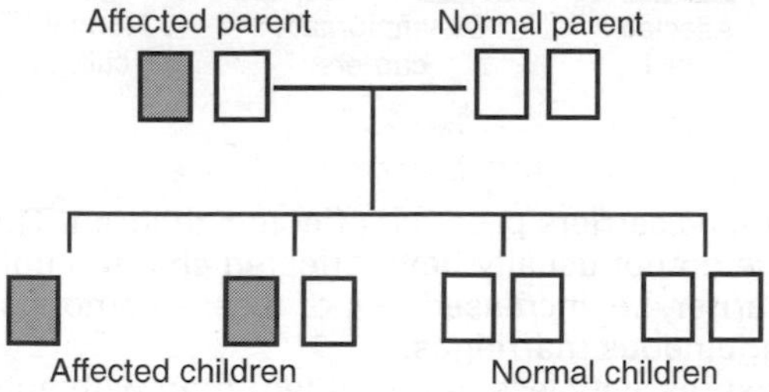

Fig. 1.10

AUTOSOMAL RECESSIVE INHERITANCE

Approximately 1000 conditions described (generally 'metabolic-type' disorders), for example:

α_1-antitrypsin deficiency
Agammaglobulinaemia
Albinism
Congenital adrenal hyperplasia
Cystic fibrosis
Most inborn errors of metabolism (e.g. galactosaemia, glycogen storage diseases, homocystinuria, phenylketonuria, lipidoses and mucopolysaccharidoses)
Congenital erythropoietic porphyria
Haemoglobinopathies (e.g. sickle cell disease and thalassaemias)
Wilson's disease
Xeroderma pigmentosa
Limb-girdle muscular dystrophy
Werdnig–Hoffman disease
Infantile polycystic disease

Summary

1. Both sexes are equally affected.
2. Heterozygotes are phenotypically unaffected, i.e. carrier state exists.
3. When both parents carry the gene, 1:4 children are affected and 2:4 children are carriers (Fig. 1.11)

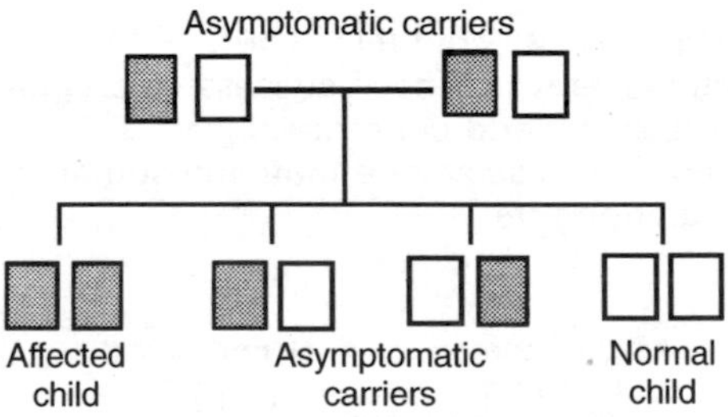

Fig. 1.11

4. Asymptomatic carriers produce affected children. Those with the disease do not usually have affected children unless they marry a carrier, i.e. increased risk of disease amongst offspring of consanguineous marriages.
5. Variable expressivity less of a problem than with autosomal dominant inheritance.

Table 1.4 Ethnic associations with autosomal recessive diseases

Disease	*Ethnic groups*
Beta-thalassaemia	Mediterraneans, Thais, Blacks, Middle East populations, Indians, Chinese
Sickle cell disease	US and African Blacks, Asian Indians, Mediterraneans (especially Greeks) and Middle East populations
Tay–Sachs disease	Ashkenazi Jews
Gaucher disease	Ashkenazi Jews
Bloom syndrome	Ashkenazi Jews
Adrenogenital syndrome	Eskimos
Severe combined immunodeficiency	Apache Indians
Cystic fibrosis	Caucasians
Albinism	Hopi Indians

SEX-LINKED DOMINANT INHERITANCE

Rare e.g. vitamin D-resistant rickets (X-linked).

Summary

1. Affects both sexes, but females more than males.
2. All children of affected homozygous females are affected.
3. Females pass the trait to half their sons and half their daughters.
4. All daughters of affected males are affected, but none of their sons.

SEX-LINKED RECESSIVE INHERITANCE

Approximately 200 conditions described (almost exclusively X-linked), for example:

Colour blindness
Nephrogenic diabetes insipidus
Glucose-6-phosphate dehydrogenase deficiency
Wiscott–Aldrich syndrome
Complete testicular feminization syndrome
Haemophilia A (VIII) and B (IX)
Lesch–Nyhan syndrome (hypoxanthine guanine phosphoribosyl transferase deficiency)
Duchenne muscular dystrophy
Becker's muscular dystrophy
Immunodeficiencies: agammaglobulinaemia and severe combined immunodeficiency
Ichthyosis
Fabry's disease
Hunter's syndrome.

Summary

1. Affected cases are usually males carrying the gene and homozygous females (rare).

2. Half the sons of carriers are affected, and half the daughters are carriers.
3. No male-to-male transmission: condition is transmitted by carrier women who produce affected boys, normal boys, carrier girls and normal girls with equal frequency (Fig. 1.12).
4. Affected males can have only normal sons and carrier daughters.
5. Affected cases have affected brothers and affected maternal uncles.

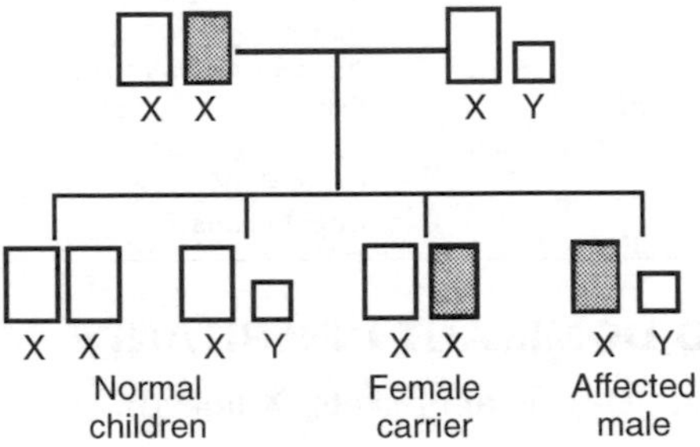

Fig. 1.12

SUMMARY OF INHERITANCE IN MUSCULAR DYSTROPHIES (Table 1.5)

Table 1.5 Inheritance in muscular dystrophies

Muscular dystrophy	*Inheritance*	*Presentation*
Duchenne	X-linked recessive	Most common, presents early
Becker	X-linked recessive	Milder, presents later
Limb-girdle (Erb)	Autosomal recessive	Less common
Facio-scapulo-humeral-peroneal	Autosomal dominant	Long course
Distal myopathy (Welander)	Autosomal dominant	Late onset
Ocular myopathy	Autosomal dominant	Retinopathy or dysphagia may also be present

MITOCHONDRIAL INHERITANCE

The mitochondrial genome is circular and approximately 16.5 kb in length. It encodes genes for the mitochondrial respiratory chain and for some species of transfer RNA. Mitochondrial genetic disorders are mostly rare and complex neurological conditions e.g. mitochondrial encephalopathy, lactic acidosis and stroke-like episodes (MELAS).

1. Mitochondrial DNA (mtDNA) mutates 10 times more frequently than nuclear DNA; as there are no introns, a mutation will invariably strike a coding sequence.

2. Maternal inheritance: no mitochondria are transferred from spermatozoa at fertilization.
3. Normal and mutant mtDNA may coexist within one cell (heteroplasmy).
4. Poor genotype–phenotype correlation.
5. Several phenotypes have been shown to be due to mtDNA mutations:
   — sensorineural deafness
   — diabetes mellitus
   — optic atrophy
   — chronic progressive external ophthalmoplegia
   — stroke in young people
   — myopathy
   — lactic acidosis
   — cardiomyopathy and cardiac conduction defects
   — pigmentary retinopathy.

TRINUCLEOTIDE REPEAT DISEASES

A number of mainly neurological genetic diseases are caused by a mutation that is an expansion of a repetitive sequence of three nucleotides. This arrangement appears to be prone to instability and has therefore become known as a dynamic mutation.

1. Conditions include Huntington's disease, myotonic dystrophy, fragile X syndrome, Friedrlech's ataxia, X-linked bulbospinal neuronopathy (Kennedy's syndrome), spinocerebellar ataxias (at least seven variants).
2. Mutant alleles arise from a population with repeats at the upper end of normal range which are prone to instability.
3. Disease severity worsens with an earlier age of onset in successive generations (genetic anticipation).
4. The length of the expansion continues to increase as cells divide throughout life (somatic instability).
5. Trinucleotide repeats either lie in the 5′ non-coding region of genes where they disrupt gene transcription because they cause steric hindrance of RNA polymerase or they code for the amino acid glutamine (CAG) and appear to produce a toxic protein which forms intracellular inclusion bodies.

MOLECULAR BASIS OF SINGLE-GENE DISORDERS

Autosomal dominant

Achondroplasia Disorder of skeletal development due to mutations in the fibroblast growth factor receptor type 3. Almost all patients have mutations at the same site in the protein.
Polycystic kidney disease Leading genetic cause of renal failure in adults and accounts for 10% of end stage renal disease. Causative gene in the vast majority of cases (*ADPKD1*) is called

polycystin and is believed to be involved in the establishment of epithelial cell polarity in development.
Myotonic dystrophy One of the trinucleotide repeat disorders (see above). The mutation is an expansion in the 3′ untranslated region of a protein kinase (dystrophia myotonica protein kinase), although the mechanism whereby this leads to the phenotype is still controversial.
Familial hypercholesterolaemia One of the few inborn errors of metabolism inherited as a dominant trait. Due to mutations which disrupt the synthesis, function or recycling of the low density lipoprotein receptor, there is poor uptake of LDL-bound cholesterol and high serum levels.
Marfan's syndrome Results from mutations in a gene called *fibrillin*, the protein product of which is the major component of extracellular microfibrils and is widely distributed in connective tissue throughout the body.
Neurofibromatosis (NF1) The progressive accumulation of nerve sheath tumours is caused by mutations in a tumour supressor gene called *neurofibromin*; a GTPase-activating protein (GAP) which enhances the inactivation of growth-promoting signals. 30–50% are due to new mutations. NF2 is a different disorder which is characterized by the development of bilateral acoustic neuromas.
Familial breast cancer Mutations in at least two genes (*BRCA-1* and *2*) give rise to familial breast cancer, often in association with ovarian tumours.

Autosomal recessive

α_1-Antitrypsin deficiency One of the most common hereditary diseases affecting Caucasians. The prime function of the enzyme is to inhibit neutrophil elastase and it is one of the serpin superfamily of protease inhibitors.
Cystic fibrosis The defective gene encodes a protein called the cystic fibrosis transmembrane conductance regulator (CFTR), which is involved in the regulation of ion flux through chloride channels and in mucin production. The opening of the protein is mediated by ATP binding. Over 70% of the mutations in Caucasians are due to a deletion of three nucleotides (encoding a phenylalanine residue) at position 508 (ΔF 508).
Wilson's disease Due to mutations in a copper-binding protein, which is probably important for binding copper to the transport protein, caeruloplasmin.

X-linked

Duchenne dystrophy A genetic disease due to mutations in a protein called *dystrophin*, which is part of a large complex of membrane-associated proteins, defects in most of which can cause forms of muscular dystrophy. Out-of-frame deletions lead to the production of a nonsense protein which is completely without functionality. In-frame deletions lead to the formation of a truncated protein with partial function, and to the milder *Becker dystrophy*.

PRENATAL AND POSTNATAL DIAGNOSIS

PRENATAL: INDICATIONS

1. Women aged over 35 years.
2. Raised maternal serum alphafetoprotein.
3. Strong family history of neural tube defects, e.g. previous affected child.
4. Strong family history of chromosomal abnormality.
5. Carriers of X-linked recessive diseases who have decided to terminate male fetuses.
6. Known carriers of prenatally diagnosable biochemical disorders, e.g. creatine kinase in Duchenne muscular dystrophy, phenylalanine tolerance test in phenylketonuria, alphafetoprotein in neural tube defects.
7. Conditions for which genetic prediction using DNA analysis is available, e.g. alpha- and beta-thalassaemia, cystic fibrosis, fragile X syndrome, haemophilia A, Huntington disease, muscular dystrophy (Duchenne and Becker), myotonic dystrophy, spinal muscular atrophy.

Amniocentesis

- Performed at about 16 weeks' gestation.
- Risk to fetus approximately 1%.

Chorionic villus sampling

- Performed at 8–10 weeks' gestation.
- Involves aspiration via a cannula inserted through the cervix under ultrasound guidance.
- Chorionic villi can be used for chromosomal analysis, fetal DNA analysis and certain biochemical investigations.
- Risk of causing miscarriage is approximately 2–3%.

POSTNATAL DIAGNOSIS

Guthrie test

- Performed between 6th and 14th day of life.
- Screens routinely for phenylketonuria, TSH level and histidinaemia. Also: galactosaemia, glucose-6-phosphate dehydrogenase deficiency and hyperleucinaemia (maple syrup urine disease).

POLYGENIC INHERITANCE

- Observed phenotype is due to the additive effect of many different gene loci.
- The genetic liability of individuals to develop a disease of multifactorial aetiology has a normal distribution, and the condition occurs when a certain threshold is exceeded (Fig. 1.13).

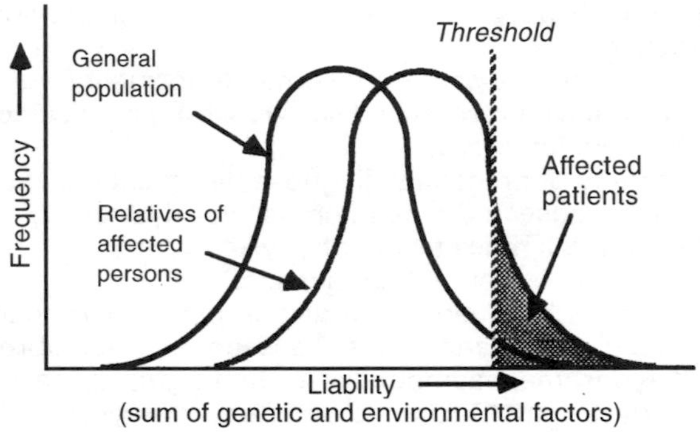

Fig. 1.13

Examples

(i) Congenital malformations

Neural tube defects:
  Spina bifida (2 per 1500 births).
  Anencephaly (2 per 1000 births). Risk after first, second and third affected child is 1:20, 1:8 and 1:4, respectively.
Congenital heart disease (6 per 1000 births)
Cleft lip ± cleft palate (1 per 1000 births)
Pyloric stenosis (3 per 1000 births; M:F ratio = 5:1)
Congenital dislocation of hip (1 per 1000 births; M:F ratio = 1:8)
Hirschsprung disease (M:F ratio = 3:1)

(ii) Common adult diseases

Diabetes mellitus
Schizophrenia
Manic depression
Breast cancer (a small proportion of cases are due to single-gene mutations: *BRCA-1* and *BRCA-2*)
Rheumatoid arthritis
Epilepsy
Multiple sclerosis

REGULATION OF GENE EXPRESSION

- 80 000 genes in the human genome.
- Each cell typically expresses 16 000–20 000 genes.
- Expression is regulated by transcription factors; proteins which bind to DNA at the 5′ end of genes (the promoter; Fig. 1.14) initiate transcription of genes.
- Some genes have a fundamental biological role and will be expressed in all cells at all times ('housekeeping genes').

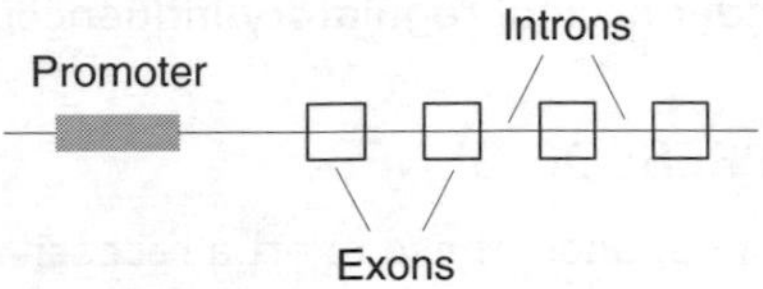

Fig. 1.14

THE SOMATIC EVOLUTION OF CANCER

- Cancer cells are a clonal population of cells. The malignant phenotype arises from the accumulation of mutations in multiple genes.
- It is a combination of three types of genetic mutation (inherited, spontaneous and environmentally determined) which leads to cancer. Therefore cancer evolution is a complex, multifactorial process.
- Most tumours show visible abnormalities of chromosome banding on light microscopy, suggesting that as tumours develop they become more bizarre and more prone to genetic error.
- In contrast to other types of genetic disorders, for most cancers the genetic mutations are not inherited but arise in somatic cells during adulthood as a result of exposure to environmental carcinogens. Multiple mutations are usually involved.
- These mutations (inherited and acquired) commonly involve three types of genes: tumour suppressors, oncogenes and genes involved in DNA-repair mechanisms.

ONCOGENES

- Oncogenes when expressed, lead to loss of growth control by a dominant gain of function mutation (i.e. only one copy needs to be mutated for cancer to occur)
- **Protooncogenes**, found in the normal human genome and expressed in normal tissue have a central role in the signal-transduction pathways that control cell growth and differentiation.

- May be growth factors, growth factor receptors, G-proteins, second messengers or transcription factors.
- ***ras*** is a small G-protein which is one of the most commonly mutated genes in solid tumours. It acts to promote cell growth and division.
- **c-*myc***, is a transcription factor which commits the cell to go into mitosis, is overexpressed in Burkitt's lymphoma because of a translocation which juxtaposes it next to the immunoglobulin heavy-chain promoter.
- In the Philadelphia chromosome in CML, a *bcr-abl* fusion gene product is created by a translocation. This protein is a kinase which is not under normal regulatory influences.

TUMOUR SUPPRESSOR GENES

- In contrast to oncogenes, these exert a **recessive** effect, such that both copies must be mutated before tumorigenesis occurs. Mutation results in loss of function.
- These genes normally function to inhibit the cell cycle and therefore, when inactivated, lead to loss of growth control.
- Many tumour types have been studied for loss of heterozygosity of chromosome 13 and elsewhere, to identify the location of tumour suppressor genes. Over 20 have been identified; retinoblastoma, p53 and adenomatous polyposis coli genes have been cloned.
- Retinoblastoma is the commonest malignant eye tumour in childhood. All of the bilateral and 15% of the unilateral cases are inherited as an autosomal dominant trait. The gene for this trait is localized to the proximal long arm of chromosome 13 (13q14).
- **p53** is a protein which occupies a pivotal role in the cell cycle and is the most commonly mutated gene in tumours (e.g. breast, colon). It encodes a transcription factor, the normal function of which is to downregulate the cell cycle. Inactivation of p53 is the primary defect in the **Li–Fraumeni** syndrome (a dominantly inherited monogenic cancer syndrome, characterized by breast carcinoma, sarcomas, brain and other tumours); p53 is a central regulator of **apoptosis**.

APOPTOSIS

This is the morphological description of cells undergoing programmed cell death, a process whereby unwanted cells are removed by the activation of specific genetic pathways.

Features

- Cell shrinkage
- Compaction of chromatin
- Nuclear blebbing

- Formation of apoptotic bodies
- Phagocytosis.

Functions of apoptosis

- Elimination of cells in embryological development (e.g. motor neurones).
- Induction of tolerance to self antigens by removal of autoreactive T-lymphocytes.
- Removal of virally infected cells.
- Removal of cells which have undergone DNA damage.

Principal mediators

p53: A tumour supressor gene which inhibits mitosis and drives apoptosis in cells in which DNA has been damaged. Mutation correlates with poor prognosis in tumours.
bcl-2: A strong negative regulator of apoptosis. If it is overexpressed in tumours, cells have a prolonged survival.
fas (CD95): A cellular receptor which, when activated, is directly coupled to the activation of intracellular proteases which lead to apoptosis.
caspases: Present in all cells and, unless inhibited, lead to the morphological changes of apoptosis.

Diseases of excess apoptosis

- Neurodegeneration
- HIV disease (CD4+ cells die through programmed cell death).

Diseases of insufficient apoptosis

- Cancer
- Autoimmunity.

IMMUNOGENETICS

THE MAJOR HISTOCOMPATIBILITY COMPLEX

- The major histocompatibility complex (MHC) in humans is located on the short arm of chromosome 6, and carries the genes determining the histocompatibility antigens, termed human leucocyte antigens (HLA), specific to each individual.
- Responsible for tissue rejection and some other immunological functions.

HLA ANTIGENS

- Several distinct loci coding for the major histocompatibility antigens (HLA-A, -B, -C, -DR, -DQ and -DP antigens) and some complement components (Fig. 1.15).

Map of the HLA loci and their genes

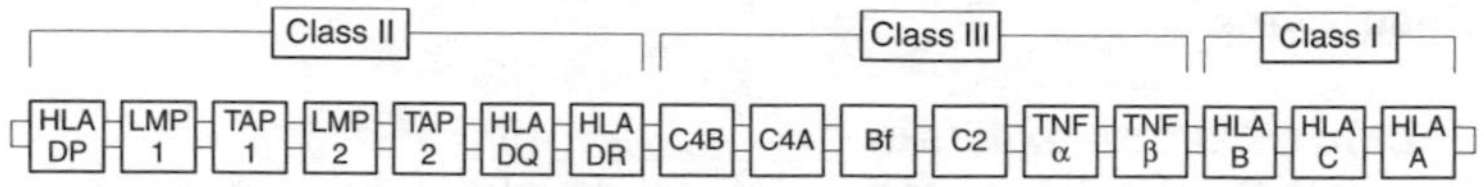

HLA = human leucocyte antigen
LMP = latent membrane protein
TAP = transporter associated with antigen processing
TNF = tumour necrosis factor

Fig. 1.15

- Each locus has several alleles: (20 alleles at the A locus, 30 at the B and at least 10 at the C and DR loci).
- 3 classes of MHC gene products:
  1. Class I antigens are coded for by HLA-A, -B, -C genes. They are present on all nucleated cells, and determine graft rejection.
  2. Class II antigens are coded for by HLA-D, -DR, -DP and -DQ genes. They are only present on monocytes/macrophages, B lymphocytes and occasionally activated T lymphocytes. They act as receptors for the presentation of antigen to helper T cells (immune response genes).
  3. Class III antigens are associated with certain complement components (e.g. C2, C4 and C3b receptor). Not involved in either immune response or graft rejection.
- I region: A region of the MHC where immune response (Ir) genes are located and plasma membrane (Ia) molecules are encoded.
- Ir genes: Genes that control the ability of helper T cells to develop a specific immune response to antigen.
- Ia: Histocompatibility antigen found primarily on B cells, but also on some macrophages and T cells.
- Each parent and child will have 50% of HLA antigens in common.
- Non-identical siblings have:
  1:4 chance of sharing all four HLA antigens
  2:4 chance of sharing two antigens
  1:4 chance of sharing no antigens.

CLASSIFICATION OF DISEASES ASSOCIATED WITH HLA

Certain diseases are associated with particular HLA antigens (Table 1.6). This may be due to:

1. Linkage disequilibrium (i.e. allelic association) with an unidentified disease susceptibility gene, e.g. an immune response gene, or may
2. Reflect the function of the specific HLA antigen.

Table 1.6 Diseases associated with HLA

HLA antigen	*Disease*	*Relative risk**
A3	Haemochromatosis	9
B5	Bechet's disease	6
B27	Ankylosing spondylitis	90
	Reiter's syndrome	37
	Psoriatic arthritis	4
	Acute anterior uveitis	3
DR2	Multiple sclerosis	4
	Pernicious anaemia	1.7
	Narcolepsy	1.4
	Juvenile-onset diabetes mellitus	4
DR3	Dermatitis herpetiformis	15
	Coeliac disease	11
	Sjogren's syndrome	10
	1° biliary cirrhosis	8
	Chronic active hepatitis	7
	Addison's disease	6
	Systemic lupus erythematosis	6
	Grave's disease	4
	Hashimoto's thyroiditis	3.5
	Insulin-dependent diabetes mellitus	3
	Myasthenia gravis	2
DR4	Insulin-dependent diabetes mellitus	6
	Rheumatoid arthritis	4
DR5	Pernicious anaemia	9
DR7	Coeliac disease	5

*Relative risk is the factor of increased risk for developing the disease among individuals with the HLA antigen. If there is no association, the relative risk is 1.

ETHNIC GROUPS AND GENETIC DISEASE

Table 1.7 Ethnic groups and genetic disease

Group	*Associated disease*
Scandinavians	α_1-antitrypsin and lecithin cholesterol acyl transferase (LCAT) deficiency
Northern Europeans	Cystic fibrosis
Ashkenazi Jews	Tay–Sachs disease
Sephardic Jews and Armenians	Familial Mediterranean fever
Eskimos	Congenital adrenal hyperplasia and pseudocholinesterase deficiency
Mediterranean races	β-thalassaemia, glucose-6-phosphate dehydrogenase deficiency and familial Mediterranean fever
Chinese	Glucose-6-phosphate dehydrogenase deficiency
Africans	Haemoglobinopathies especially sickle cell disease, alpha- and beta-thalassaemias
South African whites	Porphyria variegata

2. Microbiology

CHAPTER CONTENTS

Table 2.1 Comparison of bacteria, rickettsiae, chlamydiae and viruses

Characteristics	*Bacteria*	*Rickettsiae*	*Chlamydiae*	*Viruses*
1. Obligate intracellular parasite	–	+	+	+
2. Contains both DNA and RNA	+	+	+	–
3. Visible with light microscope	+	+	–	–
4. Contains muramic acid in cell wall	+	+	+	–
5. Independent metabolic activity	+	+	+	–
6. Synthesizes ATP	+	+	–	–
7. Susceptible to antibacterial antibiotics	+	+	+	–

PROCARYOTIC PATHOGENIC BACTERIA

BOX 2.1 GENERAL CHARACTERISTICS

In general:

• All cocci are Gram-positive.	Exceptions: Neisseria
• All rods are Gram-negative.	Exceptions: Bacillus, Clostridia and Corynebacterium
• All pathogens are facultative anaerobes.	Exceptions: Clostridia and Bacteriodes (obligate anaerobes)

ENDOTOXINS AND EXOTOXINS

Table 2.2 Comparison of exotoxins and endotoxins

Exotoxins	*Endotoxins*
Mainly produced by Gram-positive bacteria	Lipopolysaccharides – part of Gram-negative cell wall
Heat-labile proteins	Heat-stable
High potency	Liberated when Gram-negative bacteria lyse
Strong antigenicity	Non-specific effect
Neutralized by antitoxin	
Often possess specific mechanisms of action	

Endotoxins (lipopolysaccharides; LPS)

- Important in the pathogenesis of Gram-negative septic shock (endotoxic shock), e.g. *Salmonella, E. coli, Proteus* and *Klebsiella*.
- The LPS molecule activates the complement and cytokine pathways, releasing activated components which increase vascular permeability and result in shock. The clotting and fibrinolytic cascades are also activated, resulting in disseminated intravascular coagulation.

Exotoxins (extracellular)

- Produced by most Gram-positive bacteria, e.g. *C. diphtheria, Cl. welchii, tetanus* and *botulinum, B. anthracis*, and *Staph. aureus*; but also a few Gram-negative bacteria, e.g. *V. cholera* and *Shigella*.
- *Botulinus toxin* produced by *Cl. botulinum* affects motor neurons, blocking release of acetylcholine at synapses and neuromuscular junctions and resulting in motor paralyses (e.g. dysphagia, respiratory arrest).

- *Diphtheria toxin* produced by *Corynebacterium diphtheriae* inhibits protein synthesis and causes necrosis of epithelium, heart muscle, kidney and nerve tissues.
- *Cholera toxin* produced by *Vibrio cholera* binds to ganglioside receptors of the small intestine epithelial cells, and results in increased adenylate cyclase activity with massive hypersecretion of chloride and water into the lumen.

BACTERIAL CHARACTERISTICS, DISEASES AND RESERVOIRS OF INFECTIONS

Bacterial characteristics, the diseases produced in man and the reservoirs of infection are presented in Tables 2.3–2.12.

Table 2.3 Gram-positive bacilli

Genus and species	*Characteristics*	*Diseases produced in man*	*Reservoir of infections*
1. Corynebacterium *C. Diphtheria*	• Aerobic, non-spore-forming • Catalase +ve • Non-haemolytic • Toxin production	• Diphtheria (non-invasive infection) • Diphtheria can cause prosthetic device infections	• Nasopharynx of case or carrier
2. Listeria *L. monocytogenes*	• Aerobic • Haemolytic • Often in pairs	• Meningoencephalitis, chiefly in neonates and immunocompromised patients	• Widely distributed in animals and man
3. Bacillus *B. anthracis*	• Aerobic, spore-forming	• Cutaneous and pulmonary anthrax	• Anthrax in animals (cattle and sheep) • Occasional human infection
B. cereus	• Enterotoxins	• Food poisoning	• Contaminated fried rice
4. Clostridium *Cl. welchii (perfringens)*	• Anaerobic, spore-forming • α-haemolytic toxin	• Food poisoning and gas gangrene • Sometimes associated with diabetes	• Soil and intestinal flora of man and animals
Cl. oedematiens and *Cl. Septicum*	• Anaerobic, spore-forming	• Gas gangrene	• Soil and dust • Faeces of man and animals
Cl. tetani	• Anaerobic, spore-forming	• Tetanus	• Intestinal flora of man and animals • Soil and dust
Cl. botulinum	• Anaerobic, spore-forming • Heat-labile neurotoxin	• Botulism • Mild watery diarrhoea	• Soil and dust • Badly canned food

Table 2.3 *(cont.)*

Genus and species	*Characteristics*	*Diseases produced in man*	*Reservoir of infections*
Cl. difficile	• Anaerobic, spore-forming • Toxigenic strains produce exotoxins A and B.* • Non-toxigenic strains are not usually pathogenic	• Pseudomembraneous colitis	• Commonest enteropathogen in hospital patients • Source of infection may be endogenous, exogenous from the environment or directly from a carrier • Carriage rates in healthy volunteers vary from 0 to 15%. • Spores can be found on the hands of patients and staff, as well as on beds and floors
Mycobacterium *M. tuberculosis* (human type) and *M. bovis* (bovine type)	• Aerobic • Rod-shaped • Acid- and alcohol-fast (requires Lowenstein–Jensen medium for culture)	• Pulmonary TB • TB of lymph nodes, intestine, bones and joints • Meningitis and genitourinary infection	• Lungs of man, cattle and birds
Atypical mycobacteria (opportunistic) e.g. *M. ulcerans* *M. kansasii*		• Skin ulcers (tropics) • Chest disease	
M. marinum *M. chelonei* and		• Granulomatous skin lesions associated with cleaning fish tanks and swimming pools • Cutaneous abscesses; occasionally disseminated infection in the immunocompromised	
M. avium-intracellulare		• Cervical lymphadenopathy in children; chest infection and invasive infections in AIDS patients	
M. leprae	• Cannot be cultured in vivo	• Leprosy	

*Toxin A is an enterotoxin, thought to bind to mucosal receptors which enter the cell and cause fluid secretion and mucosal damage. Toxin B is a cytotoxin which also binds to specific membrane receptors, but is 1000 times more potent in tisuue cultures than toxin A.

Table 2.4 Gram-positive cocci

Genus and species	*Characteristics*	*Diseases produced in man*	*Reservoir of infections*
Streptococcus *Str. viridans* (α-haemolysis)	• Facultative anaerobes*, some microaerophilic • In chains • Catalase –ve	• Dental abscess • Subacute bacterial endocarditis	• Commensal in mouth
Str. mutans		• ?Dental caries	
Str. pyogenes (β-haemolysis)† Lancefield Group *A*	• Grouped by carbohydrate antigens • In chains • Catalase –ve • Production of haemolytic exotoxins, e.g. streptokinase, hyaluronidase and DNAase	• Acute tonsillitis, wound infections, puerperal sepsis, otitis media, scarlet fever, rheumatic fever and glomerulonephritis • Skin and soft tissue infections, e.g. pyoderma, impetigo, erysipelas, acute cellulitis • Toxic shock syndrome • Necrotizing fasciitis‡	• Nose and throat of case and carrier
Lancefield Group *B*		• Septicaemia (without focus), meningitis • Important pathogen in neonatal period	
Lancefield Group *C*		• Pharyngitis, cellulitis	
Str. faecalis (Lancefield Group *D*)	• In short chains or pairs	• Urinary tract infections, wound infections and cholecystitis	• Commensal of large intestine
Lancefield Group *G*		• Cellulitis	

Table 2.4 *(cont.)*

Genus and species	*Characteristics*	*Diseases produced in man*	*Reservoir of infections*
Str. pneumoniae (pneumococcus) (α-haemolysis)	• Diplococcus • Heavily encapsulated	• Lobar pneumonia, infections of eye and ear, purulent meningitis and sinusitis • More frequent in splenectomized patients	• Commensal of upper respiratory tract
Str. milleri		• Deep abscesses, especially liver, lung and brain	
Staphylococcus			
Staph. aureus (β-haemolysis) (Table 2.5)	• Coagulase +ve (most strains) and catalase –ve • In clumps • Phage typing identifies virulent strains • Six types of enterotoxin are known (see Table 2.5)	• Superficial infections, including boils and carbuncles, scalded skin syndrome in neonates and toxic shock syndrome, wound infections, osteomyelitis, bronchopneumonia, endocarditis, vascular catheter infections, septicaemia, pseudomembraneous colitis, and food poisoning	• Colonizes nose and perineum of carriers • Contaminated salads and milk
Staph. saprophyticus (epidermis, albus and micrococcus)	• Coagulase +ve and catalase –ve • In clumps	• Infection of indwelling cannulae, other prosthetic device infections, endocarditis, and urinary tract infections	• Contaminated salads and milk

*Facultative organisms can grow with or without air.

†Streptolysin-O is an oxygen-labile haemolysin. Anti-streptolysin-O (ASO) appears within 1–2 weeks of infection, reaches a maximum at 3–5 weeks and disappears within 6–12 months.

‡Several factors predispose to infection, including penetrating injuries, surgical procedures, cuts, burns, varicella infection, and childbirth.

Table 2.5 Toxin production associated with *Staph. aureus*

*Toxin**	*Effect*
Enterotoxins	Released into foods resulting in food poisoning
Exfoliative or epidermolytic	Scalded skin syndrome, producing peeling of layers of epidermis
Haemolysins	Lyse erythrocytes
Leucocidins	Lyse leucocytes and macrophages
Toxic shock syndrome	Vascular collapse, rash with desquamation

*Toxin production varies between strains of *Staph. aureus*.

Table 2.6 Gram-negative pyogenic cocci

Genus and species	*Characteristics*	*Diseases produced in man*	*Reservoir of infections*
Neisseria *N. meningitides* (meningococcus)	• Both aerobic • Both diplococcus • Need enriched medium and CO_2 for culture • Serogroups A and C are commonest worldwide	• Acute meningitis • Septicaemia	• Commensal in nasopharynx (carriage rate in general population is approx. 25%), • Transmission is via respiratory route — More common in the winter weather, and has two peaks of incidence, in infancy and teenage years — Predisposing factors are influenza infection, smoking and complement C5 and C9 deficiencies
N. gonorrheae (gonococcus)	• In the UK, group B is the most common	• Gonorrhea, ophthalmia neonatorum, suppurative urethritis in the male, acute cervicitis in the female, pelvic inflammatory disease, suppurative arthritis and endocarditis	

Table 2.7 Gram-negative bacteria

Genus and species	*Characteristics*	*Diseases produced in man*	*Reservoir of infections*
Parvobacteria *Moraxella catarrhalis*		• Lower respiratory tract infections	
Haemophilus *H. influenzae*	• Facultative anaerobe • Encapsulated • Needs factors V and X for growth	• Chronic bronchitis, bronchopneumonia, acute epiglottis and purulent meningitis in children	• Commensal in nasopharynx
H. parainfluenzae		• Exacerbations of chronic lung disease	
H. aegyptius (Koch–Weeks) bacillus)	• Aerobic	• A form of conjunctivitis	• Conjunctiva of a case
H. ducreyi	• Aerobic	• Genital ulcers, chancroid	
Bordetella *Bord. pertussis*	• Very fragile • Small coccobacillus • Needs Bordet–Gengou agar and CO_2 for culture	• Whooping cough	• Nasopharynx of a case
Brucella (i) *Br. abortus* (ii) *Br. melitensis** (iii) *Br. suis* (iv) *Br. canis*	• Non-spore-forming, aerobic • All are small coccobacilli • Need CO_2 for culture	• Brucellosis	• Disease in (i) cattle (ii) goats, sheep (iii) pigs and (iv) dogs • Secondary human infection. • Consumption of unpasteurized milk

*Most common worldwide.

Table 2.7 *(contd.)*

Genus and species	*Characteristics*	*Diseases produced in man*	*Reservoir of infections*
Yersinnia *Y. pestis*	• Aerobic	• Bubonic plague, pneumonic plague	• Rats: fleas transfer infection to man
Y. enterocolitica		• Gastroenteritis (invasive infection)	
Pasteurella *P. multocida*	• Aerobic	• Wound sepsis following a bite	• Dogs and cats
Legionella *L. pneumophila*	• Fastidious organism • Exotoxin • Demonstrated with difficulty in in tissues, using a silver stain	• Nosocomial pneumonia • Pontiac fever	• Air-conditioning units

Table 2.8 Gram-negative bacilli: Vibrios

Genus and species	*Characteristics*	*Diseases produced in man*	*Reservoir of infections*
Vibrio			
V. cholerae (classic and Eltor types)	• Aerobic, curved, motile rods	• Cholera (non-invasive infection)	• Human cases and carriers • Endemic disease in India and
Bangladesh			
V. parahaemolyticus	• Salt-dependent • Haemotoxins	• Food poisoning	• Warm sea-water; seafood, especially shellfish
Campylobacter			
C. fetus subspecies	• Microaerophilic	• Acute bloody diarrhoea	• Disease in wide range of animals

Table 2.9 Gram-negative bacteria: the enterobacteriae (non-spore-forming rods)

Genus and species	*Characteristics*	*Diseases produced in man*	*Reservoir of infections*
Escherichia *Esch. coli*	• Aerobic • Lactose fermenter • Many antigenic types • Enterotoxins	• Urinary tract and wound infections, peritonitis, cholecystitis, septicaemia, infantile gastroenteritis (some strains), neonatal meningitis and traveller's diarrhoea	• Commensal in large bowel • Contaminated meat, milk and water
E. coli 0157:H7 (first described in 1983)	• Serotype is designated by somatic (O) and flagellar (H) antigens • Produces shigella-like toxin • Vascular damage may lead to leakage of toxins, e.g. lipopolysaccharide, into circulation, which may initiate complications, e.g. haemolytic-uraemic syndrome (HUS) and thrombotic thrombocytopaenic purpura (TTP)	• Asymptomatic infection • Non-bloody or bloody diarrhoea • Haemolytic-uraemic syndrome in approx. 6% of cases • Thrombotic thrombocytopaenic purpura	• Contaminated ground beef, raw milk and water
Klebsiella *K. aerogenoses*	• Aerobic • Lactose fermenter • Heavily encapsulated	• Urinary tract and wound infections, otitis media and meningitis	
K. pneumoniae		• Pneumonia	• Saprophytic in water; also commensal in respiratory tract and intestine of man and animals

Table 2.9 *(cont.)*

Genus and species	*Characteristics*	*Diseases produced in man*	*Reservoir of infections*
Proteus *Pr. mirabilis* and other species	• Aerobic • Non-lactose fermenters • Swarming growth on agar medium	• Urinary tract and wound infections	• Commensal in large bowel • Occasionally pathogenic
Salmonella *S. typhi** and *S. paratyphi A, B* and *C*	• Aerobic • Non-lactose fermenters • Enterotoxins	• Typhoid fever, septicaemia and paratyphoid fever (the enteric fevers) • Food poisoning	• Contaminated food and water • Small bowel and gallbladder of cases and carriers
S. enteriditis and other species		• Food poisoning	• Cattle, poultry and pigs
Shigella *Sh. flexneri* *Sh. boydii* *Sh. sonnei* and *Sh. dysenteriae*	• Non-lactose fermenters • Endotoxin and exotoxin production	• Bacillary dysentery	• Human cases and carriers
Pseudomonas *Ps. aeroginosa*	• Aerobic • Non-lactose fermenting • Produces pigments: fluorescein and pyocyanin	• Hospital-acquired infections, pneumonia in ventilated patients, urinary tract and wound infections and septicaemia	
Ps. pseudomallei	• Diagnosed by blood or pus cultures and serology • Resistant to aminoglycosides†	• 4 presentations of melioidosis — acute — subacute — chronic — subclinical • Pulmonary involvement is commonest site • May be chronic with suppurative abscesses at several sites	• Endemic in South-East Asia (Thailand, Southern China), Central and South America, and Northern Australia • Direct contact with contaminated soil or water • Sporadic cases occur in temperate climates among travellers to endemic areas

Table 2.9 *(cont.)*

Genus and species	*Characteristics*	*Diseases produced in man*	*Reservoir of infections*
Ps. cepacia	• Slow growing on conventional solid media	• Lower respiratory tract infection in cystic fibrosis patients	• Environmental bacillus
Stenotrophomonas maltophilia	• Used to be classified as member of *Pseudomonas* group	• Hospital-acquired infections Often multiply antibiotic-resistant	• Also found in human intestines
Bacteroides			
B. fragilis and other species	• Anaerobic, non-spore-forming	• Appendicitis, peritonitis, wound infection, brain abscess, septicaemia and postoperative bacteraemic shock	• Commensal in intestine of man and animals • Present in vaginal flora and mouth
Fusobacterium *F. fusiforme*	• Anaerobic, non-spore-forming	• 'Vincent's' angina, gingivitis and stomatitis are associated with this organism and *Borr. vincenti*	• Commensal in mouth and intestine
Acinetobacter	• Strict anaerobes	• Hospital-acquired infections • Hospital outbreaks, particularly chest infections, occur in intensive care units	

**Widal test*
'O' (somatic) antigen appears on the 10th day of infection; antibody titres fall soon after infection.
'H' (flagellar) antigen appears late in the disease; antibodies are more specific and persist for long periods.
'V' (surface) antigen is measure of virulence; antibodies are present in about 75% of carriers.

Table 2.10 Gram-negative bacteria: the spirochaetes

Genus and species	*Characteristics*	*Diseases produced in man*	*Reservoir of infections*
Borrelia			
Borr. vincenti	• Aerobic • Long with loose spirals	• 'Vincent's' infections of gums or throat	• Commensal of mouth
Borr. recurrentis	• Anaerobic	• European relapsing fever	• Louse-borne
Borr. duttoni	• Anaerobic	• West African relapsing fever	• Tick-borne
Borr. burgdorfi	• Anaerobic	• Lyme disease	• Tick-borne
Helicobacter pylori (discovered in 1984)	• Spiral organism • Invasive tests require endoscopy (histology, culture and urease-based tests) • Non-invasive *H. pylori* antibody tests are >85% sensitive	• Peptic ulcer disease • Gastric carcinoma • Gastric lymphoma	• 50% prevalence in Western countries (higher in developing countries) • Prevalence increases with age • Transmission is thought to occur by the faecal–oral or oral–oral route, and is associated with close contact and poor sanitation.
Treponema			
Tr. pallidum	• Anaerobic • Short with tight spirals, and motile	• Syphilis	• Infected human cases • Sexually transmitted
Tr. pertenue	• Anaerobic	• Yaws	
Tr. carateum	• Anaerobic	• Pinta	
Leptospira			
Lepto. ictero-haemorrhagica	• Anaerobic • Fine, tight spirals with hooked ends	• Weil's disease	• Rodents
Lepto. canicola	• Anaerobic	• Canicola fever	• Dogs and pigs

Table 2.11 Gram-negative bacteria: the rickettsiae

Genus and species	*Characteristics*	*Diseases produced in man*	*Reservoir of infections*
Rickettsia	• Very small obligate intracellular bacteria • Positive Weil–Felix reaction, except *R. burnetti*		
R. prowazeki		• Epidemic typhus fever	• Louse-borne
R. mooseri		• Endemic typhus	• Rat flea-borne
R. rickettsii		• Rocky Mountain spotted fever	• Tick-borne (wood and dog tick)
R. tsutsugmushi		• Scrub-typhus	• Mite-borne
R. burnetti (*Coxiella burnetti*)		• Q fever (atypical pneumonia, endocarditis)	• Disease in cattle, sheep and goats
Ehrlichia chafeensis		• Human ehrlichiosis • Human granulocyte ehrlichiosis	• Tick-borne
Mycoplasma			
M. pneumoniae	• Very small, obligate intracellular bacteria, with no rigid cell wall • Special enriched media for culture	• Primary atypical pneumonia, upper respiratory tract infection • CNS complications e.g. Guillain–Barré syndrome	• Human cases and carriers • Droplet spread
Ureaplasma urealyticum	• Related genus that hydrolyses urea	• Urethritis • Endocarditis • Pelvic inflammatory disease	
M. hominis		• Pyelonephritis • Pelvic inflammatory disease • Post-abortal and post-partum fever	• Colonization with genital mycoplasmas occurs through sexual contact

Table 2.11 *(cont.)*

Genus and species	*Characteristics*	*Diseases produced in man*	*Reservoir of infections*
Chlamydia			
C. psittaci	• Very small spheres • Obligate intracellular bacteria	• Psittacosis	• Sick birds and their infectious excreta • Droplet spread
C. trachomatis	• Very small spheres • Obligate intracellular bacteria • Serotypes		
	— A, C	• Trachoma	• Man
	— D–K	• Cervicitis, conjunctivitis, urethritis, proctitis, pneumonia	• Man
	— L1, L2, L3	• Lymphogranuloma venereum	• Man
		• Urethritis • Possible cause of pelvic inflammatory disease, and opportunistic infections in the immunocompromised host (arteritis and meningitis)	
C. pneumoniae		• Atypical pneumonia	

Table 2.12 Higher bacteria

Genus and species	*Characteristics*	*Diseases produced in man*	*Reservoir of infections*
Actinomyces *A. israelii*	• Anaerobic • Branching filaments	• Actinomycosis, abscess in cervicofacial region, (occasionally in abdomen and chest)	• Commensal in mouth
Nocardia *N. asteroides*	• Anaerobic • Branching filaments	• Opportunistic infection • Pulmonary and systemic nocardiosis	• Saprophytic in soil

ANTIBACTERIAL CHEMOTHERAPY

SPECTRA OF ACTIVITY AND SITES OF ACTION

These are presented in Tables 2.13 and 2.14.

Table 2.13 Antibacterial chemotherapy: spectra of activity

Antibiotic	*Spectrum of activity*
Penicillins (penicillinase-sensitive)	*Gram +ve cocci* *Staph. aureus* (non-penicillinase-producing strains) *Strep. pneumoniae, Strep. viridans* and β-haemolytic strep. *Gram –ve cocci* *N. meningitides* and *gonorrhoeae* *Gram +ve bacilli* *B. anthracis, Cl. tetani* *Resistant organisms* Penicillinase-producing staphylococci *Strep. faecalis* *N. gonorrhoeae* (some strains) *H. influenzae* *E. coli* *Klebsiella* sp. *Proteus* sp. *Pseudomonas aeroginosa* *Bacteroides fragilis* *Mycoplasma pneumonia* (lacks a cell wall)
Flucloxacillin/methicillin (penicillinase-resistant)	Penicillinase-producing staphylococci*
Amoxicillin/ampicillin (penicillinase-sensitive)	Similar spectrum to penicillins Also effective against some Gram –ve organisms, e.g. *E. coli, H. influenzae, Brucella* and *Salmonella* species

Table 2.13 *(cont.)*

Antibiotic	*Spectrum of activity*
Carbenicillin/piperacillin (penicillinase-sensitive)	Broad spectrum Severe infections due to sensitive Gram +ve, –ve and anaerobic bacteria Also *Pseudomonas aeroginosa*
Cephalosporins *1st generation* cephaloridine cephalexin cephradine *2nd generation* cefotoxin cefuroxime *3rd generation* cefotaxime	1st generation has a similar spectrum to penicillins 2nd and 3rd generation have a broader spectrum and are active against some Gram –ve bacteria, e.g. *E. coli, Salmonella* and *Klebsiella* 3rd generation also active against anaerobic species, and are very resistant to β-lactamase
Aminoglycosides amikacin gentamicin neomycin tobramycin	Serious Gram –ve infections, e.g. *E. coli, Pseudomonas, H. influenzae* Some strains of *Staph. aureus*
Tetracycline (longer-acting analogues are demeclocycline and doxycycline)	*Brucella, Chlamydia, Mycoplasma* and *Rickettsiae* (Q fever) However, *Proteus, Pseudomonas* and many *Staph.* and *Strep.* strains are resistant
Chloramphenicol	Typhoid and paratyphoid infections *H. influenzae meningitis* *Klebsiella* sp. *Rickettsia* sp. *Chlamydia* sp.
Erythromycin (macrolide antibiotic)	Similar spectrum to penicillins *Mycoplasma* sp. Diphtheria carriers *Legionella pneumophila* *Chlamydia* sp. *Campylobacter* sp.
Sulphonamides/ co-trimoxazole/ trimethoprim	Severe urinary tract infections and chronic bronchitis *Salmonella* infections *Brucella* sp. *Pneumocystis carinii* *Toxoplasma gondii*
Rifampicin	Gram +ve and –ve bacteria *Mycobacterium tuberculosis*

*Most strains of *Staph. aureus* are sensitive to cloxacillin, cephalosporins and gentamicin; 50% of strains in the community and 85% in hospitals are resistant to benzylpenicillin.

Table 2.14 Sites of action of antibacterials

Site of action	*Examples of antibacterials*
Cell wall	Penicillins Cephalosporins Vancomycin
Cell membrane	Polymyxins
Protein synthesis	Aminoglycosides Chloramphenicol Fusidic acid Macrolides Tetracyclines
DNA synthesis	Sulphonamides Trimethoprim Quinolones
RNA synthesis	Rifampicin

BACTERICIDAL AND BACTERIOSTATIC DRUGS (Table 2.15)

Bactericidal drugs kill bacteria; these are preferable if the host is immunocompromised.
Bacteriostatic drugs stop bacterial division; bacteria are eliminated by the host's defences.

Table 2.15 Bactericidal and bacteriostatic drugs

Bactericidals	*Bacteriostatics*
Penicillins	Tetracyclines
Cephalosporins	Chloramphenicol*
Aminoglycosides	Sulphonamides
Nitrofurantoin	Erythromycin
Co-trimoxazole	Trimethoprim
Metronidazole	PAS
Isoniazid	Novobiocin
Quinolones (ciprofloxacin, norfloxacin)	Clindamycin
Rifampicin	

*Bactericidal against some bacteria e.g. *Strep. pneumoniae, H. influenzae.*

BOX 2.2 DRUGS IN COMBINATION

In general:

- The combination of a bacteriostatic drug with a bactericidal drug results in *antagonism*, e.g. penicillin with chloramphenicol or tetracycline.
- Bactericidal drugs in combination tend to be *synergistic*, e.g. aminoglycosides with penicillin.
- Synergism is unusual when two bacteriostatic drugs are used in combination.

ANTIBIOTIC RESISTANCE

- Natural resistance
- Acquired resistance arises either by:
  1. Emergence of pre-existent resistant mutant pathogens (e.g. penicillinase-resistant) through selective pressure, or by
  2. New mutation through several possible mechanisms.
     (a) *Transformation* – direct uptake of genetic material liberated from another cell.
     (b) *Conjugation* – genetic exchange between two bacterial strains with transfer of a resistance (R) factor or plasmid, which is dependent on cell-to-cell contact, e.g. development of gentamicin resistance.
     (c) *Transduction* – transfer of genetic material from one cell to another by means of a viral vector or bacteriophage, e.g., development of penicillin resistance by *Staph. aureus*
     (d) *Transfection* – infection of a cell with isolated DNA or RNA from a virus or virus vector.

Enzyme-mediated resistance is the most important form of acquired resistance seen in clinical isolates, and is generally plasmid-mediated.
Hospital multiply-resistant organisms, include *E. coli*, *Klebsiella* and methicillin-resistant *Staph. aureus* (MRSA), which also has variable resistance to the aminoglycosides.

VIRUSES

STRUCTURE OF THE VIRION (Fig. 2.1)

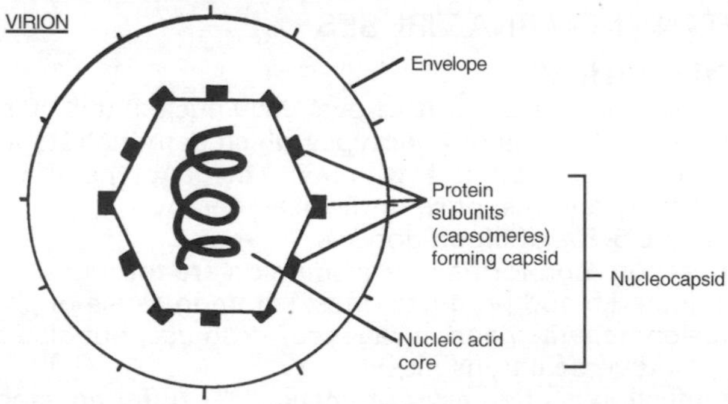

Fig. 2.1

VIRAL REPLICATION AND SITES OF ACTION OF ANTIVIRAL DRUGS (Fig. 2.2)

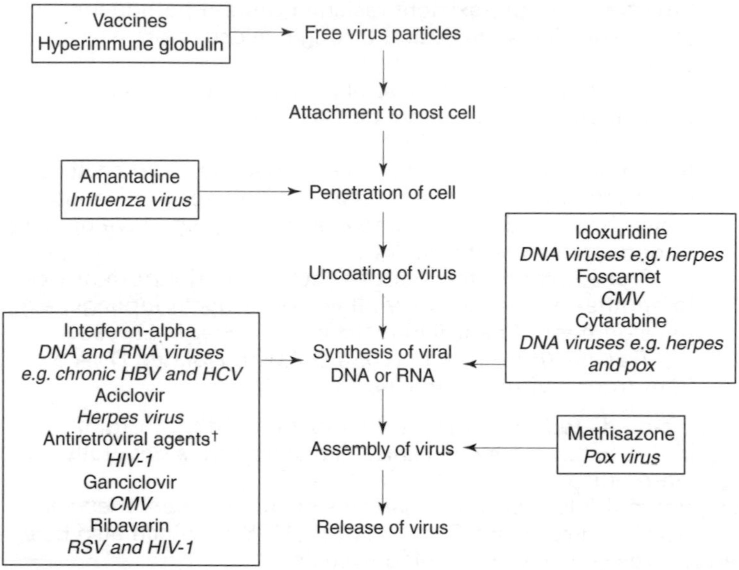

† Nucleoside reverse transcriptase inhibitors (NRTI) e.g. ZDV, ddI, ddc, 3TC, d4T
Non-nucleoside reverse transcriptase inhibitors (NNRTI) e.g. nevaripine, delavirdine

Fig. 2.2

RNA-CONTAINING VIRUSES (Table 2.16)

IMPORTANT NEW RNA VIRUSES

Hepatitis C (HCV)

- Positive stranded RNA virus of over 9000 nucleotides. It is classified into two major genotypes which demonstrate a geographical variation in distribution. The genotype affects pathogenicity and response to medical therapy.
- Present in 0.5–8% of blood donors.
- The most common forms of transmission are through contaminated blood products (most common cause of post-transfusion hepatitis) and intravenous drug use, but also sexual contact and vertical transmission.
- Acute infection is often asymptomatic; 25% suffer an icteric illness; 60% of patients have a chronic course; 20% will develop cirrhosis after 20 years, and 15% of these will develop hepatocellular carcinoma.

Table 2.16 RNA-containing viruses

RNA-containing viruses	*Main diseases produced in man*
Picornaviruses	
A. Enteroviruses:	Usually subclinical
Polio (3 types)	Poliomyelitis, aseptic meningitis
Coxsackie A (23 types)	Aseptic meningitis, herpangina, conjunctivitis
Coxsackie B (6 types)	Pleurodynia, myocarditis, aseptic meningitis and encephalitis
Enterovirus 70	Pandemic conjunctivitis
Enterovirus 72	
ECHO (31 types)	Aseptic meningitis, conjunctivitis
B. Hepatovirus	Hepatitis C
C. Rhinoviruses (>100 serotypes)	Common cold
Orthomyxoviruses and paramyxoviruses	
Influenza A, B, C, parainfluenza	Upper respiratory tract infections, influenza, Reye's syndrome
Mumps	Mumps, occasionally meningitis
Measles	Measles, encephalomyelitis, subacute sclerosing panencephalitis
Respiratory syncytial virus (RSV)	Bronchiolitis
Reoviruses	
Reovirus	Upper respiratory tract infections
Rotavirus	Infantile diarrhoea
Togaviruses	
Alphaviruses*	Encephalitides in the US (St Louis, Western and Eastern equine viruses)
Flaviviruses*	Yellow fever, dengue fever
Rubivirus	Rubella
Hepatitis C virus (HCV)	Hepatitis
Arenaviruses	
Lassa fever	Lassa fever
Lymphocytic choriomeningitis	Aseptic meningitis in man
Toroviruses	Marburg and Ebola fever
Retroviruses	
Human immunodeficiency virus (HIV) 1 and 2	ARC and AIDS (see p. 101) Spectrum of HIV-related neurological disease,
Human T-cell lymphotrophic virus (HTLV) HTLV-I	Adult T-cell leukaemia, tropical spastic paraparesis
HTLV-II	T-cell hairy leukaemia
Rhabdoviruses	
Rabies	Rabies
Calciviruses, astroviruses and small round viruses (SRVs)	
Hepatitis E	Hepatitis
Norwalk virus	Gastroenteritis
Astrovirus	Gastroenteritis

*Formerly known as arboviruses.

- Diagnosis uses second- and third-generation antibody assays. The polymerase chain reaction can also be used to detect the presence of hepatitis C RNA. A vaccine has not been developed.

Hepatitis D (HDV)

- Defective RNA virus which can only replicate in HBV-infected cells.
- Transmission is by infected blood and sexual intercourse.
- HDV accentuates HBV infection, resulting in more severe liver disease.
- Diagnosis is by HDV antibody (or rarely antigen) detection.
- No vaccines available at present.

Hepatitis E (HEV)

- 27.34 nm diameter unenveloped, single-stranded RNA virus.
- True incidence unknown, but approximately 2% of blood donors are seropositive.
- Most outbreaks and sporadic cases have occurred in developing countries, e.g. China, India, Pakistan and Mexico. Hepatitis E can also be transmitted vertically and by the faecal–oral route. No animal hosts have been identified.
- Incubation period is 2–9 weeks. The majority of cases experience a self-limiting hepatitis. Severe fulminant hepatitis may occur in pregnant women.

Human immunodeficiency virus (HIV)

- HIV-I (formerly HLTV-III) is a retrovirus containing single-stranded RNA.
- The proviral genome consists of the *gag, pol* and *env* genes (Table 2.17), at least five regulatory genes and long terminal redundancies (LTRs) at each end.
- See also pages 101–102.

Table 2.17 Principal components of HIV

Genes	*Products*
Structural	
env	gp160 (gp120 + gp41)
gag	Core proteins (p24, p17, p15)
Enzymes	
pol	Reverse transcriptase, protease, integrase, ribonuclease
Regulatory	
tat, *rev*, *nef*	Activating and regulatory proteins

Figure 2.3 shows the immunological and virological pattern of response following HIV infection.

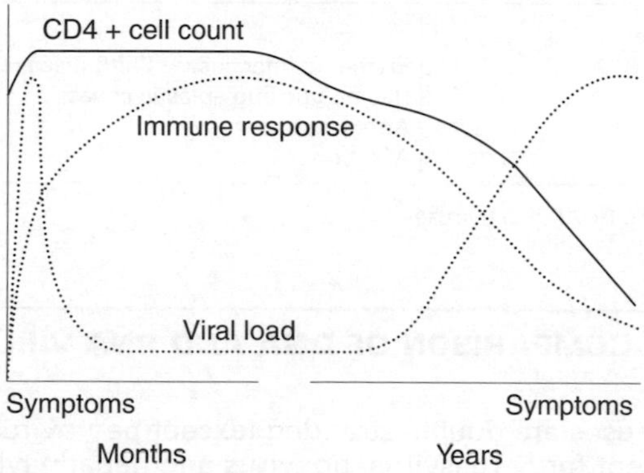

Fig. 2.3

DNA-CONTAINING VIRUSES (Table 2.18)

Table 2.18 DNA-containing viruses*

DNA-containing viruses	*Main diseases caused in man*
H Herpesviruses	
Herpes simplex (HSV) I and II	Stomatitis, cold sores, keratoconjunctivitis, genital herpes, neonatal herpes, aseptic meningitis and encephalitis
Varicella-zoster (VZV)	Chicken pox, herpes zoster
Epstein–Barr virus (EBV)	Infectious mononucleosis, also possibly Burkitt's lymphoma and nasopharyngeal carcinoma
Cytomegalovirus (CMV)	Cytomegalic inclusion disease, pneumonitis, retinitis and colitis Intrauterine infection
H Hepadnaviruses	
Hepatitis B	Hepatitis
A Adenoviruses	
(41 serotypes)	Upper respiratory tract infections, epidemic keratoconjunctivitis, diarrhoea
P Papovaviruses	
Papilloma virus	Warts
Polyoma (BK and JC viruses)	Progressive multifocal leucoencephalopathy
P Pox viruses	
Variola	Smallpox
Vaccinia	Vaccinia
Molluscum contagiosum	Molluscum contagiosum
Orf	Pustular dermatitis

Table 2.18 *(cont.)*

DNA-containing viruses	*Main diseases caused in man*
P Parvoviruses Parvovirus B19	 Erythema infectiosum ('fifth disease') Haemolytic and aplastic crises Arthropathy Abortion

*Mnemonic – the HHAPPP(Y) viruses.

BOX 2.3 COMPARISON OF DNA AND RNA VIRUSES

In general:
All DNA viruses are double-stranded (except parvovirus) and naked (except for herpesvirus, poxvirus and hepadnavirus). All RNA viruses are single-stranded (except reovirus) and enveloped (except for picornavirus and reovirus).

HUMAN SLOW VIRUS INFECTIONS (Table 2.19)

Table 2.19 Human slow virus infections

Virus/agent	*Disease*
Measles	Subacute sclerosing panencephalitis (SSPE)
Papovavirus (JC virus)	Progressive multifocal leucoencephalopathy (PML) HIV encephalopathy
Rubella	Progressive rubella panencephalitis (PRP)
Retrovirus	Acquired immunodeficiency syndrome (AIDS)
Prion disease*	Kuru Creutzfeldt–Jakob disease (CJD)
?Measles virus	Multiple sclerosis

*Proteinacious infectious particle: virus-like particle, but with no nucleic acid content.

Prion diseases (transmissible spongiform encephalopathies)

- Rare.
- Present classically with rapidly progressive neurodegeneration, cognitive impairment, ataxia, myoclonus and motor dysfunction.
- May be genetic, sporadic or infectious. Iatrogenic transmission of CJD has been well documented following human growth hormone therapy and corneal transplantation, but not following

blood transfusion. It remains controversial as to how CJD is transmitted from cattle with bovine spongiform encephalopathy.

- The pathogenic prion-related protein (PrP) is encoded by the PRNP gene on chromosome 20. It is protease-resistant and accumulates in the brain. In the familial forms, mutations of the PRNP gene are found.
- Histologically these diseases resemble amyloidoses, in which the host-encoded protein acquires a beta sheet conformation producing amyloid which accumulates and causes vacuolar degeneration of neurons.

ONCOGENIC VIRUSES (Table 2.20)

- May possess either RNA or DNA.
- Invasion of the host cell results in recombination with the host genome, causing permanent infection of the cell. These transformed cells differ from normal cells in that they have lost their capacity for contact inhibition.
- The RNA viruses become integrated by an RNA-dependent DNA polymerase (reverse transcriptase).

Table 2.20 Oncogenic viruses

Virus	*Disease*
Pox virus	Molluscum contagiosum
Hepatitis B	Liver cancer
EBV	Burkitt's lymphoma (in malaria-infested parts of Africa), and other lymphomas in immunosuppression; nasopharyngeal carcinomas (S. China)
Human papilloma virus (HPV 16, 18 and others)	Warts, genital warts, cervical, vulval, penile, anal and perianal carcinoma, and ?skin cancer (HPV types 5, 8, 14, 17, 20)
HTLV-I	Adult T-cell leukaemia
HHV 8	Kaposi's sarcoma
Adenovirus, SV40	Malignant neoplasms in mice

IMPORTANT SEROLOGICAL TESTS

1. HEPATITIS B SEROLOGY (Table 2.21)

Hepatitis B (HB)

- Part double-stranded, 42-mm enveloped particle with inner 27-mm core particle (Dane particle)
- Three viral antigens:
  1. Surface antigen (HBsAg) leading to production of HBsAb.

Table 2.21 Interpretation of hepatitis B serum antigen and antibody markers

HBsAg	*Anti-HBs*	*Anti-HBc*	*Interpretation*
+	–	–	Early acute disease – patient is considered infectious
+		+	Acute disease or chronic carrier – patient is considered infectious
–	+	+	Convalescing from the disease or immune
–	+	+	Immune via disease or vaccination
–	–	+	Recent disease. Serum taken after HBsAg disappeared and before anti-HBs – patient is considered infectious

2. Core antigen in Dane particles (HBcAg) leading to production of HBcAb.
3. DNA polymerase-associated 'e' antigen (HBeAg) is formed as the result of the breakdown of core antigen released from infected liver cells. Marker of infectivity.

- Whole particle and surface antigen present in serum, saliva and semen.

2. HIV SEROLOGY

- Serum antibody to HIV may appear between 2 weeks and 1 year after infection (most commonly 1–3 months after infection).
- An enzyme-linked immunoabsorbent assay (ELISA) is used to screen for HIV antibody. When a positive test is obtained, it should be confirmed with a Western blot or further Elisa assay.
- The Western blot measures patient antibody to specific HIV proteins (see p. 101). Combining these two tests, the false-positive rate is 1 in 135 200.

3. SYPHILIS SEROLOGY

Non-treponemal tests

These detect an antibody-like substance (not a specific antitreponemal antibody) which appears more commonly and in high titre in treponemal disease. Relatively insensitive in primary/late syphilis.

1. Venereal disease research laboratory (VDRL) test: antibody detected by a flocculation reaction.
2. Rapid plasma reagin (RPR).

Treponemal tests

These are more specific.

1. Treponema pallidum haemagglutination test (TPHA).
2. Treponema pallidum immobilization test (TPI).
3. Fluorescent treponemal antibody absorption test (FTA-ABS): most sensitive test for syphilis; positive early in the disease.

Interpretation of results

- If treatment is early in primary infection, then serological tests may remain negative.
- If treated during the secondary stage when serology is usually positive, non-treponemal tests revert to negative within a year, but treponemal tests usually remain positive for years.
- Treatment in the late stages may not affect the serological reactions.
- Non-treponemal tests positive and treponemal tests negative: classic biologic false-positive reaction, such as with acute viral illness, collagen vascular disease and pregnancy.

FUNGI

Table 2.22 Important fungal infections

Genus	*Main diseases produced in man*
Dermatophytes	
Epidermophyton	• Tinea of foot, groin and nail
Microsporum	• Tinea of head and body
Tricophyton	• Tinea of head, body and nails ('athlete's foot')
Malassezia	• Pityriasis versicolor
Pathogenic yeasts	
Candida	• Candidiasis, oral thrush, oesophagitis, vulvovaginitis and skin disease • Causes septicaemia with endocarditis and meningitis in immunocompromised persons
Torulopsis	• Oropharyngitis, vulvovaginitis, septicaemia and endocarditis
Cryptococcus	• Meningitis, lung, skin and bone infection
Dimorphic fungi (i.e. grow as moulds and yeasts)	
Blastomyces	• N. American blastomycosis: primary infection of lungs, and sometimes skin. Also S. American sp.
Coccidioides	• Coccidioidomycosis: usually a benign infection of the lungs; rarely disseminated spread. Occurs in Central and S. America
Histoplasma	• Acute or chronic pulmonary infection • Disseminated histoplasmosis with granulomata especially in lymphoreticular organs. Meningitis and endocarditis may also occur. Found in USA
Miscellaneous fungal infections	
Aspergillus	• Primary infection usually of the lung: asthma. • Systemic infection: aspergillosis
Mucor and rhizopus	• Phycomycosis: local infection of nose, paranasal sinuses, lungs and gastrointestinal tract may lead to systemic infection and meningitis

ANTIFUNGAL CHEMOTHERAPY

- *Amphotericin B* is the drug of choice for all agents listed, except for candida (nystatin).
- *Griseofulvin* is the drug of choice for dermatophytes but is ineffective against aspergillus.
- *Ketoconazole* is recommended for blastomycosis, coccidioidomycosis and candida.
- *Miconazole* is recommended for coccidioidomycosis, cryptococcus and candida.
- *Fluconazole* is used to treat candidiasis and cryptococcal meningitis.
- *5-Flucytosine* is used mainly in the treatment of cryptococcus in combination with amphotericin B.

PARASITES

Table 2.23 Important parasitic infections

Genus	*Mode of infection*	*Main disease produced in man*
Taenia solium (pork tapeworm)	Via ingestion of ova	Enteritis
Enterobius vermicularis (threadworms)	"	Pruritis ani
Ascaris lumbricoides (roundworms)	"	Enteritis, pneumonitis, ileal and biliary obstruction, acute cholangitis
Toxocara canis	"	Visceral larvae migrans, toxocariasis (hepatosplenomegaly, chorioretinitis and CNS mass lesions)
Echinococcus granulosa	"	Pulmonary and hydatid disease
Entamoeba histolytica	Via ingestion of cyst	Amoebiasis, amoebic liver abscess
Naegleria and Acanthamoeba	"	Meningitis
Cryptosporidium parvum	"	Cryptosporidiosis
Isospora belli	"	Diarrhoea
Giardia lamblia	"	Giardiasis, malabsorption
Toxoplasma gondii	"	Widespread, usually asymptomatic infection, encephalitis in immunocompromised Also intrauterine infection
Trichinella spiralis	Via ingestion of larvae	Trichinosis (myalgia and eosinophilia)

Table 2.23 *(cont.)*

Genus	*Mode of infection*	*Main disease produced in man*
Taenia saginata (beef tapeworm)	Via ingestion of larvae	Enteritis
Taenia solium	"	Enteritis and cysticercosis (focal lesions in skeletal and cardiac muscle, subcutaneous tissue and brain)
Diphyllobothrium latum	"	Enteritis and vitamin B_{12} deficiency
Ancylostoma duodenale (hookworm)	Via larval penetration of skin	Enteritis and iron deficiency anemia
Schistosoma mansoni	Via cercarial penetration of skin	Enteric schistosomiasis, hepatic fibrosis (S. America, Caribbean, Africa and Middle East)
Schistosoma japonicum		Enteric schistosomiasis, precancerous bladder inflammation (Far East)
Plasmodium falciparum, vivax and ovale	Via bite of arthropod vector	Malaria, blackwater fever (falciparum)
Leishmania		
L. Donovani	"	Visceral leishmaniasis (Africa, Asia)
L. tropica } *L. major* }	" "	Cutaneous leishmaniasis (Africa, Asia, Mediterranean)
L. braziliensis	"	Mucutaneous leishmaniasis
Onchocerca volvulus	"	Onchocerciasis ('river blindness')
Wuchereria bancrofti	"	Lymphadenitis and elephantiasis
Trichomonas vaginalis	Via direct contact	Silent venereal infection in females and males, or acute vaginitis in females and acute urethritis in males
Pneumocystis carinii	Via inhalation	Pneumonitis in premature infants and immunosuppressed adults (e.g. AIDS)

Plasmodial infection (Table 2.24)

Table 2.24 Plasmodial infection in humans

Species	*Fever cycle (h)*	*Clinical condition*
Plasmodium falciparum malaria	36–48	Malignant tertian
Plasmodium malariae	72	Quartan malaria
Plasmodium ovale	36–48	Benign tertian malaria
Plasmodium vivax	36–48	Benign tertian malaria

Life cycle of Plasmodium species (see Fig. 2.4)

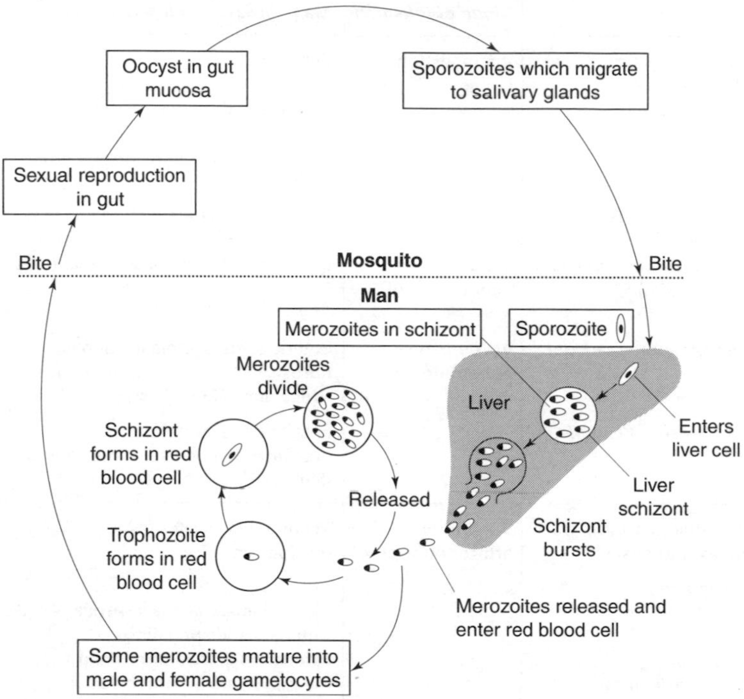

Fig. 2.4

1. The Anopheles mosquito is the intermediate host. It is infected by blood-borne gametocytes from man.
2. These develop in the mosquito and sporozoites are formed which pass into the blood stream of man when bitten.
3. The sporozoites pass to the liver where they develop into merozoites which are then released into the blood stream.
4. These are taken up by the erythrocytes where they develop and divide (schizogony). This coincides with the clinical attack of malaria following rupture of erythrocytes, and is the phase most susceptible to treatment.
5. Some gametocytes are formed which are released into the blood where they can reinfect the mosquito.

ANTIPARASITE CHEMOTHERAPY

Table 2.25 Antiparasite chemotherapy

Organism	*Drug*
Nematodes *(roundworms)* *Trichinella spiralis* *Enterobius vermicularis* *Ancylostoma duodenale* *Ascaris lumbricoides*	Mebendazole
Cestodes *(tapeworms)* *Taenia saginata* *Taenia solium* *Echinococcus granulosa* *Diphyllobothrium latum*	Niclosamide
Trematodes *(blood flukes)* *Schistosoma mansoni, japonicum and haematobium*	Praziquantel
Protozoa	
Entamoeba histolytica *Giardia lamblia* *Trichomonas vaginalis*	Metronidazole, Tinidazole
Plasmodium spp.	4-aminoquinolines, e.g. chloroquine, block nucleic acid synthesis by the malarial parasites in their erythrocyte forms. Used as suppressive treatment and for clinical attack. Diaminopyridamines, e.g. pyrimethamine, inhibit dihydrofolate reductase and so block the synthesis of folic acid. Effective against the erythrocyte form and formation of sporozoites.
Toxoplasma gondii	Pyrimethamine and sulphadiazine
Pneumocystis carinii	Trimethoprim and sulphamethoxazole, pentamidine
Filariasis	Diethylcarbamazine, Ivermectin
Trypanosomiasis	Suramin, pentamidine and melasoprol (for CNS disease)
Leishmaniasis	Sodium stibogluconate, pentamidine

OPPORTUNISTIC PATHOGENS

Common examples of these are presented in Table 2.25.

Table 2.25 Common opportunistic pathogens

Bacteria	*Staphylococcus aureus* Coagulase-negative staphylococci *Mycobacterium avium-intracellulare* Enterobacteriaceae
Fungi	*Candida* species *Aspergillus* species *Pneumocystis carinii*
Protozoa	Toxoplasma
Parasites	*Strongyloides stercoralis*
Viruses	Herpes simplex viruses Cytomegalovirus Varicella zoster virus Epstein–Barr virus

INCUBATION PERIODS

These are presented in Tables 2.26 and 2.27, for common infections and food poisoning.

Table 2.26 Incubation of common infections

Incubation period	*Disease*
Short: 1–7 days	Anthrax Diphtheria Gonorrhoea Meningococcus Influenza Cytomegalovirus Group A streptococci (erysipelas) Scarlet fever Bacillary dysentery
Intermediate: 7–14 days	Measles Lassa fever Whooping cough Malaria Tetanus Typhus fever Typhoid Poliomyelitis
Long: 14–21 days	Brucellosis Amoebiasis Chickenpox Rubella Mumps
Very long: >21 days	Hepatitis: A (2–6 weeks) B (2–6 months) non-A non-B (6 weeks–6 months)

Table 2.27 Food poisoning incubation periods

Organism	*Incubation period (h)*
Bacillus cereus	0.5–6.0
Campylobacter jejuni	48–120
Clostridium perfringens	12–24
Clostridium botulinum	12–36
Salmonellae	18–48
Staphylococcus aureus	1–6
Vibrio parahaemolyticus	6–36

IMMUNIZATION

VACCINES

Vaccines in clinical use are shown in Table 2.28, and live attenuated and killed vaccines are compared in Table 2.29.

Table 2.28 Vaccines in clinical use

Live attenuated bacteria	Bacillus Calmette–Guérin (BCG)
Live attenuated viruses	Measles, Mumps, Rubella } i.e. MMR
	Polio (oral)
	Varicella zoster
	Yellow fever
	Typhoid (new)
Whole killed organism	Rabies
	Polio (Salk)
	Pertussis
	Typhoid
	Cholera
	Influenza*
Subcellular fragment	
Inactivated toxin (toxoid)	Diphtheria
	Tetanus
	Cholera (new)
Capsular polysaccharide	Meningococcus (group A and C)
	Pneumococcus (23 capsular types)
	Haemophilus
	Typhoid (new)
Surface antigen	Hepatitis B recombinant-DNA-based

*Non-live subunit trivalent preparation with two A and one B subunits. Vaccination is recommended for all groups at risk, e.g. patients with diabetes, renal failure, and the immunosuppressed.

Table 2.29 Differences between live attenuated and killed vaccines

	Live attenuated	*Killed*
Immunity	Strong; localized Usually appropriate type Usually good memory May induce 'herd' immunity	May be weak May be inappropriate (e.g. antibody vs CMI) Memory variable (poor with polysaccharides)
Boosting	Usually not required	Often required
Adjuvant	Not required	Usually required
Safety	Unsafe in immunocompromised, may revert to virulence	Usually safe if properly inactivated
Storage	Depends on 'cold chain'	Usually no problem
Side-effects	Egg hypersensitivity (some viruses)	Toxicity (e.g. pertussis?)

IMMUNIZATION SCHEDULE

The ages at which immunization should take place, as recommended in the UK, are shown in Table 2.30.

CONTRAINDICATIONS

Contraindications to immunization

1. Febrile illness, intercurrent infections.
2. Hypersensitivity to egg protein contraindicates influenza vaccine; previous anaphylactic reaction to egg contraindicates influenza and yellow fever vaccines.

No live vaccine

No live vaccine should be used in cases of:

1. Immunodeficiency.
2. Immunosuppression.
3. High dose of corticosteroids.
4. Malignancy, e.g. lymphoma, leukaemia, or Hodgkin's disease.
5. Pregnancy.

Non-contraindications

The following are *not* contraindications to immunization:

1. Family history of any adverse reactions following immunization.
2. Family history of convulsions.
3. Previous history of pertussis, measles, rubella or mumps infection.
4. Prematurity.

Table 2.30 Recommended UK immunization schedule

Recommended age	*Vaccine*
Neonatal	BCG (infants of Asian mothers or with family history of active TB)
2 months	Diphtheria-tetanus-pertussis (DPT)—1st dose Oral polio vaccine (OPV)—1st dose Haemophilus influenzae b (Hib) vaccine
3 months	DPT—2nd dose OPV—2nd dose
4 months	DPT—3rd dose OPV—3rd dose
1–2 years	Measles/mumps/rubella (MMR)
5 years or at school entry	DT—booster (pertussis under review) OPV—booster MMR (if not previously given)
10–13 years	BCG (for tuberculin –ve)*
11–13 years	Rubella (girls only)
15–19 years	Rubella for seronegative women of child-bearing age Influenza† and Hepatitis B‡ for individuals in high risk groups Polio and tetanus for previously unimmunized individuals

*Other indications: contacts of known BCG cases; neonates born in households where there is active TB; immigrants from countries with a high prevalence of TB, and their children, wherever born; health workers at risk of exposure, e.g. lab. workers and veterinary staff.
†Indications: the elderly, especially those in long-term residential accommodation; children in residential accommodation who have reached the age of 4 years; those with chronic heart, lung and renal disease, or diabetes; medical nursing and ambulance staff.
‡Indications: health workers in direct contact with carriers or other high-risk patients; renal dialysis patients; sexual partners of infected carriers; drug addicts; homosexuals and their sexual partners. Meningococcus used in epidemics; pneumococcus in elderly or splenectomized patients; varicella zoster in leukaemic children.

5. Stable neurological conditions, e.g. cerebral palsy or Down's syndrome.
6. Asthma, eczema or hay fever.
7. History of jaundice after birth.
8. Over the age recommended in immunization schedule.
9. Recent or imminent surgery.
10. Replacement corticosteriods.

PREPARATIONS FOR PASSIVE IMMUNIZATION

Normal or specific immunoglobulin

- Measles, hepatitis A and B, chickenpox, tetanus, rabies, rubella and mumps.
- All used for prophylaxis and postexposure treatment (within 72 hours) except hepatitis A.

Antitoxins

- Diphtheria, gas gangrene and botulism.
- All used for prophylaxis and postexposure treatment.

STERILIZATION AND DISINFECTION

- *Sterilization*: the process by which all viable microorganisms, including spores, are removed or killed.
- *Disinfection*: the process by which most, but not all viable microorganisms are removed or killed.
- *Pasteurization*: the process used to eliminate pathogens in foods such as milk. Spores are unaffected.

The characteristics of some agents used in sterilization and disinfection are presented in Table 2.31.

Table 2.31 Agents used in sterilization and disinfection

Group	*Example*	*Bactericidal*		*Sporicidal*	*Fungicidal*	*Viricidal*	*Mycobactericidal*	*Uses*
		Gram-negative	*Gram-positive*					
Alcohols	70% ethyl alcohol	+	+	–	–	–	–	Skin antiseptic
Aldehydes	Formaldehyde	+	+	+	+	+	+	Fumigation
	Glutaraldehyde	+	+	+	+	+	+	Disinfection of fibreoptic endoscopes
Biguanides	Chlorhexidine	–	+	–	–	–	–	Hand wash; skin antiseptic
Halogens	Hypochlorites Chlorine	+	+	±	+	+	–	General environmental cleaning; blood spills; treating water
	Iodine	+	+	±	+	+	–	With alcohol; used for skin preparation; hand wash and skin ulcers
Phenolics	Phenol (carbolic acid)	±	+	–	–	–	+	Absorbed by rubber; too irritant for general use
	Hexachlorophane	–	+	–	–	–	–	Powder form for skin
	Chloroxylenols (Dettol)	–	±	–	–	–	–	application, skin disinfection
Quaternary ammonium compounds	Cetrimide	±	+	–	±	–	–	Skin disinfection
	Benzalkonium chloride	±	+	–	+	–	–	Preservative of topical preparation/antimicrobial plastic catheters

+, yes; –, no; ±, intermediate.

3. Immunology

CHAPTER CONTENTS

GLOSSARY

Adaptive immunotherapy: The transfer of immune cells for therapeutic benefit.

ADCC, antibody-dependent cellular cytotoxicity: The ability of sensitized cells to lyse other cells that have been coated by specific antibodies.

Adhesion molecule: A cell surface molecule involved in cell–cell interaction.

Adjuvant: Any foreign material introduced with an antigen to enhance its immunogenicity, e.g. killed bacteria, (mycobacteria), emulsions (Freund's adjuvant) or precipitates (alums).

Alloantibody: Antibody raised in one individual and directed against an antigen (primarily on cells) of another individual of the same species.

Allogeneic: See p. 107.

Allotypes: Antigenically dissimilar variants, e.g. of plasma proteins.

Apoptosis: Programmed cell death: a mode of cell death which occurs under physiological conditions, and is controlled by the dying cell itself ('cell suicide').

Autologous: Originating from the same individual.

β_2-microglobulin: A polypeptide which constitutes part of some membrane proteins including the class I MHC molecules.

CD markers (cluster of differentiation): Used as a prefix (and number). Cell surface molecules of lymphocytes and platelets that are distinguishable with monoclonal antibodies, and may be used to distinguish different cell populations.

Cell adhesion molecules (CAMs): A group of proteins of the immunoglobulin supergene family involved in intercellular adhesion, including ICAM-1, ICAM-2, ICAM-3, VCAM-1, MAd CAM-1 and PECAM.

Class I/II restriction: The observation that immunologically active cells will only operate effectively when they share MHC haplotypes of either the class I or class II loci.

Class switching: The process by which B cells can express a new heavy chain isotype without altering the specificity of the antibody produced. This occurs by gene rearrangement.

Clonal selection: The fundamental basis of lymphocyte activation in which antigen selectively causes activation, division and differentiation only in those cells which express receptors with which it can combine.

Colony-stimulating factors (CSFs): A group of cytokines which control the differentiation of haemopoetic stem cells.

Constant regions: The relatively invariant parts of the immunoglobulin heavy and light chains, and the α, β, γ and δ chains of the T-cell receptor.

Domain: Segments or loops on heavy and light chains formed by intrachain disulphide bonds. Each immunoglobulin domain consists of about 110 amino acids.

Epitope: Part of an antigen that binds to an antibody-combining site or a specific T-cell surface receptor, and determines specificity. Usually about 9–20 amino acids in size.

Fas ligand: The ligand that binds to the cell surface molecule Fas (CI 95) which is normally found on the surface of lymphocytes. When Fas ligand binds to its receptor, cell death (apoptosis) is triggered.

Haplotype: A set of genetic determinants coded by closely linked genes on a single chromosome.

Hapten: A substance of low molecular weight which is not itself immunogenic, but which can bind to an antibody molecule and produce a new antigenic determinant; e.g. 2,4-dinitrophenol will only evoke an antibody response when coupled with ovalbumin.

Helper (TH) cells: A functional subclass of T cells which can help generate cytotoxic T cells and cooperate with B cells in the production of antibody responses. Helper cells recognize antigen in association with class II molecules.

Heterologous: Originating from a different individual or different inbred line.

Heterophile antigen: Antigen which occurs in tissues of many different species and is therefore highly cross-reactive, e.g. Paul–Bunnell antigen which reacts with both sheep and beef erythrocytes.

HLA: See p. 31.

Idiotype: Unique antigenic determinant on the antigen-binding region of an immunoglobulin molecule.

Hypervariable regions: Amino acid sequences within the variable regions of heavy and light immunoglobulin chains and of the T-cell receptor which show the most variablilty and contribute most to the antigen-binding site.

Immunoglobulin subclass: Immunoglobulin of the same class that is detectable in the constant heavy chain region, and differs in electrophoretic mobility and antigenic determinant, and function, e.g. IgG1, IgG2, IgG3 and IgG4.

Integrins: One of the ‘families’ of adhesion molecules, some of which interact with CAMs, and others with components of the extracellular matrix.

Isologous: Originating from the same individual or member of the same inbred strain.

Isotype: The class or subclass of an immunoglobulin common to all members of that species. Each isotype is encoded by a separate immunoglobulin constant region gene sequence that is carried by all members of a species.

Killer (K) cells: Type of cytotoxic lymphocyte that is able to mediate antibody-dependent cellular cytotoxicity (ADCC).

Langerhans' cells: Antigen-presenting cells of the skin which emigrate to local lymph nodes to become dendritic cells; they are very active in presenting antigen to T cells.

Mixed lymphocyte reaction (MLR): Proliferative response when lymphocytes from two genetically different (i.e. allogeneic) persons are mixed in cell culture. A vital test in matching donor and recipient prior to bone marrow transplantation.

Natural killer (NK) cells: Type of cytotoxic lymphocyte that has the intrinsic ability to recognize and destroy virally infected cells and some tumour cells.

Superantigens: Antigens (often bacterial, e.g. staphylococcal enterotoxins) which bind to the MHC outside the peptide-binding groove and stimulate all or most of the T cells bearing particular T-cell receptor V regions. Antigens must normally be processed in order to trigger the T-cell receptor. Superantigens are not processed but bind directly to class II and Vβ.

Suppressor (TS) cell: Functionally defined populations of T cells which reduce the immune responses of other T cells or B cells, or switch the response into a different pathway to that under investigation.

Syngeneic: See p. 107.

Titre: The highest dilution of a given substance, e.g. antibody, that will still produce a reaction with another substance, e.g. antigen.

T-cell receptor: The T-cell antigen receptor consists of either an αβ dimer (TCR-2) or a γδ dimer (TCR-1) associated with the CD3 molecular complex.

T-dependent/ T-independent antigens: T-dependent antigens require immune recognition by both T and B cells to produce an immune reponse. T-independent antigens can directly stimulate B cells to produce specific antibody.

Tumour necrosis factor (TNF): See p. 83.

THE IMMUNE RESPONSE SYSTEM

CELLS INVOLVED IN THE IMMUNE RESPONSE

ANTIGEN-PROCESSING CELLS

- Include macrophages, monocytes or their derivatives (microglial cells, Kupffer cells and skin Langerhans cells).
- Characterized by their ability to phagocytose, internalize and process antigen.
- Possess Ia antigen, Fc receptors and C3b receptors and produce interleukin I.

COMPARISON OF B AND T LYMPHOCYTES

B lymphocytes (See also Immunoglobulins, pp. 88–92)

Functions:	Humoral immunity – antibody production; control of pyogenic bacteria; prevention of blood-borne infections; neutralization of toxins.
% of total lymphocytes:	12%; mainly fixed.
Site of production:	Produced in germinal centre of lymph nodes and spleen.
Assessment of function:	Serum specific immunoglobulin levels; specific antibodies; immunoglobulin response to pokeweed mitogen; endotoxin and EBV.

T lymphocytes

Functions:	Cell-mediated immunity; protection against intracellular organisms, protozoa and fungi; graft rejection; control of neoplasms.
% of total lymphocytes:	70–80%; mainly circulating; long-lived memory cells.
Site of production:	Produced in paracortical region of lymph nodes and spleen.
Assessment of function:	Delayed hypersensitivity skin reactions using candida, mumps and purified protein derivative (PPD); active sensitization with dinitrochlorobenzene (DNCP); lymphocyte transformation: mitogenic response to phytohaemagglutinin (PHA) and concanavalin-A; mixed lymphocyte reaction (MLR); lymphokine release.
Identified by:	T-cell surface phenotypes identified by reaction with monoclonal Abs (Table 3.1)

Table 3.1 T-cell surface antigens and CD markers (see also Fig. 3.1)

Surface antigen	*% of peripheral T cells*	*HLA restriction*	*Function*
T3 (CD3)	All		
T4 (CD4)	65	Class II MHC	TH and TDH cells
T8 (CD8)	35	Class I MHC	TS and TC cells

CD, cluster of differentiation; MHC, major histocompatibility complex; TH, helper T cells; TDH, delayed hypersensitivity T cells; TS, suppressor T cells; TC, cytotoxic T cells (see below).

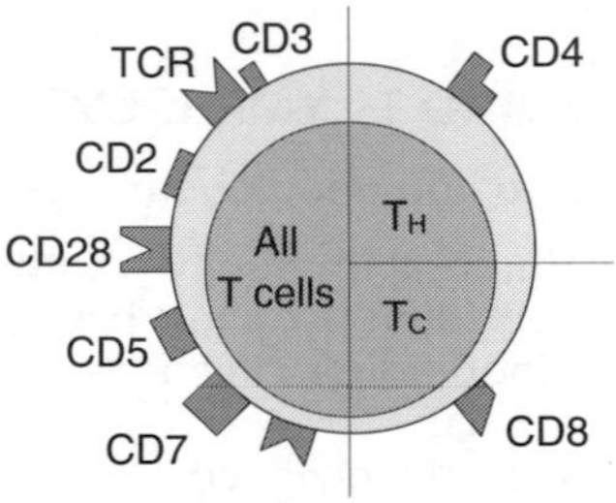

Fig. 3.1

T-cell subpopulations

Regulatory and effector T cells

Regulatory cells:

1. TH, helper T cells: recognize antigen by means of the T-cell receptors in association with macrophage receptors. Activate B cells and other T lymphocytes and produce cytokines.
2. TS, suppressor T cells: interfere with the development of an immune response, either directly or via suppressor factors.

Effector cells:

3. Tc, cytotoxic T cells: regulate the immune response and can lyse cells, e.g. viral or tumour antigens. Interleukin-2 (IL-2) is responsible for the generation of cytotoxic T cells.
4. TDH, delayed hypersensitivity T cells: release mediators that cause an inflammatory response attracting macrophages, neutrophils and other lymphocytes to the site.

T-cell antigen receptor (TCR)

TCR is a disulphide-linked heterodimeric glycoprotein that enables T cells to recognize a diverse array of antigens. It is associated at the cell surface with a complex of polypeptides known collectively as CD3.

- T cells can be divided into different subsets based on the expression of one or other T-cell receptor (TCR-1 or TCR-2).

- TCR-1 cells are thought to have a restricted repertoire and to be mainly non-MHC restricted.
- TCR-2 cells express either CD4 or CD8 which determines whether they see antigen in association with MHC class II or I molecules.

TH_1 and TH_2 populations

- MHC class II-restricted T cells can also be subdivided into TH_1 and TH_2 populations based on their profiles of cyokine production.
- The T-cell TH_1 profile is associated with production of IL-2, tumour necrosis factor (TNF)-β and interferon (IFN)-γ and is driven by IL-12.
- The TH_2 profile is associated with IL-4, IL-5, IL-6 and IL-13 and is driven by IL-10.
- TH_1 cytokines are involved in helping cell-mediated immunity and the TH_2 cytokines mediate humoral immunity (Fig. 3.2).

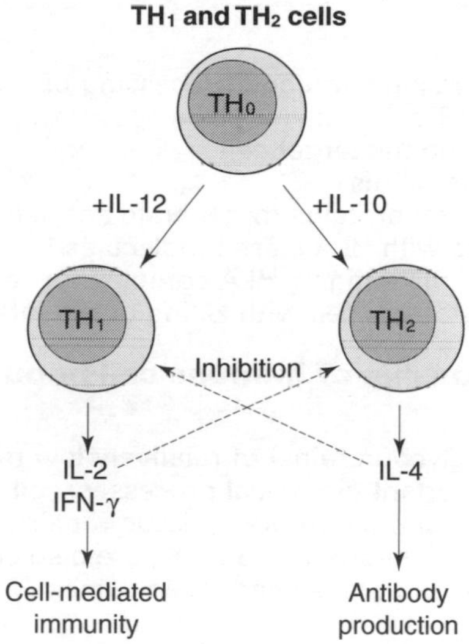

Fig. 3.2

T-cell recognition of an antigen

- T cells recognize antigens that originate within other cells, such as viral peptides from infected cells.
- T cells bind specifically to antigenic peptides presented on the surface of infected cells by molecules encoded by the MHC.
- The T cells use their specific receptors (TCRs) to recognize the unique combinations of MHC molecule plus antigenic peptide (Fig. 3.3).

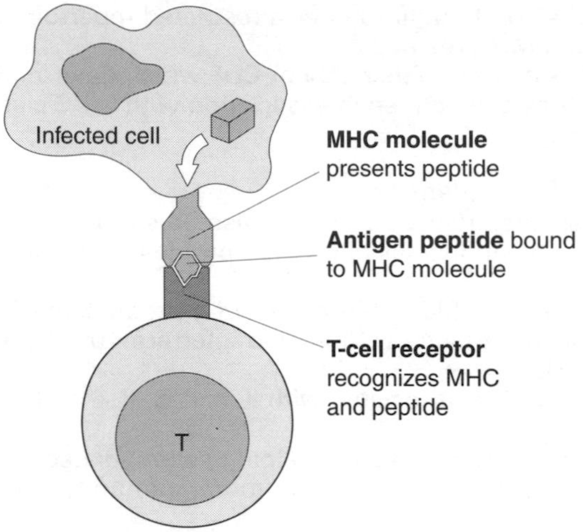

Fig. 3.3

The stages in the recognition and processing of a virally infected cell by a cytotoxic T cell are:

1. Entry of virus into the target cell.
2. Replication of the virus.
3. Processing of viral proteins to generate antigenic determinants which associate with HLA class I molecules.
4. Presentation of the antigen–HLA complex for recognition by a specific CD8 cytotoxic cell with killing of the infected cell.

The interrelationship of immune cell populations (Fig. 3.4)

Cytokines

Proteins (usually glycoproteins) of relatively low molecular weight. They regulate important biological processes: cell growth, cell activation, inflammation, immunity, tissue repair and fibrosis. Some cytokines, e.g. interleukin-8 (IL-8), are also chemotactic for specific cell types, and are termed 'chemokines'.

1. Interferons (IFNs) (see Table 3.2)

These glycoproteins are produced by virus-infected cells.

- Three species of interferon:
  1. alpha-interferon (IFN-α) produced by human leucocytes.
  2. beta-interferon (IFN-β) produced by human fibroblasts.
  3. gamma-interferon (IFN-γ) produced by human T lymphocytes in response to antigenic stimulation.
- Properties:
  1. prevent viral replication
  2. anti-tumour activity
  3. activate macrophages and natural killer (NK) cells.

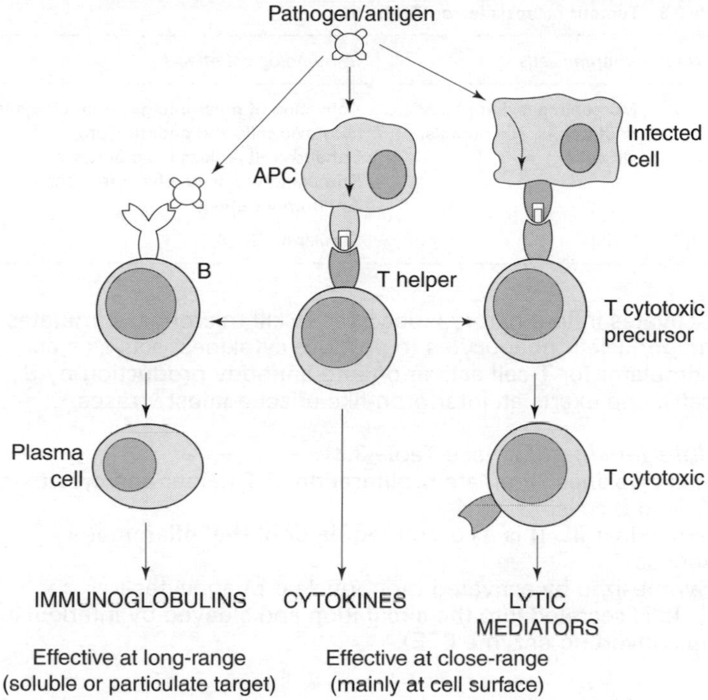

APC = antigen presenting cell

Fig. 3.4

Table 3.2 Interferons (IFNs)

Cytokine	*Immune cells*	*Immunological effects*
IFN-α, β	T and B cells, monocytes or macrophages	Antiviral activity Stimulation of macrophages and large granular lymphocytes (LGL) Enhanced HLA class I expression
IFN-γ	T and LGL	Antiviral activity Stimulation of macrophages and endothelium Enhanced HLA class I and class II expression Suppression of TH_2 cells

2. Tumour necrosis factor (TNF) (see Table 3.3)

- The principal mediator of the host response to Gram-negative bacteria. May also play a role in the response to other infectious organisms, and is a key cytokine in the pathogenesis of multi-organ failure.

Table 3.3 Tumour necrosis factor (TNF)

Cytokine	*Immune cells*	*Immunological effects*
TNF-α	Macrophages, lymphocytes, neutrophils, eosinophils, NK cells	Activation of macrophages, granulocytes, cytotoxic cells and endothelium Enhanced HLA class I expression Stimulation of acute phase response Anti-tumour effects
TNF-β	T cells	Similar to TNF-α

- Activates inflammatory leucocytes to kill microbes; stimulates mononuclear phagocytes to produce cytokines; acts as a co-stimulator for T-cell activation and antibody production by B cells, and exerts an interferon-like effect against viruses.

3. Interleukins (ILs) (see Table 3.4)
These cytokines stimulate proliferation of T helper and cytotoxic cells and B cells.
Interleukin-1 (IL-1) is a central regulator of the inflammatory response.
- Synthesized by activated mononuclear phagocytes.
- IL-1β is secreted into the circulation and cleaved by interleukin-1β converting enzyme (ICE).

Table 3.4 Interleukins (ILs)

Cytokine	*Immune cells*	*Immunological effects*
IL-1α, β	Monocytes/macrophages	Activation of T and B cells, macrophages, and endothelium Stimulation of acute phase response
IL-2	T cells	Proliferation and/or activation of T, B and LGL
IL-4	T and B cells, macrophages, mast cells and basophils, bone marrow stroma	Activation of B cells Differentiation of TH_2 cells and suppression of TH_1 cells
IL-5	T cells, mast cells	Development, activation and chemoattraction of eosinophils
IL-6	T cells, monocytes or macrophages	Activation of haemopoietic stem cells Differentiation of B and T cells Production of acute phase proteins
IL-8	T cells, monocytes, neutrophils	Chemoattraction of neutrophils, T cells, basophils Activation of neutrophils
IL-10	T and B cells, macrophages	Suppression of macrophage functions and TH_1 cells Activation of B cells

- $IL-1\beta$ levels in the circulation are only detectable in the following situations: after strenuous exercise, in ovulating women, sepsis, acute organ rejection, acute exacerbation of rheumatoid arthritis.
- Acts in septic shock by increasing the number of small mediator molecules such as PAF (platelet-activating factor), prostaglandins and nitric oxide which are potent vasodilators.
- The uptake of oxidized low density lipoproteins (LDL) by vascular endothelial cells results in IL-1 expression which stimulates the production of platelet-derived growth factor. IL-1 is thus likely to play a role in the formation of the atherosclerotic plaque.
- IL-1 has some host defence properties, inducing T and B lymphocytes, and reduces mortality from bacterial and fungal infection in animal models.

Interleukin-2 (IL-2) is also known as T-cell growth factor.

- Induces proliferation of other T lymphocytes; generates new cytotoxic cells, and enhances natural killer cells.

4. Colony stimulating factors (CSFs) (see Table 3.5)

- These are involved in directing the division and differentiation of bone-marrow stem cells, and the precursors of blood leucocytes.

Table 3.5 Colony stimulating factors (CSFs)

Cytokine	*Immune cells*	*Immunological effects*
G-CSF	T cells, macrophages, neutrophils	Development and activation of neutrophils
M-CSF	T cells, macrophages, neutrophils	Development and activation of monocytes/macrophages
GM-CSF	T cells, macrophages, mast cells, neutrophils, eosinophils	Differentiation of pluripotent stem cells Development of neutrophils, eosinophils and macrophages
Transforming growth factor (TGF)-β	T cells, monocytes	Inhibition of T and B cell proliferation and LGL activity

5. Chemokines

- Recently described large family of cytokines that have chemoattractant properties.
- Responsible for recruiting leucocytes to inflammatory lesions, induce release of granules from granulocytes, regulate integrin avidity and in general exhibit pro-inflammatory properties.
- Chemokines are secreted by many cell types.
- Family can be divided into α (also called CXC) and β (also called CC) subgroups. The main β chemokines are RANTES, MIPs and MCPs.
- The receptors for the chemokines are also family-specific.

NATURAL KILLER (NK) CELLS

- Functions:
  1. Recognize antigens on target, e.g. tumour cells, and lyse targets.
  2. Antibody-dependent cytotoxicity.
- Identified by: Fc receptor for IgG.

HEAT SHOCK PROTEINS

The **heat shock response** is a highly conserved and phylogenetically ancient response to tissue stress that is mediated by activation of specific genes. This leads to the production of specific heat shock proteins that alter the phenotype of the cell, and enhance its resistance to stress. Their principal function appears to be to act as molecular chaperones for damaged protein to direct it into degradation pathways such as ubiquitination.

FREE RADICALS

A **free radical** is literally any atom or molecule which contains one or more unpaired electrons, making it more reactive than the native species.

- Free radical species produced in the human body are:
  –$OOH^{\bullet}$ (peroxide radical)
  –$OH^{\bullet}$ (hydroxyl radical)
  –$O_2^{\bullet}$ (superoxide radical)
  –$NO^{\bullet}$ (nitric oxide).
- The hydroxyl radical is by far the most reactive species, but the others can generate more reactive species as breakdown products.
- When a free radical reacts with a non-radical, a chain reaction ensues which results in the formation of further free radicals and direct tissue damage by lipid peroxidation of membranes (particularly implicated in atherosclerosis and ischaemia reperfusion injury within tissues).
- Free radical scavengers bind reactive oxygen species.
- Principal dietary antioxidants:
  vitamin E
  vitamin C
  beta carotene
  flavanoids.
- Patients with dominant familial forms of amyotrophic lateral sclerosis (motor neurone disease) have mutations in the gene for Cu-Zn SOD-1, suggesting a link between failure of free radical scavenging and neurodegeneration. Protection against heart disease and cancer may be conferred by dietary antioxidants.

TRANSFORMING GROWTH FACTOR-BETA (TGF-β)

- Initiates and terminates tissue repair.
- Undergoes autoinduction.
- Released by platelets at the site of tissue injury and promotes the formation of extracellular matrix.
- Implicated in diseases of tissue fibrosis such as cirrhosis and glomerulosclerosis.

ADHESION MOLECULES (see Table 3.6)

- Involved in cell–cell communication and recognition, and controls leucocyte migration.
- They fall into families that are structurally related:
  —the cell adhesion molecules (CAMs) of the immunoglobulin superfamily (antigen presentation)
  —the cadherin superfamily (neuromuscular interaction)
  —integrins (interaction between cells and the extracellular matrix)
  —selectins (leucocyte adhesion to endothelium during inflammation).

Table 3.6 Adhesion molecules involved in lymphocyte interactions

	Receptor on lymphocyte	*Ligand on interacting cell*
T cells	CD4	HLA class II
	CD8	HLA class I
	CD28	CD80
	CD2	LFA-3
	VLA-4	VCAM-1
B cells	LFA-1	ICAM-1, -2 or -3
	CD40	CD40-ligand

LFA, lymphocyte function-associated antigen; VLA, very late antigen; ICAM, intercellular adhesion molecule; VCAM, vascular cell adhesion molecule.

NITRIC OXIDE (NO)

NO is an important transcellular messenger molecule which is involved in a diverse range of processes.

- NO is synthesized from the oxidation of nitrogen atoms in the amino acid L-arginine by the action of **NO synthase** (NOS; Fig. 3.5).
- NO acts on target cells close to its site of synthesis where it activates guanylate cyclase leading to a rise in intracellular **cGMP** which acts as a second messenger to modulate a variety of cellular processes. It has a very short half-life.
- There are at least three distinct **isoforms** of NO synthase:
  1. neuronal (constitutive) NO synthase (CNS neurotransmission, memory formation)

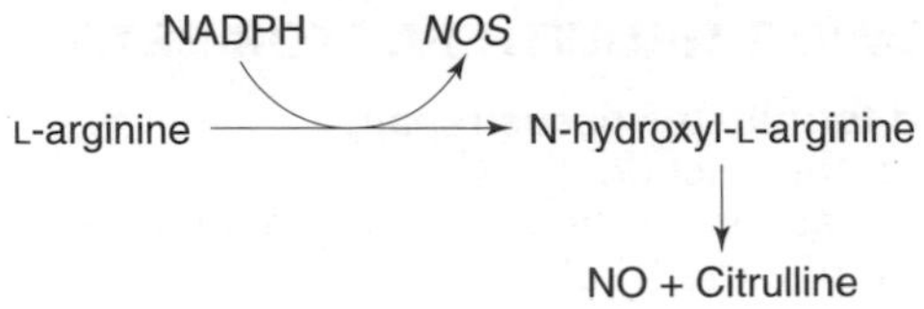

Fig. 3.5

2. endothelial (constitutive) NO synthase (vasodilator tone modulation, organ-specific microcirculatory control, e.g. kidney)
3. macrophage (inducible) NO synthase.

Pathology

- Septic shock (NO is released in massive amounts and correlates with low BP).
- Atherosclerosis (where NO synthesis may be impaired leading to tonic vasoconstriction and vasospasm).
- 1° and 2° pulmonary hypertension (inhaled NO reverses pulmonary hypertension).
- Hepatorenal syndrome and the hypertension of chronic renal failure.
- Glutamate-mediated excitotoxic cell death in the CNS such as Alzheimer's disease and also in acute brain injury such as stroke.
- Tissue damage in acute and chronic inflammation (probably by interacting with oxygen-derived free radicals).
- ARDS (adult respiratory distress syndrome).

IMMUNOGLOBULINS

PROPERTIES, FUNCTIONS AND REACTIONS

The properties and functions of the major classes of immunoglobulins are shown in Table 3.7, and the immunological reactions of IgG, IgA and IgM are summarized in Table 3.8.

STRUCTURE OF IMMUNOGLOBULIN MOLECULE

(Fig. 3.6)

- An immunoglobulin molecule is a 4-polypeptide chain structure with two heavy and two light chains linked covalently by disulphide bonds.
- Treatment of the antibody unit with papain produces:
  —two identical univalent *antigen-binding fragments* (*Fab*), each containing one antigen-binding site, and
  —one *crystallizable fragment* (*Fc*), which contains sites for complement fixation, reactivity with rheumatoid factors, skin and macrophage fixation and regulation of catabolism.

Table 3.7 Properties and functions of the major classes of immunoglobulins

Ig class	*Heavy chains*	*Molecular weight*	*% total Ig level*	*Normal plasma level*	*Function*
IgG	γ	150 000 (monomer)	80	8–16 g/l	1. Distributed in blood and interstitial fluids. 2. The major immunoglobulin of the secondary immune response.* 3. The only immunoglobulin that crosses the placenta, and therefore the major protective immunoglobulin in the neonate. Most maternally transmitted IgG has disappeared by 6 months.† 4. Opsonization, toxin neutralization and agglutination. Coats cells prior to killing by killer cells. Activates complement via classical pathway.
IgA	α	160 000 370 000 (dimer and secretory form)	13	1.4–4 g/l	1. Principal immunoglobulin in secretions of respiratory and gastrointestinal tract and in sweat, saliva, tears and colostrum. Key defence role for mucosal surfaces. 2. Polymerizes to a dimer intracellularly by binding through a cysteine-rich polypeptide (J-chain), synthesized locally by submucosal cells. 3. Secreted through epithelia as the dimer bound to a secretory transport piece, synthesized locally by epithelial cells. 4. When aggregated binds polymorphs and activates complement by the alternative pathway.
IgM	μ	900 000 (pentamer)	6	0.5–2 g/l	1. Macroglobulin made up of five monomeric immunoglobulin subunits linked by a J-chain. 2. Mainly intravascular. 3. Principal immunoglobulin of the primary immune response. 4. Does not cross the placenta. Fetal production of high levels of specific IgM in intrauterine infection may be of diagnostic significance, e.g. rubella. 5. Agglutinates and opsonizes particulate antigens. Activates complement via the classical pathway. Blood group antibodies: IgM.

Table 3.7 *(cont.)*

Ig class	*Heavy chains*	*Molecular weight*	*% total Ig level*	*Normal plasma level*	*Function*
IgD	δ	170 000 (monomer)	0.1	4–40 mg/l	1. Precise functions are unknown. 2. Nearly all immunoglobulin is present as cell surface receptor on human B cells and may be involved in B-cell activation.
IgE	ε	185 000	0.002	0.1–1.3 mg/l	1. Immediate hypersensitivity reactions: binds to mast cells and basophils via its Fc fragment, which degranulates and releases biologically active mediators, e.g. histamine, when exposed to the appropriate antigen. Possibly of benefit in controlling certain parasitic infections.

*Secondary antibody response characterized by: 1. lowering of the threshold of immunogen; 2. shortening of the lag phase; 3. a higher rate of antibody production; 4. longer persistence of antibody production.

†*Transient disease in the newborn caused by maternal IgG*: rhesus incompatibility, autoimmune thrombocytopaenia, thyrotoxicosis, myasthenia gravis, lupus erythematosus.

Table 3.8 Summary of reactions of various immunoglobulins

Reaction	*IgG*	*IgA*	*IgM*
Agglutination	+	+	++
Precipitation	+	+	+
Virus neutralization	+	+	+
Complement fixation	+++	−	+
Complement-dependent lysis	+	−	+++
Immune complex	+	−	+

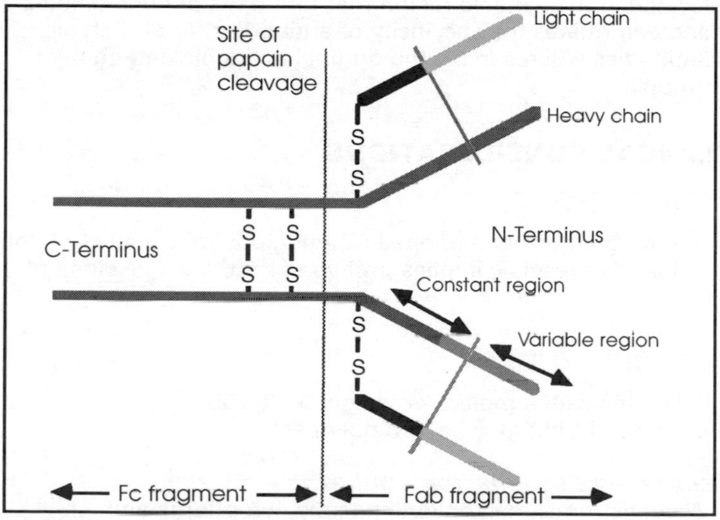

Fc, crystallizable fragment: Fab, antigen-binding fragment.

Fig. 3.6

- *Light chains*
  —Molecular weight of approximately 23 000.
  —Two types: kappa (κ) and lambda (λ). Each immunoglobulin molecule has either two κ or two λ chains.
- *Heavy chains*
  —Molecular weight of about twice that of light chains (i.e. 50 000–75 000) and twice the number of amino acids.
  —Five classes of immunoglobulin are recognized on the basis of the Fc fragment of the heavy chain, i.e. heavy chain isotypes IgG, IgA, IgM, IgD and IgE. Heavy chain classes are also divided into subclasses of molecules, e.g. IgG1, IgG2, etc.
- Both heavy and light chains consist of two regions:
  1. A *constant region* (C_H and C_L), in which the amino acid sequence of immunoglobulins of the same class is more or less identical

2. A *variable region* (V_H and V_L) where the amino acid sequence varies considerably from molecule to molecule and contributes to the antigen-binding site.

- *Isotypic* determinants are found in the constant region of the heavy chains of all molecules. These determine the heavy chain immunoglobulin class or subclass.
- *Allotypic* determinants are inherited antigenic variations that occur within a species and may be located in any region of the molecule. These allotypes are designated Gm for the gamma chain, Am for the alpha chain and Km for the kappa chain.
- *Idiotypic* determinants are unique sequences of amino acids located in the variable region that forms the antigen-binding site and determines the specificity of antibodies. Anti-idiotypic antibodies will resemble the original antigenic determinant group.

CLINICAL CONSIDERATIONS

PARAPROTEIN

- A homogenous band of one immunoglobulin, usually IgG, IgM or IgA. Its presence implies proliferation of a single clone of cells.

MACROGLOBULINS

- Globulins with a molecular weight >400 000.
- Usually IgM but may be IgM polymers.

Causes of raised macroglobulins:

- Waldenstrom's macroglobulinaemia, lymphoma and malignancies, diseases associated with a high ESR such as collagen disorders, sarcoidosis and cirrhosis.

CRYOGLOBULINS

- Immunoglobulins which precipitate when cooled to 4°C and dissolve when warmed to 37°C, so blood must be taken in a warm syringe and kept at 37°C until the serum has been separated.
- Three types:
  —Type I (25%): monoclonal cryoglobulins (IgM, IgG or IgA).
  —Type II (25%): mixed type, monoclonal protein (often rheumatoid factor) which has bound polyclonal IgG (IgM–IgG, IgG–IgG).
  —Type III (50%): mixed polyclonal type (IgM–IgG, IgM–IgG–IgA).
- May cause Raynaud's phenomenon and cutaneous vasculitis if present in high concentrations.
- Cryoglobulinaemia: two-thirds may be associated with diseases

causing a paraproteinaemia, e.g. lymphoma, myeloma, SLE, rheumatoid arthritis and chronic infection, e.g. hepatitis C. One-third are idiopathic.

COLD AGGLUTININS

- Specific IgM antibodies capable of agglutinating human red blood cells between 0°C and 4°C.
- Found in mycoplasma pneumoniae, infectious mononucleosis, listeriosis and coxsackie infections, malaria, trypanosomiasis and acquired haemolytic anaemia (Coombs test positive).

MONOCLONAL ANTIBODIES

- Myeloma cells are fused with plasma cells prepared from an immunized mouse or rat to produce a hybrid myeloma cell or 'hybridoma', which may then produce monoclonal antibodies.
- 'Humanized' antibodies (produced by enzymatic cleavage of the immunogenic mouse Fc portion) are preferable because of the potentially serious side-effects of administering mouse antibodies as therapeutic agents.

Uses

1. Lymphocyte subset determination and detection of HLA antigens.
2. Viral detection and subtyping; parasite identification.
3. Assays of peptide hormones, e.g. ACTH and PTH.
4. Identification of surface markers of cells in biopsy material, e.g. markers for transplant antigens and bacterial serotypes.
5. Histological typing of neoplasms, e.g. lymphomas, APUDomas and leukaemias.
6. Affinity chromatography to isolate and purify material, e.g., vaccines and interferon, where the amino acid sequence varies considerably from molecule to molecule.
7. Therapeutic: anti-tumour effect (e.g. anti-idiotype to surface immunoglobulin B-cell lymphoma), immunosuppression (e.g. treatment of graft-versus-host disease and graft rejection with OKT3 and drug toxicity (e.g. reversal of digitalis intoxication).
8. Targeting of drugs to specific tissue sites.
9. Conjugated to radioisotopes for imaging.

COMPLEMENT

THE COMPLEMENT SYSTEM

- Comprises at least nine plasma proteins and some regulatory factors, that mediate several functions of the inflammatory process.

- Synthesized by macrophages or hepatocytes.
- Usually circulate in an inactive form as proenzymes.
- Heat-labile.

COMPLEMENT PATHWAYS (Fig. 3.7)

A cascade of sequential activation converts each proenzyme into its active state and amplifies the response. Activation may occur via two main pathways.

1. Classical pathway, mediated by IgG, IgG2, IgG3 or IgM antibody.
2. Alternative pathway, initiated by certain antigens (lipopolysaccharide, endotoxin) and IgA complexes.

Functions

1. Opsonization, chemotaxis and immune adherence
2. Acceleration of acute inflammation
3. Immune cytolysis
4. Virus neutralization.

COMPLEMENT DEFICIENCIES

- Raised levels of all complement components can occur in any inflammatory condition.
- *Low* complement levels occur in certain diseases and may correlate with disease activity, e.g., post-streptococcal glomerulonephritis, SLE nephritis, infectious endocarditis, nephritis, membranoproliferative glomerulonephritis, serum sickness, liver disease, septicaemia and disseminated intravascular coagulation.

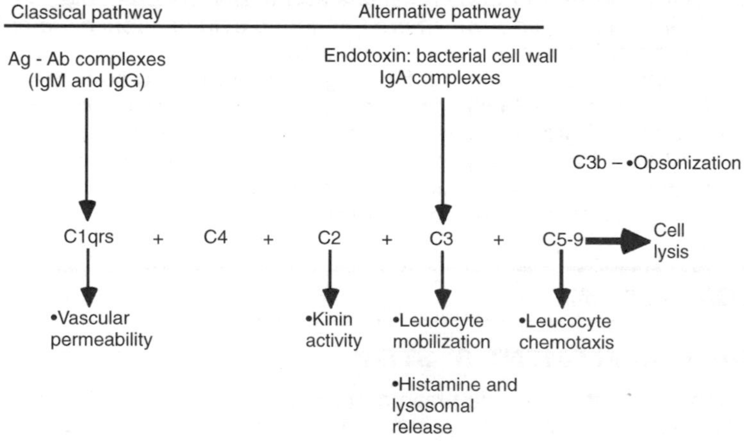

Fig. 3.7

Inherited deficiencies

Inherited deficiencies of certain groups of components are associated with characteristic clinical syndromes:

1. C1 inhibitor deficiency with hereditary angioneurotic oedema (due to uncontrolled complement activation).
2. C2, C4 deficiency with immune complex disease, e.g. Henoch–Schonlein purpura, glomerulonephritis, SLE.
3. C3 deficiency with recurrent bacterial infection.
4. C5–9 deficiency with recurrent bacterial infections, especially Neisseria.

HYPERSENSITIVITY

CLASSIFICATION

See Table 3.9.

Table 3.9 Classification of hypersensitivity

Type	*Mechanism*	*Result*	*Disease*
Type I Anaphylactic	Antigen reacts with IgE (reaginic) antibody bound to mast cells	Release of vasoactive substances* Vasodilation and chemotaxis	Anaphylactic shock, e.g. bee and wasp venom Atopic diseases, e.g. asthma, hay fever and rhinitis Drug allergies
Type II Cell-bound†	Circulating antibody (IgG or IgM) reacts with antigen on cell surface	Complement activation Phagocytosis Promotion of killer cell cytotoxicity Cell lysis	Transfusion reactions and rhesus incompatibility Autoimmune haemolytic anaemia Myasthenia gravis Post-streptococcal glomerulonephritis Myxoedema and thyrotoxicosis Idiopathic thrombocytopaenic purpura Goodpasture's syndrome Drug-induced disease (mainly haematological effects)
Stimulatory	Some IgG antibodies stimulate the cells against which they are directed	TSH receptor antibody results in prolonged hypersecretion of thyroid hormone	Graves' disease
Type III Immune complex†	Free antigen and antibody (IgG or IgM) combine in the presence of complement, and precipitate as immune complexes	Platelet aggregation Complement activation Activation of clotting factor XII, leading to fibrin and plasmin formation Damage to small blood vessels	Immune complex diseases:‡ *1. Exogenous antigens* Serum sickness Drug-induced haemolytic anaemia and thrombocytopaenia, e.g. quinine, quinidine and phenacetin Hypersensitivity pneumonitis, e.g. farmer's lung

Table 3.9 *(cont.)*

Type	*Mechanism*	*Result*	*Disease*
			2. Microbial antigens Post-streptococcal glomerulonephritis Glomerulonephritis associated with endocarditis Syphilis Quartan malaria Schistosomiasis *3. Autologous antigens* SLE, rheumatoid arthritis, mixed cryoglobulinaemia
Type IV Cell-mediated or delayed hyper-sensitivity	Sensitized T-lymphocytes are stimulated by an appropiate antigen	Lymphokine release	Tuberculin skin reaction and tuberculosis (systemic reaction = Koch phenomenon) Tuberculoid-leprosy Contact dermatitis Graft rejection (late) and GVHD Tumour immunity

*Histamine, kinins, platelet-activating factor (PAF), leucotriene-C4 (LTC4) and leucotriene-D4 (LTD4), prostaglandins, thromboxanes and chemotactic factors (eosinophil chemotactic factor of anaphylaxis (ECF-A), neutrophil chemotactic factor (NCF)). †Complement dependent. ‡Immune complex diseases successfully treated by plasma exchange include: SLE, rapidly progressive glomerulonephritis, Wegener's granulomatosis, polyarteritis nodosa, mixed essential cryoglobulinaemia, cutaneous vasculitis.

Skin testing

- *Type I* (Prick test)
  An urticarial weal and flare develops within 20 minutes and resolves within 2 hours.
- *Type II* (Intradermal injection)
  An ill-defined weal develops over several hours, is maximal at 5–7 hours and resolves within 24 hours.
- *Type IV* (Intradermal or patch test; delayed hypersensitivity)
  An indurated area develops within 2–4 days and resolves over several days.

IMMUNODEFICIENCY

PRIMARY IMMUNODEFICIENCY

B-CELL DISORDERS

- Pathogens are pyogenic bacteria (e.g. staphylococci, streptococci, H. influenzae and pneumococci), yeasts, giardia and campylobacter.
- Treated with gammaglobulin.

1. Bruton's congenital agammaglobulinaemia
- Rare, X-linked inheritance
- Presents in male infants at about 6 months with recurrent pyogenic and gastrointestinal infections.
- Increased incidence of autoimmune disorders and lymphoreticular malignancies.
- No circulating B cells: very reduced IgG and no IgM, A, D, E.
- Normal T-cell function, i.e. normal delayed hypersensitivity.

2. Common variable immunodeficiency (CVID)
- Incidence of 10 per million. Acquired at any age and in either sex.
- Heterogeneous collection of conditions.
- Presents in late childhood or adult life with recurrent pulmonary infections and chronic diarrhoea. Characterized by high incidence of autoimmune disorders.
- Low serum immunoglobulin levels: cell-mediated immunity normal in 60%.

3. Dysgammaglobulinaemia
- Selective IgA deficiency is the commonest primary defect in the UK with 1:700 individuals affected.
- Usually asymptomatic but may present with recurrent respiratory tract or gastrointestinal infections, particularly if IgG_2 is reduced.
- Increased frequency of allergic respiratory and autoimmune diseases.

4. Acquired hypogammaglobulinaemia
- Presents in infancy/adulthood.
- Associated conditions include autoimmune diseases, haemolytic anaemia and thymoma. IgG <250 mg/dl:IgM may be spared. Often normal B-cell count. Variable abnormalities in cell-mediated immunity.

5. Transient hypogammaglobulinaemia of infancy
- Usually presents between 3 and 6 months of age.
- Occurs when the onset of immunoglobulin synthesis (especially IgG) is delayed beyond the norm.

T-CELL DISORDERS

- Opportunistic infections (e.g. pneumocystis carinii, fungi) severe viral and chronic bacterial infections, e.g. TB.
- Treatment by:
  1. thymus grafts
  2. bone marrow transplantation.

1. Congenital thymic aplasia (DiGeorge syndrome)
- Rare, non-familial.
- Absence of the thymus is due to a defect in the development of the 3rd and 4th branchial pouches and arches.
- Presents in infancy/adulthood with cardiovascular defects, hypoparathyroidism, convulsions and opportunistic infections.
- Variable reduction in T-cell number and function. B-cell function often normal, i.e. normal Ab levels.

2. Chronic mucocutaneous candidiasis
- Some cases are familial.
- Severe candida infection of mucous membranes, nails and skin with associated endocrine abnormalities, e.g. hypoparathyroidism.
- Negative skin testing to candida.

COMBINED B- AND T-CELL DISORDERS

- Pathogens are pyogenic bacteria, viruses, fungi, TB and pneumocystis carinii.
- Treatment by bone marrow transplantation.

1. Severe combined immunodeficiency (SCID)
- Mostly autosomal recessive inheritance: 50% are deficient in enzyme adenosine deaminase (ADA).
- Presents in first few months of life with failure to thrive, chronic diarrhoea, recurrent pneumonia and widespread candidiasis.
- Complete absence of B- and T-cell immunity.

2. Ataxic telangiectasia syndrome

- Autosomal recessive inheritance.
- Presents in infancy with cerebellar ataxia, oculocutaneous telangiectasia and recurrent sinopulmonary infections.
- Increased incidence of malignancy, especially lymphomas.
- Low IgA and IgE levels. T-cell deficiency is variable.

3. Wiskott–Aldrich syndrome

- Incidence of four per million male births: X-linked recessive inheritance.
- Presents with severe eczema, thrombocytopaenia and recurrent pyogenic infections, e.g. *Strep. pneumoniae, N. meningitidis, H. influenzae.*
- Increased incidence of tumours of lymphoreticular system.
- Low antibody levels, especially IgM, but increased IgE levels.

NEUTROPHIL DISORDERS

- Pathogens are Gram –ve (e.g. *E. coli* and *Klebsiella*) and Gram +ve (e.g. *Staph. aureus*) bacteria, some viruses and fungi (e.g. aspergillus).
- Treatment is with antibiotics.

1. Chronic granulomatous diseases

- Rare, X-linked defect in the NADPH oxidase system (occasionally autosomal recessive).
- Presents in first 2 years of life with recurrent bacterial infections, lymphadenopathy, hepatomegaly, pneumonia, osteomyelitis and abcesses. High susceptibility to aspergillus infections.
- Impaired opsonization and bactericidal activity (nitroblue tetrazolium test).
- Hypergammaglobulinaemia.
- May respond to IFN-γ treatment.

2. Chediak–Higashi syndrome

- Very rare deficiency of NADH or NADPH oxidase in the polymorphonuclear cells.
- Presents with recurrent bacterial infections (especially Neisseria), hepatosplenomegaly, lymphadenopathy and pancytopaenia. Partial oculocutaneous albinism.
- Defective neutrophil function.

3. Leucocyte adhesion deficiency

- Rare autosomal recessive defect in the biosynthesis of the β chain (CD18) common to three glycoproteins (three integrin receptors) on the surface of leucocytes.
- Usually presents with infections of skin, mouth, respiratory tract and around rectum.
- Characterized by failure of neutrophils to migrate to sites of tissue infection.

SECONDARY IMMUNODEFICIENCY

HYPOGAMMAGLOBULINAEMIA

Causes

1. Artefactual, e.g. haemodilution during IV therapy.
2. Decreased production
   (i) Severe malnutrition
   (ii) Lymphoproliferative diseases, e.g. chronic lymphatic leukaemia and myeloma
   (iii) Infection, e.g. malaria, septicaemia, trypanosomiasis
   (iv) Drugs, e.g. cytotoxic agents, gold, phenytoin, penicillamine and irradiation
   (v) Splenectomy.
3. Increased loss or catabolism
   (i) Protein-losing enteropathy and intestinal lymphangiectasia.
   (ii) Malabsorption
   (iii) Nephrotic syndrome
   (iv) Exfoliative dermatitis
   (v) Burns.

T-CELL DEFICIENCY

Causes

1. Drugs, e.g. high dose steroids, cyclophosphamide, cyclosporin.
2. Lymphoproliferative disorders, e.g. Hodgkin's disease and advanced malignancy.
3. Infections, e.g. measles, rubella, infectious mononucleosis, TB, brucellosis, leprosy; HIV-1 and -2 and secondary syphilis.
4. Protein-calorie malnutrition.
5. Other diseases, e.g. pyoderma gangrenosum, advanced rheumatoid arthritis, sarcoidosis, diabetes and alcoholism.

Acquired immunodeficiency syndrome (AIDS)

(See p. 58).

- Causative agent: HIV-1 (see p. 58).
- Syndrome first reported in 1981.
- Clinical spectrum of HIV-1 infection includes an acute mononucleosis-like seroconversion illness, asymptomatic infection, AIDS-related complex (ARC), and overt AIDS.
- AIDS is characterized by the development of severe, disseminated opportunistic infections, especially Pneumocystis carinii pneumonia, Kaposi's sarcoma and less commonly, other neoplasms.
- 90% of cases occur in persons aged 20–49 years.

Laboratory findings

- Detection of anti-HIV-I antibodies using ELISA: (sensitivity approximately 100% specificity 99%). Western blot analysis is used to confirm positive ELISA test. HIV proteins are electrophoresed and the putative serum antibody of the patient

is then reacted and read by antihuman antibody conjugated with enzyme or radioactive label.
- Reduction in absolute blood $CD4^+$ T cell counts (used in monitoring progression of disease and inversion of CD4/CD8 ratio to <0.5 (normal >1.5)).
- Reduced delayed hypersensitivity responses.
- Decreased proliferation to soluble antigens.
- Decreased synthesis of IL-2 in vitro following stimulation with antigens.
- Decreased mitogen response in vitro.
- Increased serum β2 microglobulin levels.
- Hypergammaglobulinaemia especially of IgA, IgG_1, IgG_3 and IgM.
- Moderate decrease in natural killer cell function.

Possible mechanisms of HIV-related T-cell depletion
- Virus-induced lysis
- Syncytia formation
- Immune lysis (by antibody or cellular mechanisms)
- Induction of apoptosis.

Senescence of the immune response

Depressed humoral and cellular immune response (Table 3.10). Also characterized by a loss in some T-cell functions, especially release of interleukin 2 and suppressor cells. Occurrence of autoimmune disease is increased.

HYPERGAMMAGLOBULINAEMIA

Causes of polyclonal hypergammaglobulinaemia
1. Artefactual, e.g. prolonged venous stasis before venepuncture
2. Haemoconcentration secondary to dehydration
3. Chronic infection, e.g. TB, infective endocarditis, leishmaniasis

Table 3.10 Examples of infections related to cellular and humoral deficiency

Defensive defect	*Opportunistic organism*
T-cell	Varicella zoster virus *Candida* *Toxoplasma gondii*
T- and B-cell	Varicella zoster virus *Candida* *Toxoplasma gondii* Cytomegalovirus *Pneumocystis carinii*
Neutropaenia	*Staphylococcus aureus* *Aspergillus fumigatus* Coliforms Cytomegalovirus *Pneumocystis carinii*

4. Autoimmune disease, e.g. SLE, rheumatoid arthritis
5. Ulcerative colitis and Crohn's disease
6. Sarcoidosis
7. Hepatic disease.

Commonly recognized immunoglobulin changes in liver disease (usually accompanied by a decrease in albumin) are:

IgG ↑ in: chronic active hepatitis, cryptogenic cirrhosis
IgM ↑ in: 1° biliary cirrhosis, alcoholic cirrhosis
IgA ↑ in: alcoholic cirrhosis.

Causes of monoclonal hypergammaglobulinaemia

1. Multiple myeloma, Waldenstrom's macroglobulinaemia and heavy chain disease
2. Leukaemia, lymphoma or carcinoma
3. Bence–Jones proteinuria
4. 'Benign' paraproteinaemia
5. Amyloidosis

AUTOIMMUNE DISEASE

EXPLANATORY THEORIES

1. Microbial antigens cross-reacting with host tissues induce an immune response against self.
2. Alteration of self antigens, exposing new antigenic determinants unavailable at the time of induction of fetal tolerance.
3. Attachment of foreign hapten to self molecule forming a hapten–carrier complex.
4. Deficiency of suppressor T cells.
5. Spontaneous emergence of clones of cells capable of mounting an immune response against self.

RHEUMATOID FACTOR

- Circulating immunoglobulin, usually IgM (also IgG or IgA), which is directed against the Fc fragment of the patient's own IgG.
- Detected by latex agglutination tests and sheep red cell agglutination test (SCAT) or Rose–Waaler test (see p. 110).

Rheumatoid factor is positive in 80% of cases with rheumatoid arthritis. A high titre of seropositivity is associated with systemic complications (i.e. nodules, vasculitis and neuropathy).

False positives occur in:
1. General population, rising with age, (4%).
2. Collagen vascular disease, e.g. Sjogren's syndrome (25–30%).
3. Juvenile rheumatoid arthritis (15%).

Table 3.11 Autoimmune diseases

Disease	*Auto antibody present against:*
Organ-specific	
Hashimoto's thyroiditis	Thyroglobulin, thyroid peroxidase
Graves disease	TSH receptor
Myasthenia gravis	Acetylcholine receptor
Pernicious anaemia	Gastric parietal cells, intrinsic factor
Goodpasture's syndrome	Antiglomerular and lung basement membrane
Autoimmune thrombocytopaenia	Platelets
Autoimmune haemolytic anaemia	Red blood cells
Premature ovarian failure	Corpus luteum, interstitial cells
Pemphigus	Intercellular substance of epidermis
Pemphigoid	Basement membrane
Non-organ-specific	
Primary biliary cirrhosis	Mitochondria
Rheumatoid arthritis	IgG (rheumatoid factor)
Scleroderma (CREST variant)	Centromere
Mixed connective tissue disorder	Extractable nuclear antigens
SLE	Nuclear antigens, e.g. ANA, anti-double-stranded (ds) DNA, smooth muscle antigen and IgG

4. Bacterial and viral infections (especially HIV, viral hepatitis, rubella, infectious mononucleosis and chronic infections, e.g. TB, syphilis and leprosy).
5. Infective endocarditis.
6. Chronic fibrosing lung disease.
7. Chronic liver disease.

ANTINUCLEAR ANTIBODIES (ANA) (Table 3.12)

- IgG or IgM antibody directed against a variety of nuclear constituents, e.g. DNA, RNA or nucleolar material.
- High titres occur in:
  1. SLE
  2. Other connective tissue disorders, e.g. Sjogren's syndrome, systemic sclerosis, rheumatoid arthritis.

Table 3.12 Summary of frequency of antinuclear antibodies (ANA) and rheumatoid factor (RF) in various diseases

Disease	*ANA*	*RF*
SLE	90%	20%
Rheumatoid arthritis	20%	70%
Sjogren's syndrome	70%	90%

3. Other autoimmune disease, e.g. chronic active hepatitis, myasthenia gravis.
4. Use of certain drugs (see p. 332).

- Antiribonucleoprotein (anti-RNP) antibody is seen in high titres with mixed connective tissue disorders and in lower titres with SLE and other connective tissue disorders.
- Anticentromere antibody is present in 70% of patients with CREST and 15% of patients with diffuse scleroderma.
- CREST syndrome: calcinosis, Raynaud's phenomenon, oesophageal dysfunction, sclerodactyly and telangiectasia.
- Antihistone antibody is seen in SLE and drug-induced lupus.
- Antibodies that bind *single-stranded* denatured DNA (ss-DNA) are present in 90% of patients with SLE, but also in drug-induced lupus and other connective tissue disorders.
- Antibodies to native *double-stranded* DNA (ds-DNA) are highly specific for SLE.

ANTINEUTROPHIL CYTOPLASMIC ANTIBODIES (ANCAs) (Table 3.13)

Table 3.13 Different types of antineutrophil cytoplasmic antibody (ANCA)-associated diseases and their epitopes

Type of ANCA	*Epitope*	*Disease association*
cANCA	Proteinase 3	Wegener's granulomatosis Microscopic polyangiitis (rarely)
pANCA	Myeloperoxidase	Idiopathic crescentic glomerulonephritis Microscopic polyangiitis Churg–Strauss syndrome Wegener's granulomatosis (rarely)
False-positive ANCA		Infection, HIV, bacterial endocarditis, cystic fibrosis Bronchial carcinoma, atrial myxoma Sweet's syndrome, eosinophilia–myalgia syndrome

BLOOD GROUP IMMUNOLOGY

ABO GROUP

- Complex oligosaccharides, A, B and H, are located on the surface of red blood cells. Present in the tissue fluids and secretions of approximately 75% of people.
- An individual inherits one of three ABO antigen groups (*agglutinogen*) from each parent — A, B or neither.

- Individuals also inherit antibodies (*agglutinins*) which react against red cells of groups other than their own, i.e. anti-A or anti-B, (Table 3.14).

Table 3.14

Genotype	*Phenotype*	*Agglutinogen on cell*	*Agglutinins in plasma*	*% Frequency in population*
OO	O	Nil or H substance	Anti-A, Anti-B	46
AA/AO	A	A	Anti-B	42
BB/BO	B	B	Anti-A	9
AB	AB	AB	None	3

Agglutinogen A + agglutinin anti-A → agglutination
Agglutinogen B + agglutinin anti-B → agglutination

Significant associations between ABO blood groups, secretor status and disease include peptic ulcer disease (O), duodenal ulcer (non-secretor status), gastric carcinoma (A), and pernicious anaemia (A).

Summary of principles of blood transfusion

- Blood group O is the universal donor group because there are no A or B antigens on the red cell membrane.

Therefore blood transfusion may be given thus (Fig. 3.8):

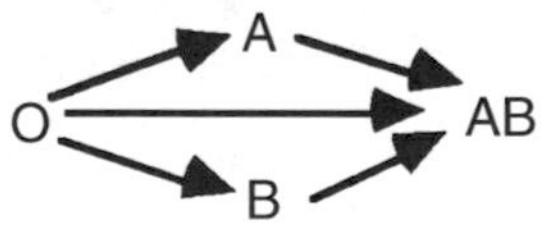

Fig. 3.8

RHESUS (CDE) GROUP

- Three further agglutinogens, C, D and E, occur in association with red cells, of which Group D is the most important agglutinogen.
- 84% of caucasians are Rhesus-positive, i.e. Rhesus (D) antigen is present on the surface of red blood cells. Africans and Japanese are generally Rhesus-negative.

RHESUS INCOMPATIBILITY

- There is no preformed Rhesus agglutinin (anti-D). A Rhesus-negative person can make anti-D only after sensitization with Rhesus-positive blood, i.e. a Rhesus-*negative* mother and a Rhesus-positive father may produce a Rhesus-*positive* fetus. If fetal red blood cells escape into the blood of the mother she produces anti-D antibodies. If these IgG antibodies cross the placenta in subsequent pregnancies, they destroy the fetal red blood cells, resulting in haemolytic disease of the newborn.
- Sensitization can be prevented by administering a single dose of anti-Rh antibodies in the form of Rh immune globulin during the postpartum period. This will destroy the fetal red blood cells, preventing maternal sensitization.

TRANSPLANTATION IMMUNOLOGY

TERMINOLOGY (Table 3.15)

Table 3.15 Summary of terms used in tissue transplantation

	Genetic term	*Transplantation*
Relationship between donor and host		
Same individual	Syngeneic (autologous)	Autograft
Identical twin	Syngeneic (isologous)	Isograft e.g. kidney transplant between monozygotic identical twins
Different individuals (same species)	Allogeneic (homologous)	Allograft e.g. cadaveric renal transplant
Different species	Xenogeneic (heterologous)	Xenograft e.g. baboon kidney transplanted into a human
Location of graft		
In a different type of tissue		Heterotopic
In the tissue from which the graft came		Isotopic e.g. corneal grafts
In same type of tissue as graft origin, but a different anatomical position		Orthotopic e.g. skin grafted from the thigh to the arm

Table 3.16 Rejection reactions

Type	*Time*	*Cause*
Hyperacute	Hours	Preformed donor circulating antibodies, and complement mismatch
Accelerated	Days	Reactivation of sensitized T cells
Acute	Days–weeks	Primary activation of T cells
Chronic	Months–years	Causes are unclear: deposition of e.g. immune complex, cellular reaction, recurrence of disease

GRAFT REJECTION

Three types of rejection reaction (Table 3.16) can take place following transplantation:

1. *Hyperacute rejection* where the recipient has preformed antibodies, occurs within hours or days. There is rapid vascular spasm, occlusion and failure of organ perfusion.
2. *Acute accelerated rejection* due to sensitized T lymphocytes and a cell-mediated immune response, occurs 10–30 days after transplantation. There is infiltration of small lymphocytes and mononuclear cells which destroy the graft.
3. *Chronic rejection* is characterized by the slow loss of tissue function over a period of months or years. May be a cellular immune response, an antibody response or a combination of the two.

GRAFT VERSUS HOST DISEASE (GVHD)

A condition resulting from an attack by the donor's immunologically reactive lymphocytes against the foreign antigens of the recipient, where there is an antigen difference between the donor and recipient. The skin, gastrointestinal tract and liver are most commonly affected. It is a major factor limiting allogeneic bone marrow transplantation in humans, but does not occur with heart or kidney transplantation.

TUMOUR IMMUNOLOGY

- Tumour cells are cells transformed by virus or by physical or chemical means. They are usually not well differentiated, proliferate uncontrollably, lack contact inhibition and have *tumour-associated antigen* (TAA) expression on their surface.

Tumour-associated antigen (TAA) (Table 3.17)

- TAA elicits both humoral and cell-mediated responses.

Table 3.17 Examples of tumour-associated antigens

Antigen	*Distribution*
Carcinoembryonic antigen (CEA)	Fetal gut cells: very small amounts on adult colonic cells but much higher on colonic tumour cells; antigen shed into serum aids early diagnosis and detection of progression
Alpha-fetoprotein	Secreted by fetal liver/yolk sac cells; serum of patients with liver or germinal cell tumours
cALL antigen (CD10)	Present on common acute lymphoblastic leukaemic cells; also on B lymphoid precursor cells in regenerating bone marrow or in fetal bone marrow

B cell involvement is characterized by:

1. Attachment of antibody to Fc receptors on macrophages and polymorphonuclear cells with phagocytosis.
2. Attachment of antibody to Fc receptors on killer cells with subsequent lysis by antibody-dependent cell cytotoxicity.
3. Activation of the classical complement cascade, causing tumour lysis.

T cell involvement is characterized by:

1. Production of lymphokines such as macrophage-activating factor (MAF) and macrophage chemotactic factor.
2. Production of tumour necrosis factor (TNF) by activated macrophages.
3. Killing of tumour cells without prior sensitization by natural killer (NK) cells.

- Tumours in immunodeficient and immunosuppressed patients (Table 3.18)
  Most of these tumours are caused by multiple factors, including virally induced pathological changes.

Table 3.18 Tumours associated with immunodeficiency and immunosuppression

Disease	*Tumour type*
Immunodeficiency	
DiGeorge syndrome	All lymphoreticular
Wiskott–Aldrich syndrome	All lymphoreticular
Ataxia telangiectasia	All lymphoreticular
Severe combined immunodeficiency (SCID)	All lymphoreticular
Chediak–Higashi syndrome	All lymphoreticular
Immunosuppression	
Organ transplants	
Azathioprine/steroids	Non-Hodgkin's lymphoma (NHL), liver cancer, Kaposi's sarcoma, cervical cancer
Cyclosporin A	Lymphoma, skin cancer, Kaposi's sarcoma
Inflammatory disease	NHL
– Rheumatoid arthritis	
– Malaria	Burkitt's lymphoma
– HIV infection	NHL, Kaposi's sarcoma

IMMUNOLOGICAL ASSAYS

Relative sensitivity of serological procedures to detect antibody

MOST SENSITIVE	│	RIA
	│	ELISA
	│	Agglutination
	│	Flocculation
LEAST SENSITIVE	↓	Precipitation

1. AGGLUTINATION ASSAYS

- Red cells or inert particles, e.g. latex, are clumped by antiserum that cross-links antigens on the surface particles.
- Examples: Coombs' antiglobulin test, Widal test, blood grouping and the Rose–Waaler test for the detection of rheumatoid factor.

COOMB'S ANTIGLOBULIN TEST

Two-stage reaction (Fig. 3.9). The direct Coombs' test is used to detect cell-bound antibody. It involves adding an antibody directed against an antiglobulin reagent, thus providing a bridge between two antibody-coated cells or particles.

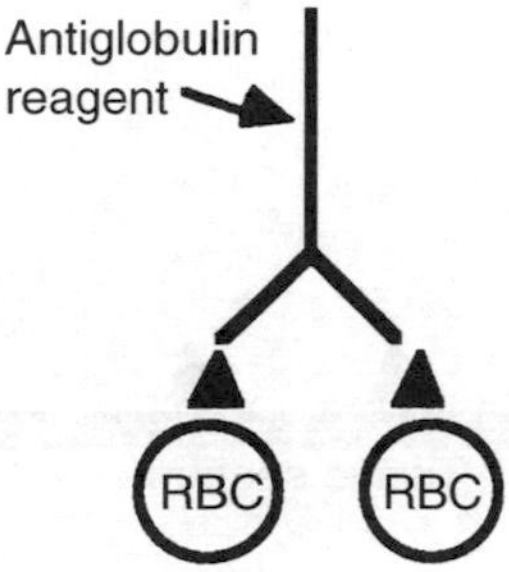

Fig. 3.9

Causes of a positive Coombs' test

1. Idiopathic acquired haemolytic anaemia and autoimmune haemolytic anaemia.
2. Haemolytic transfusion reactions.
3. Alloantibodies, e.g. haemolytic disease of the newborn.
4. SLE, lymphoma, leukaemia and carcinoma.
5. Drugs, e.g. methyldopa.

2. COMPLEMENT FIXATION TESTS

- An antigen–antibody reaction may fix complement, and the presence of a complement-fixing antibody may be detected using an indicator system.
- In the *presence* of complement-fixing antibody, complement is unavailable to lyse indicator red cells with anti-red cell antibody. In the *absence* of antibody, complement will remain unfixed and available for lysis of the indicator system.
- There are two stages to the test:
  1. Test system: patient's serum + known antigen + complement
  2. Indicator system: sheep red blood cells ± haemolysis
- Examples: tests for viral antibodies, HBsAg, anti-DNA, anti-platelet antibodies and the Wassermann reaction for syphilis.

3. IMMUNOFLUORESCENCE TESTS (Fig 3.10)

- Antigen fixed to a solid phase combines with antibody in a test serum.

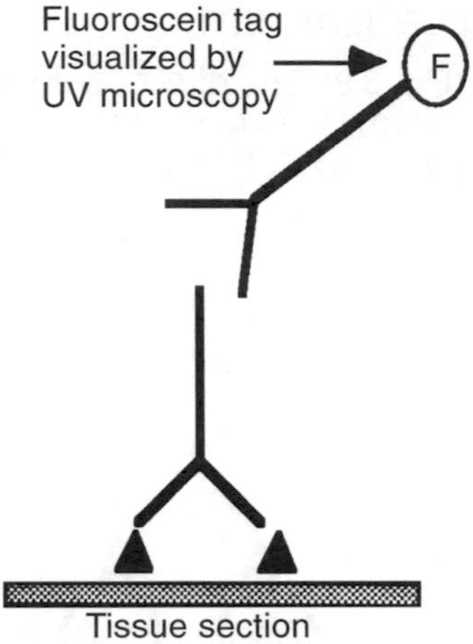

Fig. 3.10

- Anti-human antibody (IgG or IgM) labelled with fluorescein (F) is added, and the Ag–Ab complexes visualized with ultraviolet light.
- Examples: detection of organ-specific auto-antibodies (thyroid) and non-organ-specific auto-antibodies (ANA in SLE); identification of T and B cells in blood, rapid identification of microorganisms in tissues or cultures, and localization of hormones and enzymes.

4. IMMUNOENZYME ASSAYS

Example: enzyme-linked immunoabsorbent assay (ELISA) (See Note).

- Similar to 3, except label used is an enzyme, such as horse radish peroxidase, instead of fluoroscein. Enzyme will cause a colour change on the addition of a specific substrate. The intensity of the colour change is proportional to the amount of reactivity.
- Can be used to assay both antigen and antibody.
- Examples: HIV-I antibody and hepatitis B antigen.

Note: Antibody capture tests: both ELISA and RIA can be made more sensitive and specific by 'capturing' patients' IgM reacting with the virus, then adding labelled monoclonal antiviral antibody.

5. RADIOIMMUNOASSAY (RIA) (See Note above)

- Generally the most sensitive assay for antigen.
- Similar to above, except label used is a radioactive isotope, e.g. ^{125}I. Increasing known amounts of unlabelled antigen are reacted

with a constant amount of antibody, followed by labelled antigen. The bound antigen–antibody versus the free antigen ratio is determined and the amount of antigen in the unknown sample is calculated by reference to a standard curve. The partitioning of the activity indicates the concentration of the antibody in the test solution.

- Examples: assay of polypeptide hormones, anti-DNA-Ab, hepatitis B surface antigen, drugs (e.g. digoxin).

6. IMMUNODIFFUSION

- Technique for estimating antigen concentration.
- Radial immunodiffusion: antigen diffuses out of a well cut into an agar plate which has a specific antibody incorporated. The distance of the line of precipitation from the well is proportional to the concentration of antigen in the well.
- Double diffusion: solutions of antigen and antibody are placed in two adjacent wells, with antibody in the central well. The further the line of precipitation is from the latter well, the greater the concentration of antigen.
- Examples: cryptococcal antigen in CSF, carcinoembryonic antigen and alpha-fetoprotein.

4. Anatomy

CHAPTER CONTENTS

PERIPHERAL NERVOUS SYSTEM

DERMATOMES (Table 4.1)

Table 4.1 Summary of dermatomal supply

Root value	*Area innervated*
C5–T1	— the upper limb
T4	— nipple
T7	— the lower ribs
T10	— umbilical area
T12	— 'lowest' nerve of the anterior abdominal wall
L1	— inguinal region
L2, 3	— anteromedial and lateral thigh
L4, 5*	— medial border of the foot and sole, front and back of the calf up to the knee
S1*	— lateral side of the foot (fifth toe) and sole
S2	— posterior surface of the leg and thigh
S3, 4	— buttocks and perianal region

*L5 supplies the first toe; S1 supplies the fifth toe.

Dermatomes of the head and neck (Fig. 4.1)

Anterior to the auricle, the scalp is supplied by the three branches of the trigeminal nerve.
Posterior to the auricle, the scalp is supplied by the spinal cutaneous nerves from the neck.

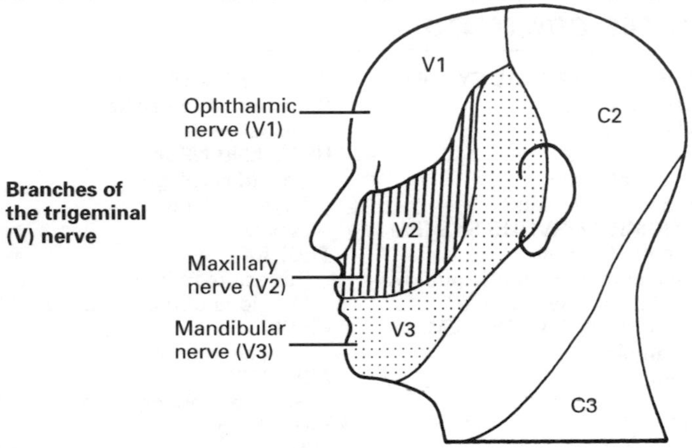

Fig. 4.1

Dermatomes in the upper limb (Fig. 4.2)

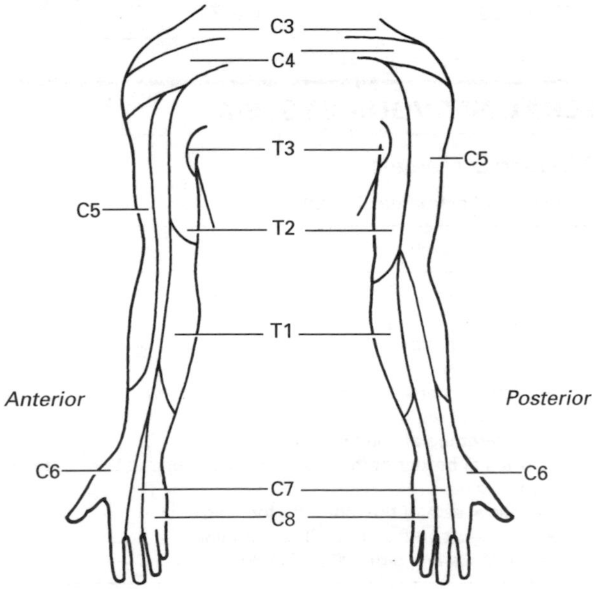

Fig. 4.2

Dermatomes in the lower limb (Fig. 4.3)

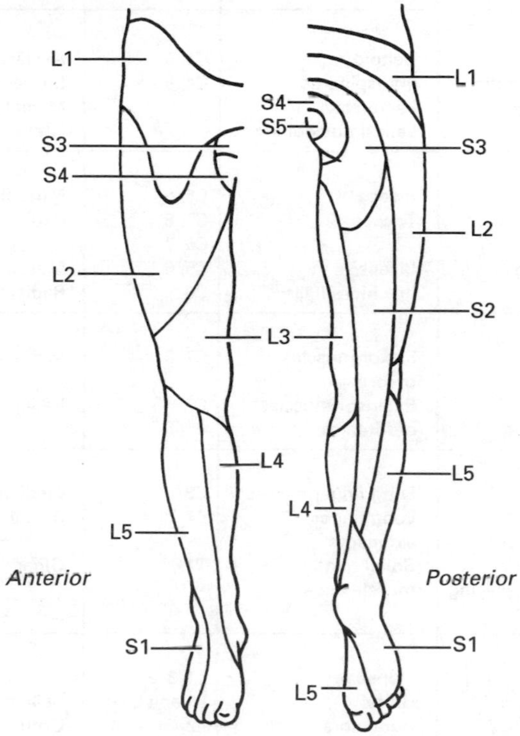

Fig. 4.3

Table 4.2 Motor root values and peripheral nerve supply of important muscle groups

Joint movement	*Muscle*	*Root value*	*Peripheral nerve*
Shoulder			
• abduction	Deltoid	C4, 5	Axillary
• external rotation	Infraspinatus	C4, 5	Suprascapular
• adduction	Pectoralis/ Latissimus dorsi	C6–8	Medial and lateral pectoral
Elbow			
• flexion	Biceps	C5, 6	Musculocutaneous
• extension	Triceps	C7, 8	Radial
• pronation		C6, 7	
• supination	Biceps/ brachioradialis	C5, 6 C6	Musculocutaneous Radial
Wrist			
• flexion	Flexor muscles of forearm	C7, 8	Median and ulnar
• dorsiflexion	Extensor muscles of forearm	C7	Radial
Finger			
• flexion	Long finger flexors	C8	Median and ulnar
• extension	Long finger extensors	C7	Radial
• opposition of thumb or splaying of fingers	Small hand muscles	T1	Ulnar
Hips			
• flexion	Iliopsoas	L1–3	—
• extension	Glutei	L5 and S1	Sciatic
• adduction	Adductors	L2, 3	Obturator
• abduction	Glutei and tensor fasciae latae	L4, 5 and S1	Sciatic
Knee			
• flexion	Hamstrings	L5 and S1, 2	Sciatic
• extension	Quadriceps	L3, 4	Femoral
Ankle			
• dorsiflexion	Anterior tibial	L4, 5	Sciatic (peroneal)
• plantar-flexion	Calf (gastrocnemius and soleus)	S1, 2	Sciatic (tibial)
• eversion	Peronei	L5 and S1	Sciatic (peroneal)
• inversion	Anterior tibial and posterior tibial	L4 L4, 5	Sciatic (peroneal) Sciatic (tibial)
Toes			
• flexion		S2, 3	
• extension	Extensor hallucis longus	L5 and S1	Sciatic (peroneal)

Note: All muscles on back of upper limb (triceps, wrist and finger extensors) are innervated by C7.

Table 4.3 Tendon jerks and abdominal reflexes

Tendon jerk	*Muscle*	*Root value*	*Peripheral nerve*
Biceps	Biceps	C5, 6	Musculocutaneous
Triceps	Triceps	C7	Radial
Supinator	Brachioradialis	C6	Radial
Finger	Long finger flexors	C8	Median and ulnar
Knee	Quadriceps	L3,4	Femoral
Ankle	Gastrocnemius	S1	Sciatic (tibial branch)
Abdominal		T8–12	
Cremasteric		L1,2	
Anal		S3,4	

SPINAL NERVES

31 pairs of spinal nerves:

- 8 cervical
- 12 thoracic
- 5 lumbar
- 5 sacral
- 1 coccygeal

CERVICAL PLEXUS (C1–4)

Phrenic nerve (C3–5)

The most important branch of the cervical plexus.

- Descends beneath sternocleidomastoid muscle, and passes in front of the subclavian artery. Right phrenic passes lateral to the superior vena cava. Left phrenic crosses the lateral aspect of the aortic arch. Both right and left nerves then descend vertically in front of the root of the lung and pass between pericardium and mediastinal pleura to the diaphragm.
- Motor fibres supply the diaphragm. Sensory fibres supply the pericardium, pleura and diaphragmatic pleura.

BRACHIAL PLEXUS

- Formed by the union of the ventral rami of the 5th to 8th cervical nerves and most of the ventral ramus of the 1st thoracic nerve.
- The three posterior divisions unite to form the posterior cord: the superior and two anterior divisions unite to form the lateral cord, and the inferior and anterior divisions form the medial cord.

Brachial plexus injuries

1. *Erb–Duchenne paralysis:* damage to C5, 6 roots.
   (i) Paralysis of the deltoid, biceps and brachialis: 'winged scapula', i.e. arm internally rotated at the shoulder and elbow extended.
   (ii) Sensory loss on the lateral aspect of shoulder and upper arm, and radial border of the forearm.

   Causes: breech presentation (with traction on the head).
2. *Klumpke's paralysis:* damage to T1 root.
   (i) Paralysis of intrinsic hand muscles: 'claw hand'.
   (ii) Sensory loss on the medial border of forearm and hand, and over medial two fingers.
   (iii) Horner's syndrome due to traction on the sympathetic chain.

   Causes: birth injury (traction with the arm extended).

Radial nerve (C5–8)

Main branch of the posterior cord of the brachial plexus (See Note).
Motor to:
Extensor muscles of the forearm, wrist, finger and thumb
Sensation:
See Fig. 4.4.

Radial nerve damage in the arm

1. Wrist drop.
2. Atrophy of triceps (if trauma occurred in the axilla), i.e. unable to extend elbow, wrist or digits.
3. Small area of anaesthesia on the dorsum of the hand between 1st and 2nd metacarpals. (See Fig. 4.4.)

Causes: fractures of neck of humerus, pressure palsy, badly placed injections, lead poisoning, and polyarteritis.

Note: The axillary nerve (C5, 6) is the smaller terminal branch, and supplies both the deltoid and teres major muscle.

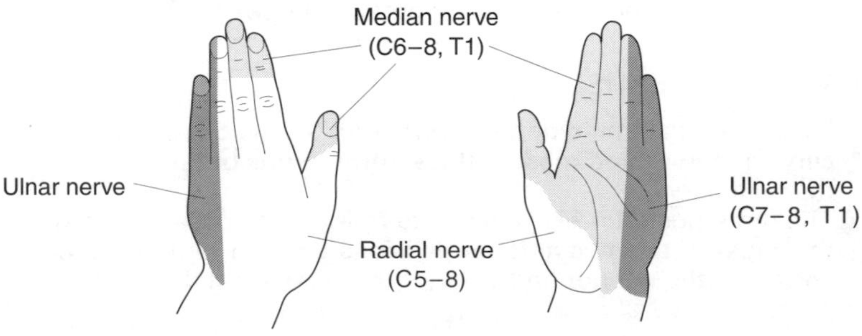

Fig. 4.4

Median nerve (C6–8, T1)

Arises from the lateral and medial cords of the brachial plexus.

Motor to:

1. Lateral 2 lumbricals (**L**),
2. Opponens pollcis (**O**), abductor pollicis brevis (**A**) and flexor pollicis brevis (**F**), i.e. the thenar eminence muscles.
3. All muscles on the flexor aspect of the forearm, apart from flexor carpi ulnaris and the ulnar half of the flexor digitorum profundus. N.B. As with the ulnar nerve, it supplies no muscles in the upper arm.

Mnemonic: **LOAF** and forearm flexors.

Sensation:

See Fig. 4.4.

Median nerve damage at the elbow

1. Pronation of forearm lost.
2. Wrist flexion weak: ulnar deviation.

Median nerve damage at the wrist

1. Paralysis and wasting of thenar muscles.
2. Paralysis of opponens pollicis.
3. Loss of sensation as shown (Fig. 4.4).

Causes: trauma, amyotrophic lateral sclerosis, heavy metal poisoning, carpal tunnel syndrome, polyarteritis nodosa, and diabetes.

Ulnar nerve (C7–8, T1)

Main continuation of the medial cord of the brachial plexus.

Motor to:

1. Medial and lateral interossei and lumbricals (**M**).
2. Adductor pollicis (**A**).
3. 1st dorsal interosseus (**F**).
4. Interossei (**I**).
5. Abductor digiti minimi and flexor digiti minimi: hypothenar muscles (**A**). (mnemonic **MAFIA**) and
6. Flexor carpi ulnaris and medial half of flexor digitorum profundus in the forearm.

i.e., it supplies all the intrinsic muscles of the hand apart from those of the thenar eminence and the 1st and 2nd lumbricals which are innervated by the median nerve. N.B. As with the median nerve, it supplies no muscles in the upper arm.

Sensation:

See Fig 4.4.

Ulnar nerve damage at the wrist

1. Wasting and paralysis of intrinsic hand muscles (apart from lateral 2 lumbricals), i.e. fingers cannot be abducted or

adducted, the thumb cannot be adducted due to paralysis of adductor pollicis: 'claw hand'. (See Note.)
2. Wasting and paralysis of hypothenar muscles.
3. Loss of sensation as shown Fig. 4.4.

Note: Distinguish from Volkmann's contracture – another claw hand deformity where ischaemia causes muscle contraction throughout the forearm.

Ulnar nerve damage at the elbow

1. Clawing less marked in the 3rd and 4th fingers due to additional paralysis of flexor digitorum profundus.
2. Radial deviation of the wrist (paralysis of flexor carpi ulnaris).

Causes: laceration at the wrist, fractures/dislocation at the elbow, pressure palsy, carpal tunnel syndrome, machine vibrating tools, polyarteritis, leprosy and lead poisoning.

LUMBOSACRAL PLEXUS

Sciatic nerve (L4, 5, S1–3)

Most important branch of lumbosacral plexus and largest nerve in the body. Terminates by dividing into medial and lateral popliteal nerves (tibial and common peroneal nerves respectively) in the proximal part of the popliteal fossa.
Motor to:
1. The hamstring muscles (biceps femoris, semimembranous and semitendinous).
2. Adductor magnus.

Sensation:
Back of thigh and distal to knee.

Sciatic nerve damage

1. Paralysis of flexion of the knee and all movement below the knee, resulting in a foot drop.
2. Sensory loss is complete below the knee, except for a small area on the medial side of the leg.
3. Ankle jerk and plantar response is lost, but knee jerk is retained.

Causes: penetrating injuries, badly placed injections, fractures of pelvis or femur, and posterior dislocation of the hip.

BRANCHES OF SCIATIC NERVE

- Medial popliteal (tibial) nerve.
- Lateral popliteal (common peroneal) nerve.

1. Medial popliteal (tibial) nerve

- Anterior divisions L4, 5 and S1–3.
- Larger of the two terminal branches of the sciatic nerve.
- Divides into medial and lateral plantar nerves.

Motor to:
1. Calf muscles (gastrocnemius, soleus, and popliteus).
2. Flexor hallucis longus and tibialis posterior.
3. Terminal plantar branches supply the intrinsic muscles and the sole of the foot.
4. Mediates the ankle and plantar reflexes.

Sensation:
Lateral aspect of the foot and 5th toe (sural nerve branch) and sensation to the sole.

Tibial nerve damage
1. Unable to plantarflex, invert the foot, or flex the toes.
2. Claw-like deformity of the toes.
3. Sensation lost to the sole of the foot.

2. Lateral popliteal (common peroneal) nerve
- Posterior divisions of L4, 5 and S1, 2.
- Passes through the popliteal fossa, winding around the head of the fibula close to biceps femoris.
- Divides into terminal branches: deep peroneal (anterior tibial) and superficial nerves.

Motor to:
1. Anterior compartment of the leg (extensor digitorum longus, extensor hallucis longus, tibialis anterior, peroneus tertius and extensor digitorum brevis); turns the foot upwards and outwards.

Sensation:
Anterolateral aspect of the lower half of the leg, including the ankle and dorsum of the foot.

Common peroneal nerve lesions
More susceptible to injury than the tibial nerve.
1. Foot drop with paralysis of dorsiflexion.
2. Paralysis of eversion and weak inversion (only with the foot in plantar flexion) and of toe extension.
3. Sensory loss to anterolateral aspect of lower half of leg.

Causes: pressure palsy, Charcot–Marie–Tooth neuropathy, fractures of tibia and fibula.

AUTONOMIC NERVOUS SYSTEM

SYMPATHETIC TRUNK

- Extends for the whole length of the spinal cord.
- Ganglia are associated with each spinal segment, except for in the cervical region where there are only three ganglia:
    1. Superior cervical ganglion (C2–4)
    2. Middle cervical ganglion (C5, 6)

Table 4.4 Sympathetic outflow (T1–L2)

Spinal segments	*Sympathetic innervation*	*Destination*
T1–T2	Via internal carotid and vertebral arteries	Head and neck Ciliary muscle and iris Blood vessels Sweat glands
T1–T4	Via cardiac and pulmonary plexuses	Heart and bronchi
T2–T7		Upper limb
T4–L2	Via coeliac, mesenteric, hypogastric and pelvic plexuses	Adrenal medulla Alimentary tract Colon and rectum Bladder and genitalia
T11–L2		Lower limb

T1–T4: relay in sympathetic ganglion.
T4–L2: do not relay in sympathetic ganglion.

3. Inferior cervical ganglion, which fuses with 1st thoracic ganglion to form the stellate ganglion (C7, 8 and T1).

Consequences of sympathectomy

1. Division of the stellate ganglion (T1) results in Horner's syndrome due to interruption of the sympathetic fibres to the eyelid and pupil.
2. 'Cervicothoracic' sympathectomy (T2–4) results in a warm, dry hand, due to interruption of sudomotor and vasoconstrictor pathways to head and upper limb.
3. 'Lumbar' sympathectomy (L2–4) results in a warm, dry and pink lower limb.

PARASYMPATHETIC (CRANIOSACRAL) OUTFLOW

- Cranial outflow supplies the visceral structures in the head via the oculomotor, facial and glossopharyngeal nerves and those in the thorax and upper abdomen via the vagus nerves.
- Sacral outflow supplies the pelvic viscera via the pelvic branches of the 2nd to 4th sacral spinal nerves.

Neurological control of bladder function

- Afferent fibres travel via parasympathetic nerves to spinal 'micturition centre' (S2, 3, 4).
- Bladder contraction initiated by parasympathetic efferents.
- Spinal 'micturition centre' normally inhibited by higher motor centre.
- An **automatic** bladder (partial emptying when bladder volume is approx. 250 ml) occurs with cord section above S2, 3, 4.
- An **autonomous** bladder (weak uncoordinated bladder

Table 4.5 Effects of sympathetic nervous system

System affected	α_1	α_2	β_1	β_2
Heart	↓ rate ↓ atrial contractility ↓ AVN conduction		↑ rate and contractility ↑ AVN conduction ↑ renin secretion	
Vessels	Little effect	Vasoconstriction of arterioles (esp. skin, abdominal viscera and coronary circulation) Constriction of systemic veins		Vasodilation of coronary arterioles and in skeletal muscle
Bronchus	Bronchoconstriction			Bronchial muscle relaxation
Gut	↑ motility; relaxation of sphincters	↓ motility		↓ motility
Urogenital	Contraction of detrusor muscles of bladder; relaxation of sphincters	Relaxation of detrusor muscles; contraction of sphincters and pregnant uterus		Relaxation of pregnant uterus
Pancreas	↑ exocrine secretion No effect on β-cells of islets	↓ exocrine secretion		↑ endocrine secretion by β-cells; lipolysis; glycogenolysis; gluconeogenesis
Eye (see Fig. 4.12)	Miosis: sphincter pupillae contracts			Mydriasis: dilator pupillae contracts
Glands		↑ secretion (lacrimal, salivary, alimentary)		↑ secretion by sweat glands

AVN, atrioventricular node.

contractions without desire to micturate occurs with lower motor neuron cord lesions at S2, 3, 4 level.
- An **atonic** bladder (distended bladder with overflow) occurs with sensory neuropathies (e.g. diabetes).

CENTRAL NERVOUS SYSTEM

BASAL GANGLIA

- Consists of the corpus striatum (caudate nucleus, putamen, globus pallidus), claustrum, amygdala and the thalamus.

MIDBRAIN

- Connects the pons and cerebellum to the diencephalon (hypothalamus and thalamus). Contains the cerebral peduncles (corticobulbar, corticospinal tracts), red nucleus, substantia nigra and the cranial nerve nuclei of III and IV and a portion of the large sensory nucleus of V.
- Ascending sensory fibres travel in the lateral and medial lemnisci.
- Descending motor fibres pass en route to pons and spinal cord.

PONS

- Lies between the medulla and midbrain and is connected to the cerebellum by the middle cerebellar peduncle.
- Upper pons: most prominent features are the pontine nuclei and the pontocerebellar fibres anteriorly.
- Lower pons: dorsal surface forms the upper part of the floor of the fourth ventricle. Contains the nuclei of the VI, VII and VIII cranial nerves. (The sensory nucleus of V is extensive, extending from the midbrain to the upper cervical level, with the most important part in the pons and the medulla. The motor nucleus of V is in the pons. The corticospinal tracts cross in the lower pons.)

MEDULLA

- Continuous through the foramen magnum with the spinal cord, and above with the pons.
- Connected to the cerebellum by the inferior cerebellar peduncle.
- Contains the nucleus ambiguus (motor to IX and X) and the solitary nucleus (sensory VIII, IX and X).
- Most prominent cranial nerve nuclei are IX, X, XI and XII.
- The dorsal column nuclei cross to form the medial lemniscus.
- Sensory decussation contains some uncrossed fibres.

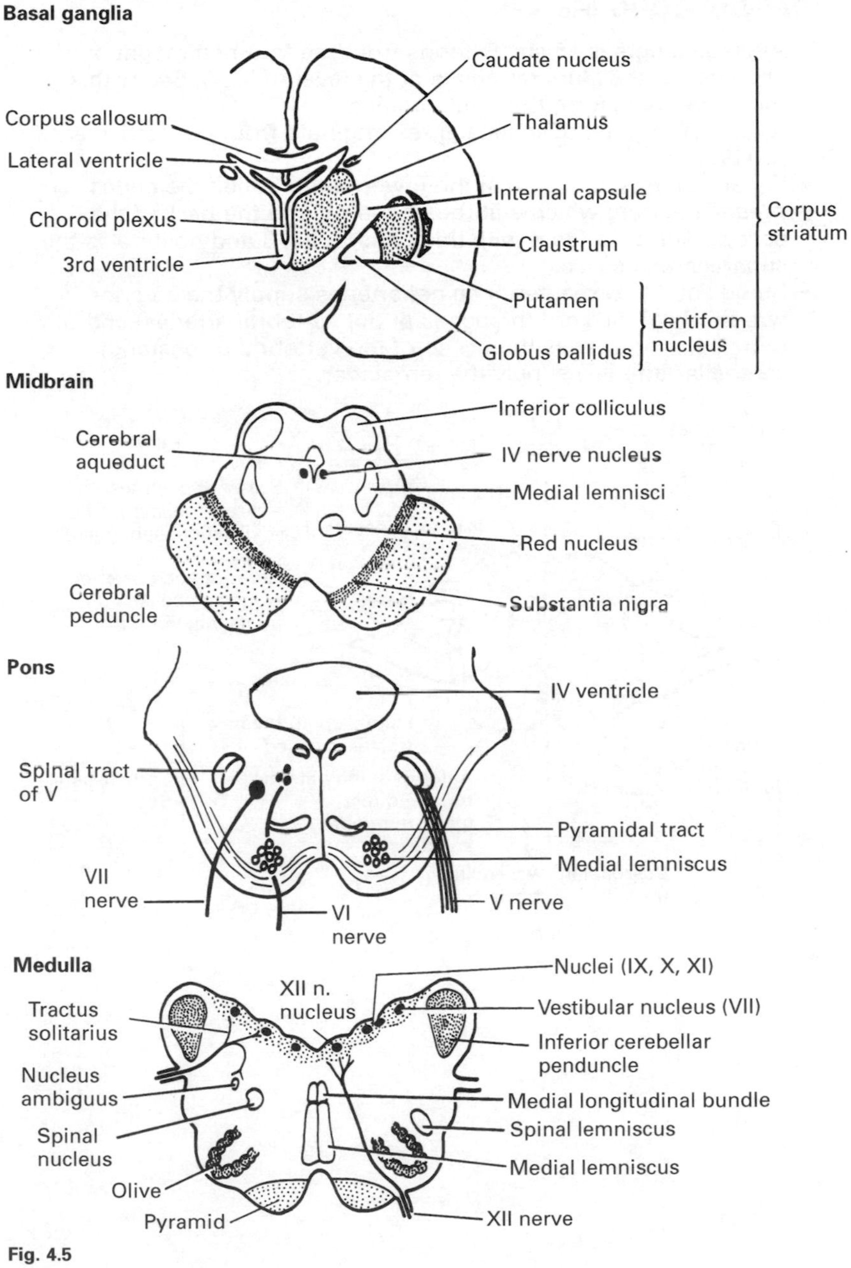
Basal ganglia
Caudate nucleus
Corpus callosum
Thalamus
Lateral ventricle
Internal capsule
Corpus striatum
Choroid plexus
Claustrum
3rd ventricle
Putamen
Lentiform nucleus
Globus pallidus
Midbrain
Inferior colliculus
Cerebral aqueduct
IV nerve nucleus
Medial lemnisci
Red nucleus
Cerebral peduncle
Substantia nigra
Pons
IV ventricle
Spinal tract of V
Pyramidal tract
Medial lemniscus
VII nerve
V nerve
VI nerve
Medulla
Nuclei (IX, X, XI)
XII n. nucleus
Tractus solitarius
Vestibular nucleus (VII)
Inferior cerebellar pendunce
Nucleus ambiguus
Medial longitudinal bundle
Spinal lemniscus
Spinal nucleus
Medial lemniscus
Olive
Pyramid
XII nerve

Fig. 4.5

SPINAL CORD (Fig. 4.6)

- Average length is 45 cm. Extends from the foramen magnum and ends in the filum terminale at the level of L2, 3. Below this the nerve roots form the cauda equina.
- A total of 31 pairs of spinal nerves originate from the cord. (see p. 119).
- Expansion of spinal cord at the lower end is called the *conus medullaris* from which a fibrous band runs to the back of the coccyx. The dura fuses with this band at S2, 3 and obliterates the subarachnoid space.
- Blood supply: two anterior spinal arteries supply the anterior two-thirds of the cord (branches of the vertebral arteries) and two posterior arteries (branches of the vertebral or posterior cerebellar arteries) supply the remainder.

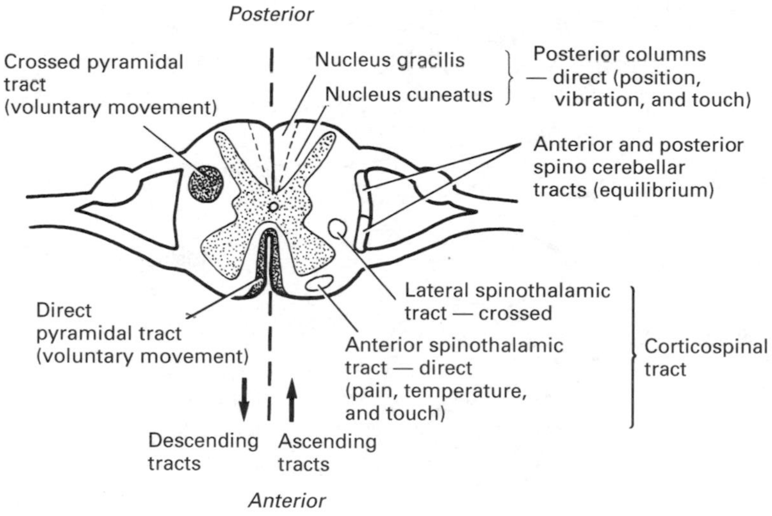

Fig. 4.6

CEREBRAL CORTEX

Arterial supply (Fig. 4.7)

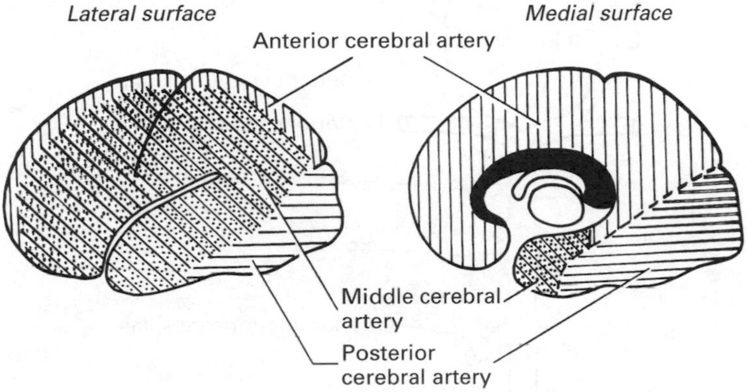

Fig. 4.7

Circle of Willis (Fig. 4.8)
Located at the base of the brain, mainly in the interpeduncular fossa.

Localization of function (Fig. 4.9)

- Lateral (Sylvian) fissure lies between the temporal, frontal and parietal lobes.
- Central sulcus runs obliquely downwards from the superior margin of the brain almost to the lateral fissure.
- The primary voluntary motor cortex lies along the posterior part of the precentral gyrus adjoining the central sulcus.
- The primary sensory cortex lies in the postcentral gyrus.
- The primary auditory area lies on the cephalic border of the superior temporal gyrus in the depths of the lateral fissure.
- The primary visual cortex lies in the calcarine fissure area of the occipital pole.
- Broca's area lies in the posterior part of the inferior frontal gyrus.
- Wernicke's area lies in the posterior part of the superior temporal lobe.

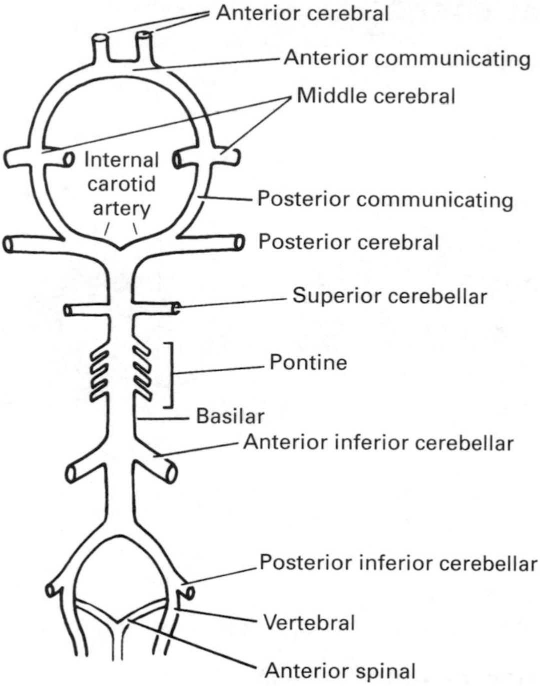
Anterior cerebral
Anterior communicating
Middle cerebral
Internal carotid artery
Posterior communicating
Posterior cerebral
Superior cerebellar
Pontine
Basilar
Anterior inferior cerebellar
Posterior inferior cerebellar
Vertebral
Anterior spinal

Fig. 4.8

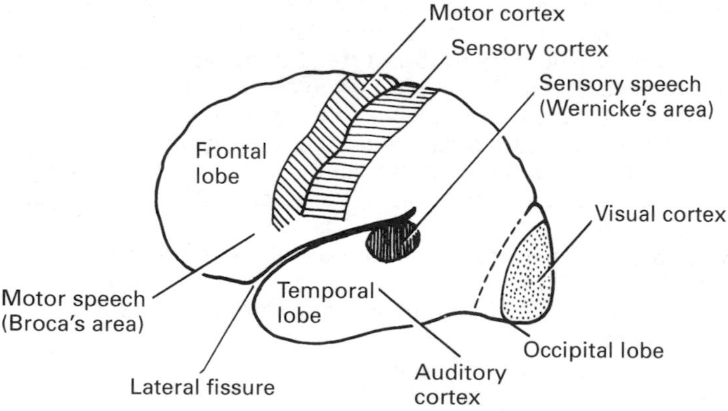
Motor cortex
Sensory cortex
Sensory speech (Wernicke's area)
Frontal lobe
Visual cortex
Motor speech (Broca's area)
Temporal lobe
Occipital lobe
Auditory cortex
Lateral fissure

Fig. 4.9

VENTRICLES OF THE BRAIN AND CEREBROSPINAL FLUID (CSF) SYSTEM

- 500–750 ml of cerebrospinal fluid (CSF) is produced per day by a process of ultrafiltration and active secretion (Fig. 4.10). The total volume of CSF is 100–150 ml.

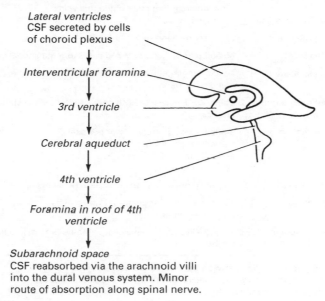

Lateral ventricles
CSF secreted by cells of choroid plexus
↓
Interventricular foramina
↓
3rd ventricle
↓
Cerebral aqueduct
↓
4th ventricle
↓
Foramina in roof of 4th ventricle
↓
Subarachnoid space
CSF reabsorbed via the arachnoid villi into the dural venous system. Minor route of absorption along spinal nerve.

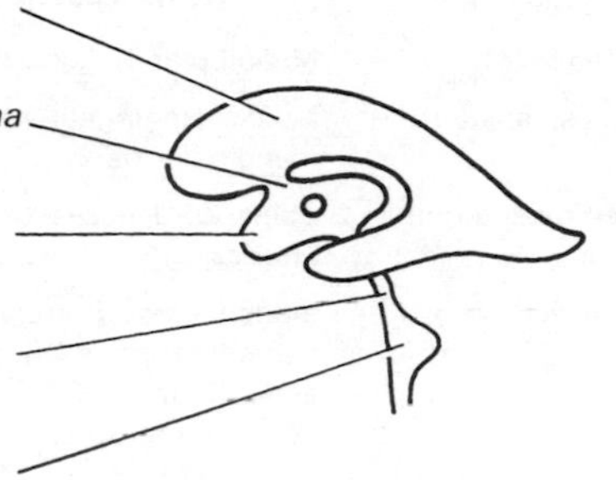

Fig. 4.10

Composition of CSF

See page 294.

Skull foramina (Table 4.6)

Base of the skull forms three fossae that contain the brain and meninges.

- Anterior fossa contains the frontal lobes.
- Middle fossa contains the hypothalamus and temporal lobes.
- Posterior fossa contains the brain stem and cerebellum.

CRANIAL NERVES (Table 4.7)

Olfactory (I) nerve

Course: Olfactory cells reside in the mucosa of the superior nasal conchae and the upper part of the nasal septum. The axons pass through the cribiform plate of the ethmoid bone to reach the overlying olfactory bulb in the anterior cranial fossa. The olfactory tracts pass from the olfactory bulb to the medial surface of the cerebral hemisphere and the temporal lobes.

Table 4.6 Skull foramina and contents

Foramen	*Contents*
Optic canal	Optic (II) nerve and ophthalmic artery
Superior orbital fissure*	III, IV, VI and ophthalmic division of V cranial nerves, sympathetic nerve and ophthalmic veins
Stylomastoid foramen	VII cranial nerve
Foramen rotundum	Maxillary division of V
Foramen ovale†	Mandibular division of V and accessory meningeal artery
Foramen spinosum	Middle meningeal artery, meningeal branch of the mandibular nerve
Foramen magnum	Spinal cord, accessory (XI) nerve, vertebral and spinal arteries
Foramen lacerum	Internal carotid artery, lesser petrosal nerve (branch of IX), greater petrosal nerve (branch of VII), deep petrosal nerves (autonomic)
Jugular foramen‡	Internal jugular vein and IX, X, XI cranial nerves
Hypoglossal foramen	XII cranial nerve, meningeal branch of ascending pharyngeal artery
Internal auditory meatus	VII and VIII cranial nerves, labyrinthine (internal auditory) artery

*Forms a communication between the middle cranial fossa and the orbit.
†Communication from middle cranial fossa to the infratemporal fossa.
‡Lies lateral to the foramen magnum.

Optic (II) nerve (Fig. 4.11)

Course: Axons of ganglion cells from the retina make up the optic nerve. The optic disc is the central collecting point for these axons. The orbital portion of the nerve extends from where the optic nerve pierces the sclera to the optic foramen in the skull. It leaves the orbit through the optic foramen and then unites with the other optic nerve to form the optic chiasma.

Posterior to the optic chiasma, the nerves continue as the optic tract and synapse with the neurons in the lateral geniculate body in the thalamus. From the lateral geniculate body, the optic radiation curves backward to the occipital visual cortex.

A small number of fibres concerned with pupillary and ocular reflexes bypass the lateral geniculate body and go to the pretectal nucleus and superior colliculus in the midbrain.

Table 4.7 Summary of cranial nerves and their functions

Nerve	*Origin*	*Cranial exit*	*Type*	*Chief functions*
I. Olfactory	Nasal mucosa	Cribiform plate	Sensory	Smell
II. Optic	Retina	Optic canal	Sensory	Vision and light reflexes (direct and consensual)
III. Oculomotor	Midbrain a. III nerve nucleus b. Edinger–Westphal nucleus	Superior orbital fissure	a. Motor b. Parasympathetic	a. Motor to four extrinsic eye muscles and levator palpebrae superioris b. Motor to ciliary and sphincter pupillae muscles for light and accommodation reflexes
IV. Trochlear	Midbrain (below inferior colliculus)	Superior orbital fissure	Motor	Motor to superior oblique muscle
V. Trigeminal a. Ophthalmic b. Maxillary c. Mandibular	Pons Trigeminal ganglion and motor V nucleus	a. Superior orbital fissure b. Foramen rotundum c. Foramen ovale	a. Sensory b. Sensory c. Mixed } a,b,c	Motor to muscles of mastication and for jaw jerk Sensation from skin of face, scalp, nasal cavity, mouth and palate: corneal reflex
VI. Abducent	Pons	Superior orbital fissure	Motor	Motor to lateral rectus muscle
VII. Facial	Pons	Stylomastoid foramen	Motor, sensory (taste) and parasympathetic	Motor to muscles of facial expression, corneal reflex efferent part Secretomotor to lacrimal and salivary glands Sensation and taste from anterior two-thirds of tongue and soft palate

Table 4.7 *(cont.)*

Nerve	*Origin*	*Cranial exit*	*Type*	*Chief functions*
VIII. Vestibulocochlear a. Vestibular b. Cochlear	Pons (organ of Corti; the cochlear and spiral ganglion)	Does not leave skull Final common pathway: superior temporal gyrus	Sensory	Hearing; balance and position of head
IX. Glossopharyngeal	Medulla	Jugular foramen	Motor, sensory (taste) and parasympathetic	Motor to pharyngeal muscles (gag reflex) Secretomotor to parotid salivary gland Sensation and taste from posterior one-third of tongue, tonsil and pharynx
X. Vagus	Medulla	Jugular foramen	Motor, sensory and parasympathetic	Motor to heart, lungs and alimentary tract Motor to the muscles of the larynx, pharynx and palate Sensation from pharynx, larynx, heart, lungs and abdominal viscera
XI. Accessory (two parts: cranial and spinal)	Medulla (nucleus ambiguus) and spinal cord (cervical)	Jugular foramen	Motor	Motor to sternocleidomastoid and trapezius muscles Motor to muscles of pharynx, larynx and soft palate
XII. Hypoglossal	Medulla	Hypoglossal canal	Motor	Motor to strap muscles of neck Motor to muscles of tongue

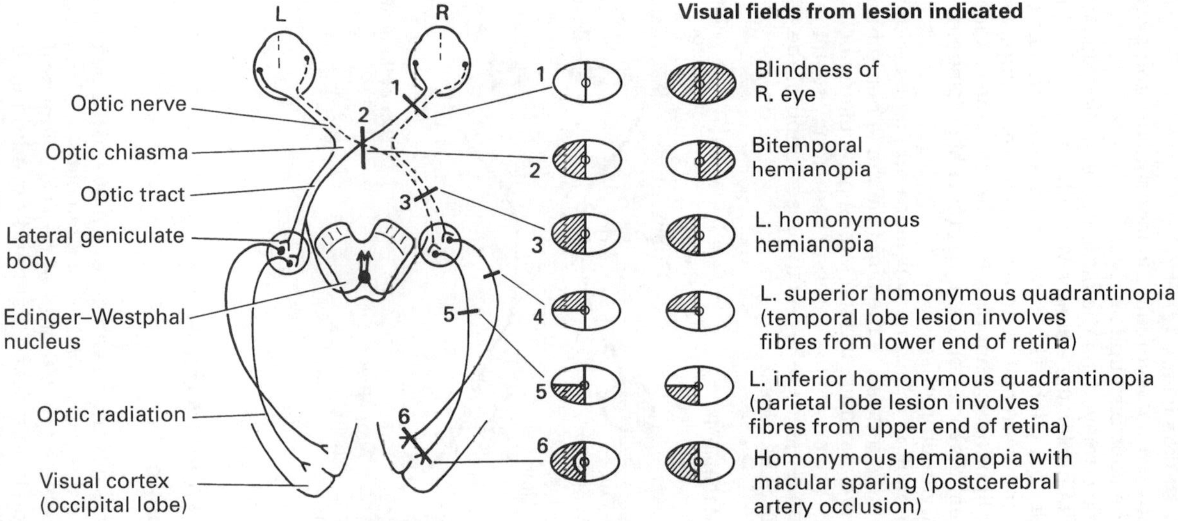

L
R
1
2
3
5
6
1
2
3
4
5
6
Optic nerve
Optic chiasma
Optic tract
Lateral geniculate body
Edinger–Westphal nucleus
Optic radiation
Visual cortex (occipital lobe)
Visual fields from lesion indicated
Blindness of R. eye
Bitemporal hemianopia
L. homonymous hemianopia
L. superior homonymous quadrantinopia (temporal lobe lesion involves fibres from lower end of retina)
L. inferior homonymous quadrantinopia (parietal lobe lesion involves fibres from upper end of retina)
Homonymous hemianopia with macular sparing (postcerebral artery occlusion)

Fig. 4.11

Pupillary reflexes (Fig. 4.12)
Balance between parasympathetic (constrictor) and sympathetic (dilator) tone controls pupil size.

1. Light reflex: relayed via the optic nerve, optic tract, lateral geniculate nuclei, the Edinger-Westphal nucleus of the III nerve and ciliary ganglion. The cortex is not involved. Lesions of the brain stem may result in an Argyl–Robertson pupil with loss of direct light reflex, but preservation of convergence reflex ('light-near dissociation') e.g. neurosyphilis, diabetes and some hereditary neuropathies.
2. Accommodation reflex: convergence originates within the cortex and is relayed to the pupil via the III nerve nuclei. The optic nerve and tract and the lateral geniculate nucleus are not involved. Lesions of the cerebral cortex may result in absence of the convergence reflex, with preservation of the light reflex, e.g. cortical blindness.

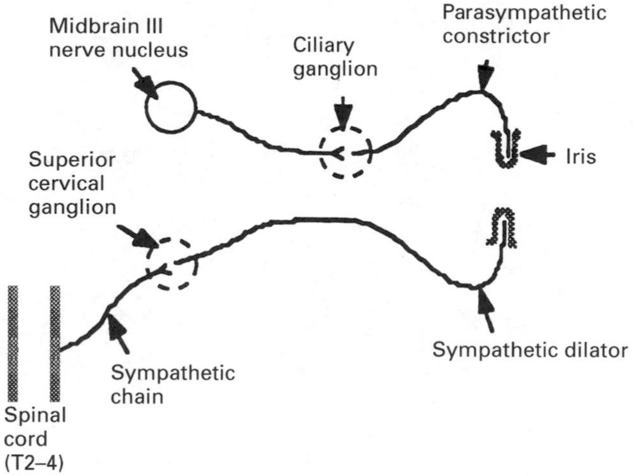

Fig. 4.12

Horner's syndrome (Fig. 4.13)

Eye movements

Vertical

- The centres governing vertical eye movements lie in the midbrain.
- Lesions of the upper midbrain cause paresis of conjugate upward gaze, often with loss of pupillary light and accommodation reflexes (Parinaud's syndrome); e.g. encephalitis, tumours around the IIIrd ventricle, midbrain or pineal body, Wernicke's encephalopathy or infarction.
- Disturbances of vertical gaze also seen with progressive supranuclear palsy, Huntington's chorea, hydrocephalus and vascular syndromes.

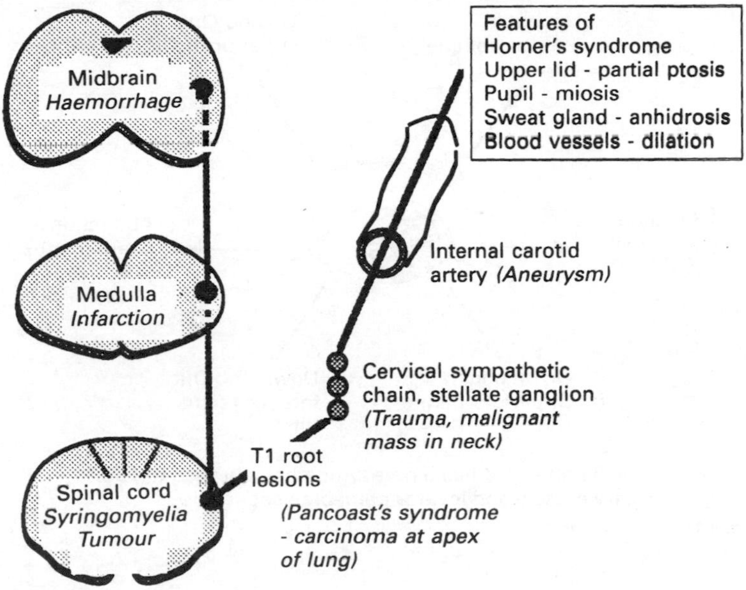

Fig. 4.13

Horizontal

- Centre is located in prepontine reticular formation in the pons.

Lesions

- Internuclear ophthalmoplegia: ipsilateral adduction weakness, contralateral abduction nystagmus, caused by a medial longitudinal fasiculus lesion.
- Wernicke's encephalopathy: weakness of abduction, gaze-evoked nystagmus, internuclear ophthalmoplegia, horizontal and vertical gaze palsies.

Frontal eye fields

- Responsible for contralateral horizontal saccades.
  1. Unilateral obliteration will lead to gaze deviation *toward* the affected side.
  2. A seizure causing hyperactivity in that area will cause gaze deviation *away* from the affected side.

Oculomotor (III) nerve (Fig. 4.14)
Course: The nerve emerges from the anterior aspect of the midbrain medial to the cerebral peduncle. It passes forward in the subarachnoid space to pierce the dura mater, and lies in the lateral wall of the cavernous sinus, close to the IV and VI nerves and the ophthalmic branch of the trigeminal nerve. The nerve enters the orbit through the superior orbital fissure.

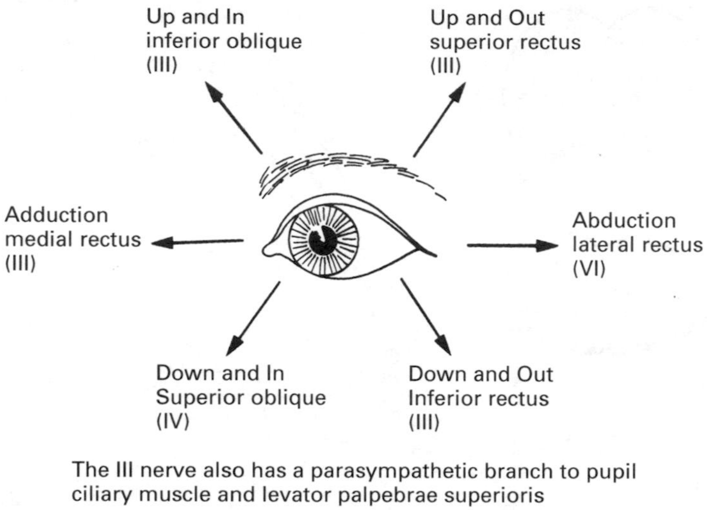

Fig. 4.14

Complete IIIrd nerve lesion

1. Ptosis: paralysis of levator palpebrae superioris.
2. Mydriasis: dilator action of sympathetic fibres unopposed.
3. Deviation of eye laterally and downwards: unopposed action of superior oblique and lateral rectus.
4. Loss of accommodation-convergence and light reflexes due to paralysis of constrictor pupillae.

Causes: vascular lesions (*Weber's syndrome*), and aneurysm of the posterior communicating artery. An isolated IIIrd nerve lesion is associated with diabetes, encephalitis and meningitis (especially due to TB, sarcoid and syphilis).

Trochlear (IV) nerve (Fig. 4.14)
Course: The nerve emerges from the posterior aspect of the midbrain, just below the inferior colliculi. It passes forward in the subarachnoid space to pierce the dura mater and then lies in the wall of the cavernous sinus, just below the oculomotor nerve. The nerve enters the orbit through the superior orbital fissure.

IVth nerve lesions

1. Rare, but most commonly seen after trauma.
2. Two images appear at an angle when the affected eye is abducted, and one above the other when the other eye is adducted. Diplopia typically occurs when looking downward and medially, e.g. descending stairs.

Trigeminal (V) nerve

Course: This is the largest of the cranial nerves. The trigeminal nerve emerges from the pons by a large sensory and a small motor root. The nerve passes forward out of the posterior cranial fossa, and on reaching the petrous part of the temporal bone in the middle cranial fossa, the large sensory root expands to form the trigeminal ganglion. Impulses reach the ganglion via its three divisions; the ophthalmic, maxillary and mandibular nerves.
The ophthalmic nerve passes through the superior orbital fissure. The maxillary nerve leaves the middle cranial fossa through the foramen rotundum, passes through the pterygopalatine fossa and the inferior orbital fissure, and crosses the floor of the orbit to emerge through the infraorbital foramen. The mandibular nerve leaves the skull via the foramen ovale.
The motor root is situated below the sensory ganglion and is completely separate from it. It passes independently out of the cranial cavity to join the mandibular division and supplies eight muscles; the muscles of mastication, the tensor tympani, the tensor veli palatini, the myelohyoid and the anterior belly of digastric.

Vth nerve lesions

1. Damage to the central organization of sensory innervation results in sensory loss, of an 'onion' skin distribution, with loss or dissociation starting over the angle of the jaw and cheek and spreading across the face.
2. Unilateral paralysis of the muscles of mastication: jaw deviates to the affected side.

Causes: brain stem vascular lesion, intrinsic brain stem tumours, syringomyelia, herpes zoster, trigeminal neuralgia, acoustic neuroma, cavernous sinus lesions, multiple sclerosis.

Abducent (VI) nerve (Fig. 4.14)

Course: Emerges from the anterior surface of the brain, in the groove between the lower border of the pons and the medulla oblongata. It runs upwards, forwards and laterally in the subarachnoid space, and traverses the cavernous sinus, lying at first lateral and then inferolateral to the internal carotid artery. The nerve enters the orbital cavity through the medial part of the superior orbital fissure.

VIth nerve lesions

1. Convergent squint with failure of abduction.
2. Diplopia is maximal on looking to the affected side.

Causes: osteitis (*Gradenigo's syndrome*), acoustic neuroma, aneurysm, meningitis, raised intracranial pressure (as a false localizing sign).

Facial (VII) nerve (Fig. 4.15)

Course: Consists of three roots, a large motor root and a small mixed sensory and parasympathetic root (*nervous intermedius*) which arise from the lateral surface of the brain stem close to the lower border of the pons. Leaving the brainstem, it accompanies the VIII nerve through the internal acoustic meatus. It then traverses the facial canal within the temporal bone, to emerge from the skull at the stylomastoid foramen, where it divides into terminal muscular branches in the substance of the parotid gland.

Branches

1. Greater petrosal nerve: mixed nerve with parasympathetic fibres to the lacrimal gland and sensory fibres to the geniculate ganglion.
2. Nerve to stapedius muscle.

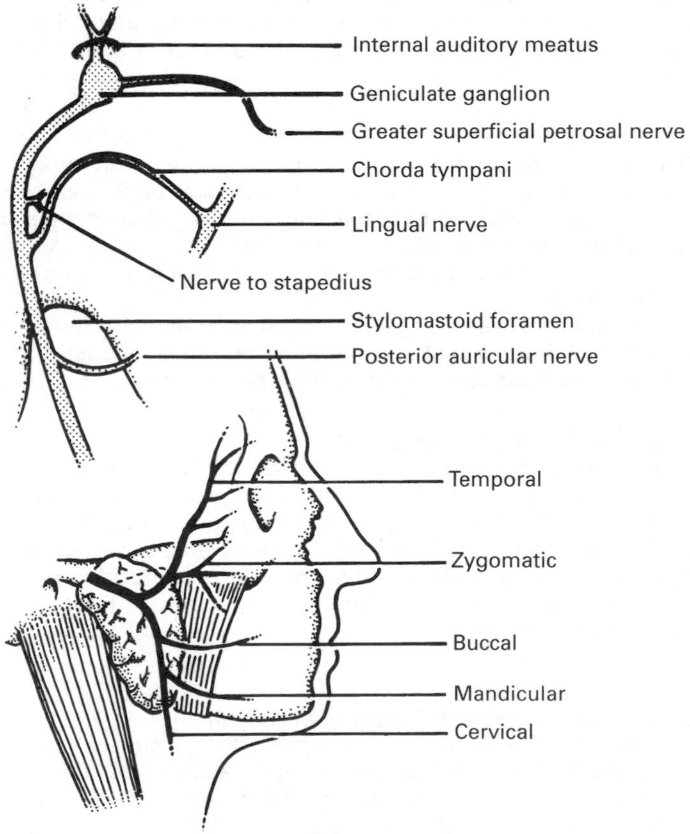

Fig. 4.15

3. Chorda tympani nerve: taste fibres to the anterior two-thirds of the tongue. Parasympathetic fibres are secretomotor to the submandibular and sublingual glands.
4. Muscular branches to all muscles of facial expression: temporal, zygomatic, buccal, mandibular and cervical.

VIIth nerve lesions

1. Supranuclear (i.e. upper motor neuron lesions): e.g. cerebrovascular accident. Sparing of forehead muscles which receive bilateral cortical fibres.
2. Nuclear: bulbar paralysis e.g. polio.
3. Infranuclear: e.g. Bell's palsy, acoustic neuroma, fractures of the temporal bone, and invasion by a malignant parotid tumour.

   } Lower motor neuron lesion. Complete facial paralysis (i.e. affects all the muscles of one side of face).

   If the intracranial part of the nerve is involved, there is:
   (i) loss of taste over the anterior two-thirds of the tongue, due to chorda tympani nerve involvement.
   (ii) hyperacusis due to paralysis of the stapedius muscle.
   (iii) decreased secretion from the lacrimal, submandibular and sublingual glands.

Vestibulocochlear (VIII) nerve

Course: Consists of two sets of sensory fibres. Cochlear nerve consists of the central processes of the bipolar neurons which have their cell bodies in the petrous temporal bone. The peripheral processes of the vestibular nerve are distributed to the semicircular canals, the utricle and the saccule. The vestibular and cochlear components enter the internal auditory meatus with the facial nerve and run in the petrous temporal bone to the inner ear.

Glossopharyngeal (IX) nerve

Course: Arises from the lateral aspect of the medulla just caudal to the pons. The nerve runs laterally and separates from the vagus nerve as it pierces the dura to enter the anterior compartment of the jugular foramen. Outside the foramen, it passes forward between the internal jugular vein and the internal carotid artery.

IXth nerve lesions

Rare in isolation. Interruption of all fibres results in:

1. loss of sensation, including taste, on the posterior third of the tongue;
2. unilateral loss of the gag reflex;
3. difficulty with swallowing.

Vagus (X) nerve

Course: Emerges from the anterior surface of the upper part of the medulla oblongata by 8–10 rootlets. Leaves the skull via the jugular foremen with the IX, and XI cranial nerves. Passes vertically downwards to the root of the neck, lying in the posterior part of the carotid sheath between the internal jugular vein and first the internal and then the common carotid artery.

Branches

1. In the neck; *pharyngeal, superior laryngeal* and *cardiac nerves.* Below the level of the subclavian artery, the nerve has a different course on each side:

- *Right vagus:* The recurrent laryngeal nerve is given off as it crosses the subclavian artery. Below this the nerve descends through the superior mediastinum posterior to the right brachiocephalic and superior vena cava and passes posterior to the lung root.
- *Left* vagus: Enters the thorax between the left common carotid and left subclavian arteries, posterior to the left brachiocephalic vein and passes posterior to the lung root. The left recurrent laryngeal nerve is given off as the vagus crosses the arch of the aorta.

2. In the thorax; *pulmonary* and *oesophageal plexuses.*

- The two vagi enter the abdomen through the oesophageal opening. The *left* vagus passes onto the anterior surface and the *right* onto the posterior surface of the stomach.

3. In the abdomen; *coeliac, hepatic* and *renal plexuses.*

Xth nerve lesions

See page 148.

Accessory (XI) nerve

Course: Consists of a spinal and cranial nerve. The spinal root passes upwards along the side of the spinal cord and joins the cranial root from the brainstem. Fibres of the cranial root travel with the nerve for a short distance and then branch to join and be distributed with the vagus nerve. The spinal root descends as a separate nerve to supply the trapezius and sternocleidomastoid muscles.

XIth nerve lesions

Paralysis of the sternocleidomastoid muscle causes weakness on turning the head away from the paralysed muscle, e.g. trauma to the base of the skull.
Usually associated with other cranial nerve lesions: IX, X and XII cranial nerves.

Hypoglossal (XII) nerve

Course: Arises from the medulla between the olive and pyramid as 10–15 rootlets. The fibres pass anterolaterally and leave the posterior cranial fossa via the hypoglossal canal just in front of the foramen magnum. Descends between the internal carotid artery and the internal jugular vein and hooks around the occipital branch of the external carotid, to lie on the hypoglossus muscle before entering the tongue.

Unilateral XIIth nerve lesions

1. Ipsilateral paralysis and wasting of the tongue muscles on the affected side.
2. Deviation of the tongue to the side of the lesion on protrusion. E.g. tumours and penetrating injuries in the neck.

Bilateral XIIth nerve lesions

1. Generalized atrophy of the tongue (with or without fasiculation).
2. Protrusion impossible and articulation disturbed e.g. motor neuron disease.

Table 4.8 Summary of sensory innervation of the tongue

Region	*Sensation*	*Taste*
Posterior one-third	IX, X	IX, X
Anterior two-thirds	Chorda tympani (VII)	Chorda tympani (VII)

PRINCIPAL VESSELS

BRANCHES OF THE AORTA

See Figure 4.16.

Common carotid artery

Surface marking: On a line from the upper border of the sternal end of the clavicle to a point midway between the apex of the mastoid and the angle of the mandible.

Course: Right common carotid and subclavian arteries originate from the brachiocephalic artery at the level of the upper part of the right sternoclavicular joint.

Left common carotid and subclavian arteries arise directly from the arch of the aorta. The former has a short intrathoracic course between the trachea and the left lung, and enters the neck opposite the left sternoclavicular joint.

Both common carotid arteries ascend in the neck under cover of the anterior border of the sternocleidomastoid muscle. Each divides at the upper margin of the thyroid cartilage, opposite the

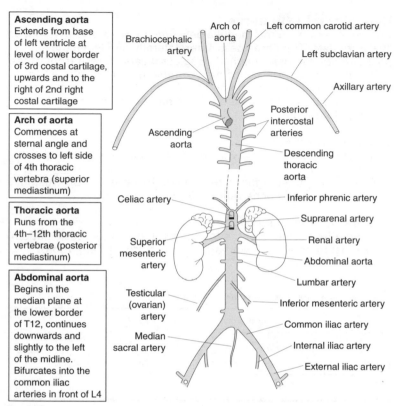

Ascending aorta
Extends from base of left ventricle at level of lower border of 3rd costal cartilage, upwards and to the right of 2nd right costal cartilage

Arch of aorta
Commences at sternal angle and crosses to left side of 4th thoracic vertebra (superior mediastinum)

Thoracic aorta
Runs from the 4th–12th thoracic vertebrae (posterior mediastinum)

Abdominal aorta
Begins in the median plane at the lower border of T12, continues downwards and slightly to the left of the midline. Bifurcates into the common iliac arteries in front of L4

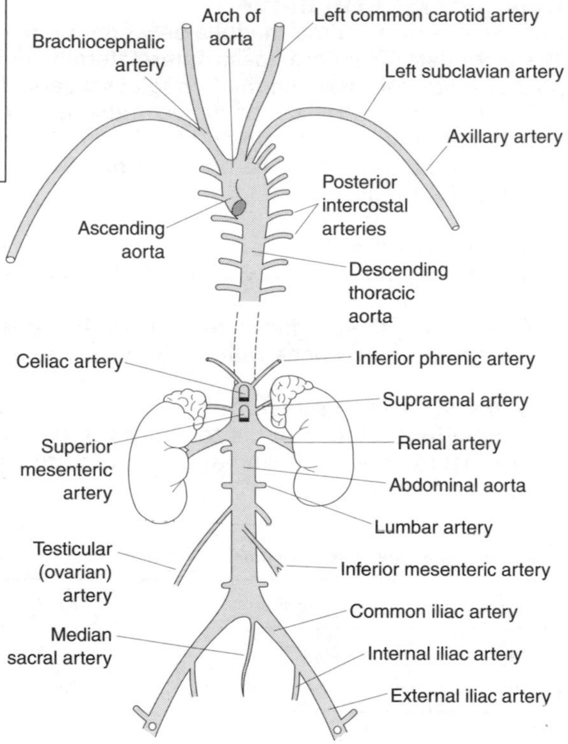

Fig. 4.16

lower border of the 3rd cervical vertebra into internal and external carotid arteries.
The carotid sinus (baroreceptor) is located at the bifurcation of the common carotid artery, and the carotid body (chemoreceptor) in the posterior wall of the sinus. Both sinus and body are innervated by the glossopharyngeal (IX) nerve.

Internal carotid artery

Supplies the major part of the cerebral hemisphere on its own side, and communicates via the circle of Willis with the opposite internal carotid artery and usually both vertebral arteries. Also supplies eye, forehead and nose.
Course: Lies within the carotid sheath posterior and then medial to the external carotid artery. Has no branches in the neck, but enters the base of the skull via the carotid canal, where it gives rise to the ophthalmic artery and bifurcates into anterior and middle cerebral arteries.

External carotid artery

Supplies the thyroid gland, tongue, throat, face, ear, scalp and dura mater. Plays no part in the arterial supply to the cerebral hemisphere. *Course:* Lies anteromedial to the internal carotid artery. Ascends lateral to the carotid sheath, glossopharyngeal nerve and pharyngeal branch of the vagus. Terminates by dividing into the superficial temporal and maxillary arteries just lateral to the temporomandibular joint.

Carotid sheath

Formed by the condensation of all three layers of deep cervical fascia.
Course: Extends from the base of the skull to the root of the neck. Lies deep to the sternocleidomastoid muscle. Contains common and internal carotid arteries, the internal jugular vein and the vagus nerves. The sympathetic trunk lies posterior to the sheath, embedded in the prevertebral layer of fascia.

Subclavian artery

Surface marking: Indicated by an arch between the medial end of the sternoclavicular joint and lateral end at the middle of the clavicle.
Course: Originates on the right from the brachiocephalic trunk and on the left from the arch of the aorta. Passes deep to the lower end of the anterior scalene muscle and becomes the axillary artery at the lateral border of the 1st rib.
Branches
Vertebral, internal thoracic, deep cervical and highest intercostal arteries and thyrocervical trunk.

PRINCIPAL VEINS

See Figure 4.17.

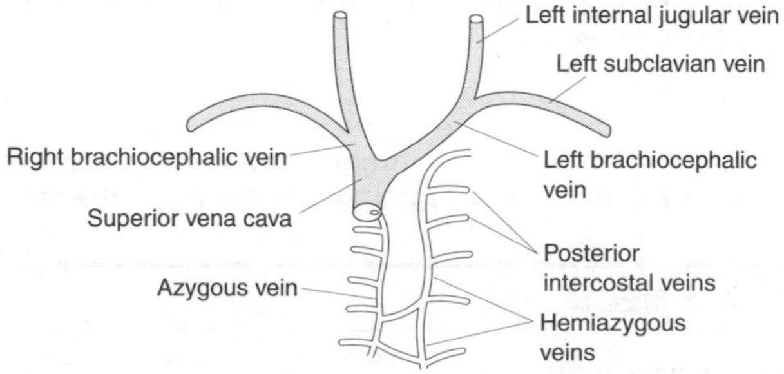

Fig. 4.17

Superior vena cava

- Formed by the right and left brachiocephalic veins at the lower border of the Ist costal cartilage.
- Drains veins of head, neck, upper extremities, thorax and azygous veins.

Course: Runs downwards behind the right border of the sternum and enters upper border of right atrium at 3rd costal cartilage.

Internal jugular vein

- Drains the cranial cavity and a few of the superficial veins of the head and neck.
- Contains valves in dilated segments at the superior and inferior ends (bulbs).

Course: Originates at the jugular foramen, descending forwards and medially within the carotid sheath to the root of the neck. Passes behind the clavicle where it joins the subclavian vein to form the brachiocephalic trunk and thence into the superior vena cava. Lies lateral first to the internal and then to the common carotid artery within the sheath.

Subclavian vein

Continuation of the axillary vein in the neck, beginning at the lateral border of the Ist rib.

Course: Passes medial, anterior and slightly inferior to the subclavian artery. Joins internal jugular vein to form the brachiocephalic vein just lateral to the sternoclavicular joint.

Inferior vena cava

- Largest vein of the body. Formed by the union of right and left common iliac veins at the level of the 5th lumbar verterbra.
- Drains veins of the abdomen, pelvis, lower extremities and azygous veins. Also receives the lumbar veins, the renal veins and the right inferior phrenic veins. The left suprarenal and testicular veins drain into the left renal vein. (N.B. Hence increased risk of varicocoele on left.)

Course: Runs to the right of the aorta, and lies anterior to the bodies of the lumbar vertebrae on the right sympathetic trunk. It extends to the central tendon of the diaphragm, and thereafter behind the bare area of the liver, before opening into the right atrium.

HEAD AND NECK

CRICOID CARTILAGE

Surface markings: Upper border marks the site of the cricothyroid membrane. Inferior border marks the beginning of trachea and oesophagus, and the level at which the common carotid may be compressed against the transverse process of the 6th vertebra.

THYROID GLAND

Structure

1. The isthmus overlies the 2nd to 4th rings of the trachea.
2. The two lateral lobes extend from the side of the thyroid cartilage downwards to the 6th tracheal ring.
3. An inconstant pyramidal lobe projects up from the isthmus.
4. Parathyroid glands lie in close relation to the posterior border of the gland.

Important relations include: Trachea and oesophagus posteriorly, and carotid sheath posteriorly and laterally.

Embryology

The thyroid develops from a thyroglossal diverticulum which pushes out from the tongue at the foramen caecum. It descends to a definitive position in the neck, and loses all connections with its origin. This development accounts for the occasional occurrence of a lingual thyroid, thyroglossal cyst or sinus and retrosternal thyroid along the path of descent.

LARYNX

Structure

1. Extends from the level of the 3rd cervical vertebra to the lower border of the 6th where it is continuous with the trachea.
2. There are nine cartilages in the laryngeal skeleton: three are single (thyroid, cricoid and epiglottis) and three are paired (arytenoid, corniculate and cuneiform).

Nerve supply

1. All intrinsic muscles of the larynx, except the cricothyroid, are innervated by the recurrent laryngeal nerve.
2. Cricothyroid muscle is supplied by the superior laryngeal nerve.

Recurrent laryngeal nerve (RLN)

This is a branch of the vagus and has a different course on each side, because of embryonic development.
Course: Right RLN arises from the vagus in the neck and passes behind the right subclavian artery.
Course: Left RLN arises from the vagus on the arch of the aorta and winds behind it.

- Both nerves then ascend between the trachea and the oesophagus and enter the larynx below the lower border of inferior constrictor.

- The recurrent nerves supply all the intrinsic laryngeal muscles, apart from the cricothyroid, and the mucosa below the vocal cords.

Recurrent laryngeal nerve lesions

1. Unilateral paralysis causes the affected cord to lie close to the midline and during phonation the unaffected cord moves across the midline to compensate. Results in dysphonia and a bovine cough.
2. Bilateral paralysis: the unopposed cricothyroids cause the cords to lie closely apposed. Results in a weak voice and stridor, especially after exertion.

Causes: Damage during thyroidectomy, thyroid carcinoma, malignant lymph nodes, broncho-oesophageal carcinoma*, aortic aneurysm* and enlarged left atrium (mitral stenosis)* (*, left RLN lesion.)

Superior laryngeal nerve

Course: This branch of vagus passes deep to the internal and external carotid arteries where it divides.
Lesions cause weakness of phonation.

With combined lesions of both the superior and recurrent laryngeal nerves the cords assume an intermediate or cadaveric position.

Muscles of the larynx (Table 4.9)

Table 4.9 Action of the muscles of the larynx

Muscle	*Action*
Cricothyroid	Lengthens, tenses and adducts
Posterior cricoarytenoid	Abducts
Lateral cricoarytenoid	Adducts
Transverse arytenoid	Adducts
Oblique arytenoid	Adducts
Thyroarytenoid	Relaxes

THORAX

Sternal angle

Surface marking: 5 cm inferior to the floor of the jugular notch at the level of T5.

Lines of pleural reflection

Surface markings: Apex of pleura is 2.5 cm above the clavicle: medial border descends from the level of the sternal angle to the 6th rib in the midline, 8th rib in the midclavicular line, 10th in the midaxillary line and 12th rib adjacent to vertebral column posteriorly (mnemonic: 6, 8, 10, 12).

Lower borders of the lungs

Surface marking: Run two rib levels higher than the pleural reflections (i.e. 4, 6, 8).

Fissures

- The right lung has three lobes and two fissures: oblique and horizontal.
- The left lung has two lobes: superior (upper) and inferior (lower).
- The lingula is the lower part of the superior lobe between the cardiac notch and the oblique fissure.

Main (oblique) fissure

- Divides the lung into upper and lower lobes.
- Extends from the 2nd thoracic spine posteriorly to 6th rib, 5 cm from the midline.

Horizontal (transverse) fissure

- Divides the upper and middle lobes of the right lung.
- Horizontal line along the 4th rib from the midline to the oblique fissure.

Trachea

Surface marking: Commences at the lower border of the cricoid cartilage (C6); bifurcates at sternal angle (T4, 5) just to the right of the midline to form right and left bronchi. At full inspiration, bifurcation is at T6. 11 cm long and 2.5 cm in diameter.

Right main bronchus

Course: Wider, shorter (2.5 cm) and more vertical than the left (i.e. foreign objects more likely to enter), and passes directly to the root of the lung of the level of T5. Right main bronchus divides into upper, middle and lower bronchus in hilar region. Left main bronchus divides into an upper (lingular) and lower lobe bronchus.

Left main bronchus

Course: 5 cm long and passes downwards and outwards below the arch of the aorta and in front of the oesophagus and descending aorta. Undivided bronchus reaches the hilum of the lung at level of T6. The structures of the root of the left lung pass in front of the descending aorta where the recurrent laryngeal nerve hooks around the aortic arch.

Divisions of right main bronchus

Division of lobar bronchi into 10 segmental bronchi within the lung – one for each bronchopulmonary segment. Azygous vein arches over right main bronchus from behind to reach the superior vena cava, and the pulmonary artery lies first below and then anterior to it. The structures of the root of the right lung pass behind the ascending aorta (see Fig. 4.18).

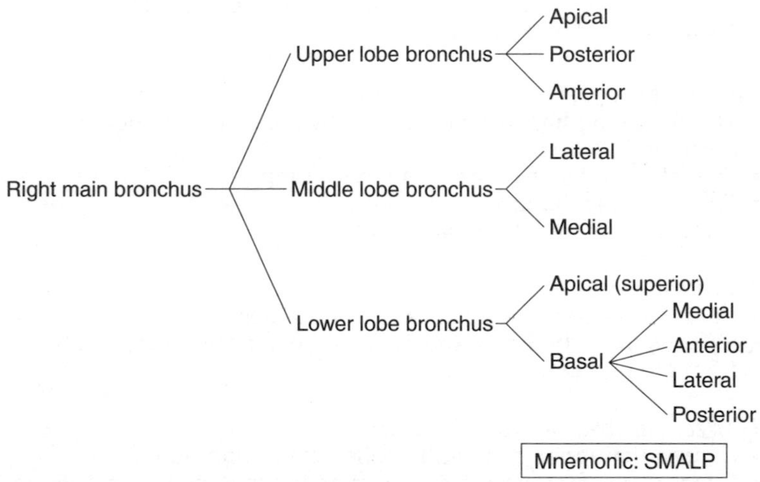

Fig. 4.18

Divisions of left main bronchus (Fig. 4.19)

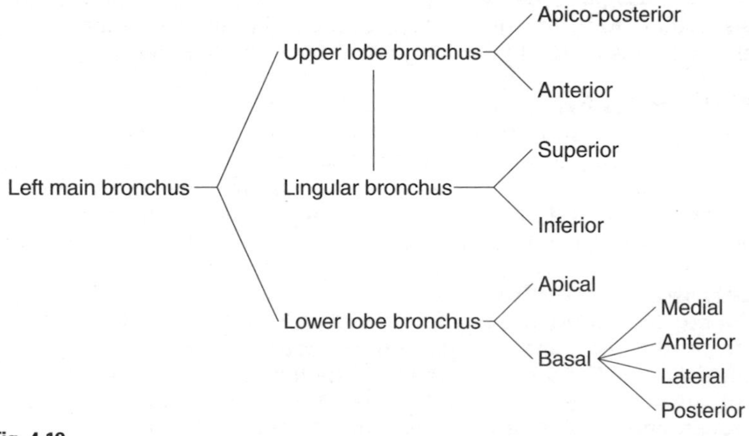

Fig. 4.19

Root of lung

Contents
1. Main bronchus
2. Pulmonary artery
3. Two pulmonary veins
4. Bronchial arteries and veins
5. Autonomic nerves
6. Lymphatics

HEART

Arterial supply

Myocardium supplied by right and left coronary arteries (Fig. 4.20).

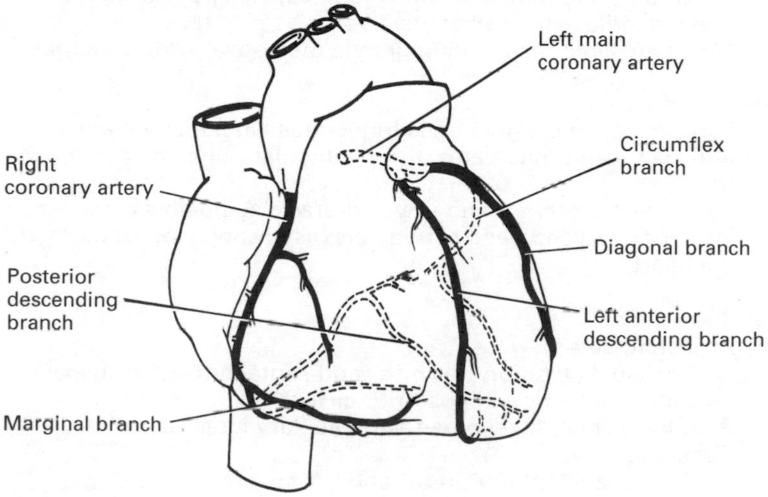

Fig. 4.20

Right coronary artery (see Note)
Supplies: The right atrium, sinoatrial node, atrioventricular node, right ventricle and posterior part of interventricular septum. Arises from the anterior aortic sinus.
Course: Runs in the atrioventricular groove, then downwards to the inferior border and around the posterior aspect in the coronary sulcus. Two main branches: *posterior descending* branch runs in the posterior interventricular groove to the apex, *marginal* branch runs along the inferior border.

Note: 20% left coronary dominance; 60% right coronary dominance; 20% equally balanced.

Left coronary artery (See Note)
Supplies: Anterior part of the left and right ventricle, anterior part of the interventricular septum, atrioventricular groove and lateral wall of the left ventricle.
Course: arises from the *posterior* aortic cusp. Two main branches: *left anterior descending* (LAD) runs in the anterior interventricular groove to the apex, and around the inferior margin to the posterior interventricular groove. The *circumflex artery* passes to the left between atria and ventricles in the coronary sulcus.
Posterior descending branch of the right coronary artery anastomoses with the anterior descending branch of the left coronary artery at apex of heart and interventricular septum.

Venous drainage

1. 90% drains into right atrium through coronary sinus via the great, middle and small cardiac veins
2. 10% drains into other chambers via the venae cordis minimae.

Nerve supply

1. Parasympathetic: right vagus innervates sinoatrial node and atria; left vagus innervates atrioventricular node and conducting tissue.
2. Sympathetic: cervical and upper thoracic sympathetic ganglia, via superficial and deep cardiac plexuses supplying all parts of the heart.

Valves

1. Atrioventricular:
   (i) Tricuspid (anterior, posterior and septal or medial cusps)
   (ii) Mitral (anterior and posterior cusps).
   Both have chordae tendinae and papillary muscles.
2. Semilunar:
   (i) Pulmonary (anterior, right and left cusps)
   (ii) Aortic (right, left and posterior cusps).

Each has a free border with a central nodule and lateral lunules.

Nodes

1. The *sinoatrial node* is supplied by the right or left coronary artery and the right vagus nerve.
2. The *atrioventricular node* is supplied by the right coronary artery and by the left vagus nerve.

Embryology

1. Formation of paired endocardial tubes in splanchnic mesoderm.
2. Differentiation of heart tube into bulbis cordis, ventricle, atrium and sinus venosus (from arterial to venous end).

3. Septation:
   (i) Interatrial from septum primum and septum secundum.
   (ii) Interventricular: muscular and membranous parts.
   (iii) Spiral aorticopulmonary: fused bulbar ridges.

The aortic arches and their derivatives

Common arterial trunk	→	Truncus arteriosus → six pairs of aortic arches (Ist, 2nd and 5th arches disappear)
3rd arches	→	Carotid arteries
Right 4th arch	→	Brachiocephalic and **right** subclavian artery
Left 4th arch	→	Aortic arch → **left** subclavian artery
6th arch	→	Right and left pulmonary arteries and ductus arteriosus

FETAL CIRCULATION (Fig. 4.21)

Sequence of events at birth

1. Expansion of lungs, causing a decrease in pulmonary vascular resistance.
   ↓
2. Increased blood flow in pulmonary arteries.
   ↓
3. Closure of umbilical artery.
   ↓
4. Reversal of flow through ductus arteriosus and closure.
   ↓
5. Increased pressure in left atrium. Closure of foramen ovale (complete in one week).
   ↓
6. Interruption of placental flow.
   ↓
7. Ductus venosus collapses.

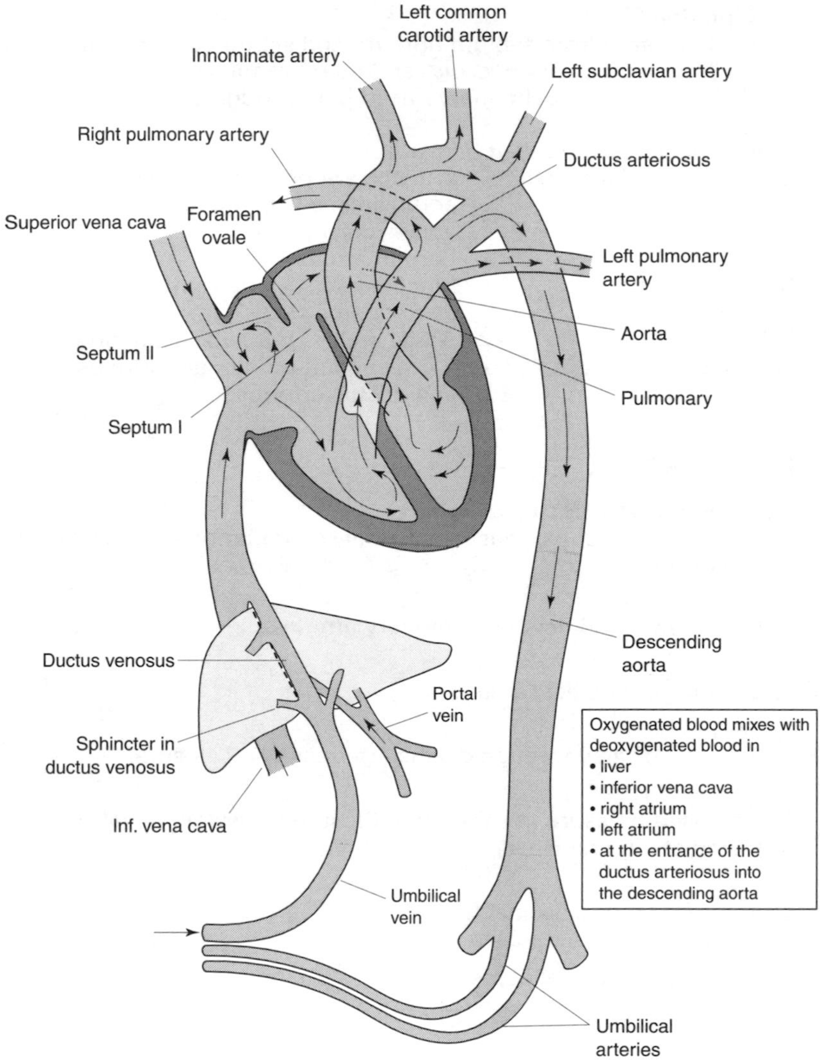
Left common carotid artery
Innominate artery
Left subclavian artery
Right pulmonary artery
Ductus arteriosus
Superior vena cava
Foramen ovale
Left pulmonary artery
Aorta
Septum II
Pulmonary
Septum I
Descending aorta
Ductus venosus
Portal vein
Sphincter in ductus venosus
Inf. vena cava
Umbilical vein
Umbilical arteries
Oxygenated blood mixes with deoxygenated blood in
• liver
• inferior vena cava
• right atrium
• left atrium
• at the entrance of the ductus arteriosus into the descending aorta

Fig. 4.21

ABDOMEN

Costal margin

Surface marking: 7th costal cartilage to the tip of the 12th rib.

Transpyloric plane

Surface marking: Level is at disc between L1 and 2.

Transumbilical plane

Surface marking: Level is at disc between L3 and 4.

Liver

Surface marking: Upper border: right 4th rib in midline to 5th space in the anterior axillary line. Lower border: tip of right 10th rib and just below left; palpable in normal subjects. Moves down on inspiration.

Spleen

Surface marking: Underlies 9th, 10th and 11th ribs posteriorly on the left side; distinct notch on inferomedial border; enlarges diagonally downwards.

Gall bladder

Surface marking: Fundus is at the tip of the 9th costal cartilage, where the lateral border of rectus abdominis cuts the costal margin.

Kidneys

Surface marking: Upper pole lies deep to the 12th rib; lower pole lies at the upper part of L3; right kidney normally 2.5 cm lower than the left, and its lower pole is normally palpable; moves slightly downwards on inspiration.

DIAPHRAGM

Openings in the diaphragm

1. Aortic opening (T12) lies just to the left of the midline. Transmits the abdominal aorta, the thoracic duct and the azygous vein.
2. Oesophageal opening (T10) transmits the oesophagus, branches of the left gastric artery and vein and the two vagi.
3. Inferior vena cava opening (T8) lies to the right of the midline in the central tendon. Transmits the inferior vena cava and the right phrenic nerve.

Nerve supply

Innervated by the phrenic nerve (C3, 4, 5) and peripherally by the lower seven intercostal nerves.

Embryology
It is formed by the fusion of the septum transversum (forming the central tendon), dorsal oesophageal mesentery, the pleuroperitoneal membranes and the body wall.

THORACIC DUCT

Drains: Whole lymphatic field below the diaphragm and the left half of the lymphatics above it.
Course: Begins at and passes superiorly from the cisterna chyli to enter the thorax through the aortic opening on the right side of the aorta, to become the thoracic duct. It ascends first behind and then to the left of the oesophagus. The duct empties into the venous system of the neck at the union of the internal jugular and subclavian veins.

OESOPHAGUS

Surface markings: Continuous with the lower end of the pharynx and extends from the lower border of the cricoid cartilage (C6) to the cardiac orifice of the stomach at the level of the 10th thoracic vertebra to the left of the midline.

Arterial supply
Inferior thyroid branch of the thyrocervical trunk, branches of the thoracic aorta, bronchial arteries and ascending branches from the left gastric and inferior phrenic artery.

Venous drainage
Lower third: Drained by the portal venous system via the gastric veins.
Middle third: Drained by the azygous system.
Upper third: Drained by the superior vena cava.

STOMACH

Blood supply
All arteries are derived directly or indirectly from the coeliac trunk. Venous drainage via the portal system.

Nerve supply
1. Parasympathetic via the vagus (motor and secretory nerve supply to the stomach):
   (i) *Anterior* vagus branches to the cardia, lesser curvature and pylorus.
   (ii) *Posterior* vagus branches to the body of the stomach, and distribution of coeliac branch to the intestine as far as the mid-transverse colon and the pancreas.

With vagotomy, neurogenic gastrin secretion is abolished, but the stomach is also rendered atonic, so vagotomy must always be accompanied by a drainage procedure, e.g. pyloroplasty.
2. Sympathetic via intrinsic nerve plexuses:
   (i) *Auerbach's* plexus lies between the circular and longitudinal muscle layers.
   (ii) *Meissner's* plexus lies in the submucosa.

DUODENUM

Course: 30 cm in length and divided into four parts.
1. The first part is intraperitoneal; the bile duct and inferior vena cava pass behind.
2. The remainder is retroperitoneal. The 2nd part of the duodenum runs round the head of the pancreas. The ampulla of Vater is situated in this part.
3. The 3rd part crosses over the inferior vena cava, the aorta and origin of the inferior mesenteric artery. The superior mesenteric artery passes anteriorly.

Arterial supply of the intestine
The gastrointestinal tract develops from the foregut, mid and hindgut. Each has its own discrete arterial supply, but with extensive anastomoses.
Foregut: The stomach and duodenum are supplied by branches of the coeliac axis arising from the aorta at T12.
Midgut: Mid-duodenum to the distal transverse colon is supplied by the superior mesenteric artery, arising from the aorta at L1.
Hindgut: Distal transverse colon to the rectum is supplied by the inferior mesenteric artery, arising from the aorta at L3.

LIVER

Blood supply (Fig. 4.22)
1. The common hepatic duct anteriorly.
2. The hepatic artery in the middle.
3. The portal vein posteriorly.

These structures lie in the free edge of the lesser omentum. The cystic artery commonly arises from the right hepatic artery in the angle between the common hepatic duct and the cystic duct.

Portal vein
Carries: Venous blood from the digestive tracts and spleen to the liver. Accompanies hepatic artery and bile duct in the free edge of the lesser omentum.
Course: Formed by the union of the superior mesenteric and splenic veins behind the neck of the pancreas. During its course it

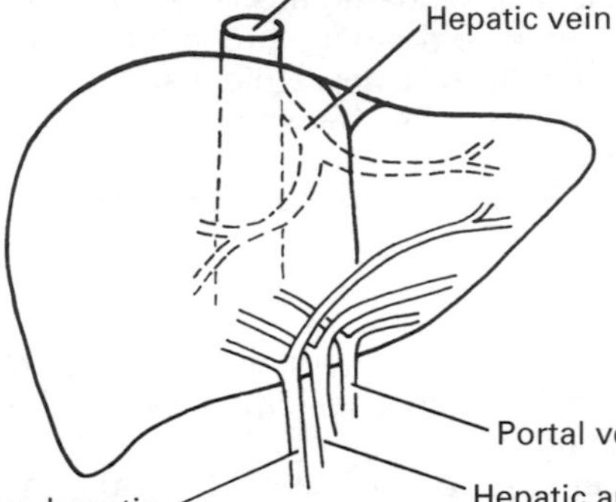

Fig. 4.22

lies behind the duodenum, gastroduodenal artery and bile duct. It passes up to the porta hepatis where it divides into right and left branches, before entering the liver with and posterior to the corresponding branches of the hepatic artery and the common hepatic ducts.

Hepatic venous portal system

Main connections between portal and systemic venous systems

1. Oesophageal branch of the left gastric veins and the oesophageal veins of the azygous system.
2. Inferior mesenteric vein of the portal system and the inferior haemorrhoidal veins draining into the internal iliac veins.
3. Portal tributaries in the mesentery and mesocolon and the retroperitoneal veins communicating with the renal, lumbar and phrenic veins.
4. Portal branches in the liver and the veins of the anterior abdominal wall via veins passing along the falciform ligament to the umbilicus.
5. Portal branches in the liver and the veins of the diaphragm across the bare area of the liver.

5. Physiology

CHAPTER CONTENTS

FLUID BALANCE

DISTRIBUTION OF WATER IN AN AVERAGE 70-KG MAN (see Fig. 5.1 opposite)

MEASUREMENT OF BODY FLUIDS

The volumes of the various fluid compartments are measured indirectly by an *indicator dilution method*. This approach requires that the introduced substance be evenly distributed in the body fluid compartment being measured.

$$\text{Volume of compartment} = \frac{\text{amount of substance introduced} - \text{amount of substance removed}}{\text{final concentration of substance in the compartment}}$$

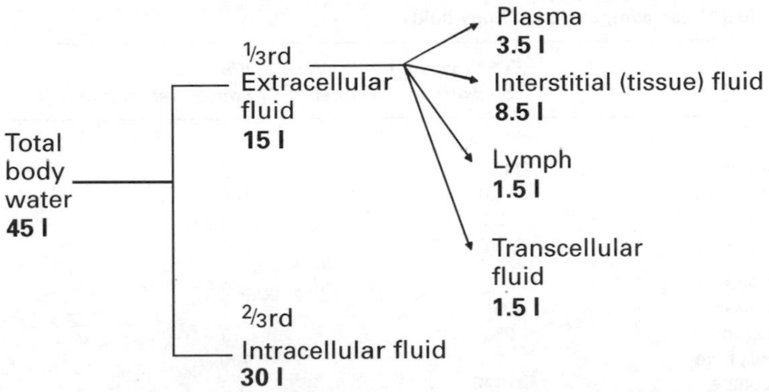

Fig. 5.1 Distribution of water in an average 70 kg man. Transcellular fluid includes digestive secretions, gut luminal fluids, bile, sweat, CSF, pleural, pericardial, synovial and intraocular fluid.

- *Total body water* (TBW) constitutes approximately 50–60% of the body weight and is measured using tritiated water (^3H_2O), or deuterium oxide (^2H_2O).
- *Extracellular fluid* (ECF) volume is measured using saccharides, e.g. inulin, mannitol or ions like thiocyanate.
- *Plasma volume* is measured using Evans Blue dye, radioiodinated serum albumin or red blood cells labelled with ^{32}P or ^{51}Cr.
- *Intracellular fluid* (ICF) volume cannot be measured directly from dilution: it is calculated from the difference between total body water and ECF volume. Similarly the interstitial fluid volume cannot be measured directly, and is calculated from the difference between the ECF volume and the plasma volume.

Control of fluid flow between plasma and interstitial compartments

- A hydrostatic pressure difference across the capillary endothelium results in fluid flow from vascular to tissue space, but the retention of proteins within the vasculature is a retarding force (plasma oncotic pressure).
- The *Starling equation* describes the relationship between hydrostatic pressure, oncotic pressure and fluid flow across a capillary membrane.

Table 5.1 Ion composition of body fluids

Ion	*ECF* (plasma) concentration (mmol/l)*	*ICF concentration (mmol/l)*
Cations		
Sodium	142	10
Potassium	4.0	145
Calcium	2.5	0.001
Magnesium	1.0	40
Anions		
Chloride	104	5
Bicarbonate	25	10
Phosphate	1.1	100
Sulphate	0.5	20
Organic anions	3.0	0
Protein†	1.1	8

*ECF: sodium and potassium are the major cations, and chloride and bicarbonate are the major anions.
†The plasma has a similar ion composition to that of the interstitial fluid except that it contains a much higher concentration of dissolved proteins.

Capillary hydrostatic pressure + tissue oncotic pressure (OUTWARD PRESSURES)	=	Interstitial fluid pressure + plasma oncotic pressure (INWARD PRESSURES)

Note: Tissue oncotic pressure: proteins in the interstitial space produce a force (generally 5–10 mmHg) causing outward filtration of fluid from the vascular space.
Interstitial pressure increases as the interstitial volume increases (oedema), which impedes further fluid filtration from the capillaries.

1. At the arterial end, the net intracapillary hydrostatic pressure (32 mmHg) exceeds the net interstitial oncotic pressure (18 mmHg), driving fluid out of the capillaries (32 – 18 = 14 mmHg)
2. At some point, the net hydrostatic pressure equals the net oncotic pressure with no net fluid movement.
3. The effective hydrostatic pressure falls to 12 mmHg on the venous side and is exceeded by the net plasma oncotic pressure (18 mmHg) and so reabsorption begins (12 – 18 = 6 mmHg). Any fluid not reabsorbed at this point is returned to the circulation by the lymphatic system. Thus filtration is favoured on the arterial side and absorption on the venous side.

OEDEMA

- A collection of excess interstitial fluid, i.e. interstitial fluid pressures become positive.

Causes

1. Increased capillary hydrostatic pressure, e.g. venous obstruction, excess blood volume, cardiac failure.
2. Decreased plasma oncotic pressure, e.g. causes of hypoproteinaemia (nephrotic syndrome, cirrhosis).
3. Increased capillary permeability, e.g. allergic, bacterial and toxic diseases.
4. Increased tissue oncotic pressure, e.g. lymphatic blockage.

OSMOLALITY

- *Osmolality* is the number of particles (osmoles) of solute dissolved in one *kg* of solution (i.e. mosmol/kg) or mosmol/l. Osmolality is usually measured directly in the laboratory or using an osmometer.
- *Osmolarity* is the number of particles dissolved in a litre of solution (i.e. mosmol/l).
- *Calculated plasma osmolarity* $\approx 2[Na^+ + K^+]$ + [glucose] + [urea]
  Plasma osmolality = 280–295 mosmol/l.
  In most cases, plasma osmolarity calculated in this way is numerically very similar to the measured osmolality.
  (Normal urine osmolality = 300–1400 mosmol/l).
  Main determinant of ECF osmolality is plasma $[Na^+]$, $[Cl^-]$ and $[HCO_3^-]$; main determinant of ICF osmolality is intracellular $[K^+]$
- *Osmotic equilibration* between the ECF and ICF is achieved by water movement between the two compartments.
- *Osmolar gap* is the disparity between the measured osmolality and the calculated osmolality. Other osmotically active substances increase measured serum osmolality without altering serum $[Na^+]$, and therefore the measured serum osmolality exceeds the calculated value.

ACID–BASE BALANCE

GLOSSARY

Acid: A proton or hydrogen ion donor. It can dissociate to yield H^+ ions and the corresponding base. A strong acid completely or almost completely dissociates in aqueous solution, e.g. hydrochloric acid. A weak acid only partially dissociates in aqueous solution, e.g. acetic acid.

Anion gap: Routine serum electrolyte determination measures most of the cations but only a few of the anions. This apparent disparity between the total cation and the total anion

concentration is called the anion gap. Anion gap ≈ $[Na^+ + K^+] - [Cl^- + HCO_3^-]$.
It is normally about 10–16 mmol/l and reflects the concentration of those anions actually present but not routinely measured, such as plasma proteins, phosphates, sulphates and organic acids.
Causes of an increased anion gap: Marked renal failure, diabetic and alcoholic ketoacidosis, lactic acidosis, ingestion of salicylate, methanol, ethylene glycol or paraldehyde.
Mild: dehydration, exogenous anions, e.g. penicillin and carbenicillin.
Causes of a decreased anion gap: Increased unmeasured cation, e.g. potassium, magnesium and calcium. Decreased unmeasured anion, e.g. hypoalbuminaemia.

Arterial blood gases: Normal ranges:
$[H^+]$ = 36–44 mmol/l
pH = 7.35–7.45
$P\text{O}_2$ = 10.6–14.0 kPa
$P\text{CO}_2$ = 4.7–6.0 kPa
Bicarbonate (actual) = 23–33 mmol/l

Base: A proton or hydrogen ion acceptor, e.g. HCO_3^- can accept H^+, thereby forming the corresponding undissociated acid, carbonic acid (H_2CO_3).

Base excess: This measures the change in the concentration of a buffer base (sum of the buffer anions of blood or plasma) from its normal value, i.e. base excess equals the observed buffer base minus the normal buffer base of whole blood. The normal range for base excess is ± 2.3 mmol/l in arterial whole blood. Metabolic acidosis is associated with a base excess below −5 mmol/l and metabolic alkalosis with a base excess above +5 mmol/l.

Henderson–Hasselbach equation: This describes the relationship of arterial pH to $P\text{aCO}_2$, bicarbonate and two constants.

$$\text{pH} = 6.1 + \log \frac{[HCO_3^-)}{0.235 \times [P\text{aCO}_2]}$$

where $P\text{aCO}_2$ is the arterial partial pressure of CO_2.

Partial pressure: The pressure of a gas in a mixture of gases which is proportional to its concentration in the mixture. The sum of the partial pressures of the constituent gases is equal to the total pressure of the mixture. The partial pressure of any gas can therefore be calculated by multiplying its percentage composition by the ambient barometric pressure.

pH: The logarithm (to the base 10) of the reciprocal of the hydrogen ion concentration. $pH = \log (1/[H^+])$ or $pH = -\log [H^+]$.
Note: A decrease in pH of 0.3 represents a twofold increase in $[H^+]$ and a decrease in pH of 1.0 represents a 10-fold increase in $[H^+]$.
Regulation of pH is achieved through control of:
(i) excretion of H^+ and reabsorption of HCO_3^- by the kidneys
(ii) excretion of CO_2 by the lungs through regulation of alveolar ventilation
(iii) buffering of H^+ by the body's buffering system.

pKa: The pH of a buffer at which half the acid molecules are undissociated and half are associated. The extent to which weak acids (or bases) dissociate in aqueous solution depends on the *dissociation constant* (pKa) for that acid or base.
pH = pKa when equimolar concentrations of weak acid and base exist.

BUFFER SYSTEMS

- The *main source of H^+* in the body is the CO_2 produced as an end-product of the oxidation of carbon compounds, e.g. glucose and fatty acids during aerobic metabolism. Control of $[H^+]$ is achieved by buffering.
- Buffers consist of a weak acid (H^+ donor) in the presence of its base (H^+ acceptor). A buffer system minimizes changes in $[H^+]$ in response to the addition of acid or base, either by binding part of the additional hydrogen ion, or by dissociating further to release hydrogen ion, e.g.:

$H^+ + Cl^-$	+	$NaHCO_3$	$\rightarrow$	H_2CO_3	+	NaCl
strong acid		buffer		weak acid		neutral salt

A buffer is most effective when the pH of the solution equals the pKa of the buffer.

IMPORTANT BUFFER SYSTEMS IN THE BODY

Table 5.2 Buffering according to body compartments

Compartment and major buffers	*% of total body buffering*
Plasma	13
Bicarbonate	
Inorganic phosphate	
Plasma proteins	
Erythrocytes	6
Haemoglobin	
Bicarbonate	
Inorganic and organic phosphate	
ICF (excluding erythrocytes)	51
Bicarbonate	
Tissue protein	
Organic phosphate in skeletal muscle	
Kidneys	30
Bicarbonate	
Inorganic phosphate	
Ammonium	

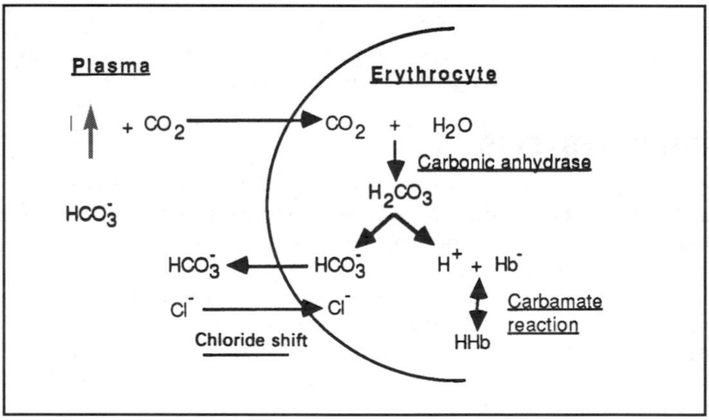

Fig. 5.2

Buffer mechanism in the erythrocytes (Fig. 5.2)

- CO_2^- is produced in the tissues, and diffuses into the erythrocytes. Carbonic acid is formed, and catalysed by carbonic anhydrase dissociates to HCO_3^- and H^+.
- Most of the HCO_3^- diffuses into the plasma in exchange for chloride (chloride shift) to maintain electrical neutrality, and is converted to CO_2 which is blown off in the lungs.

- The hydrogen ion is buffered by reduced haemoglobin (the carbamate reaction). This minimizes the rise in pH that usually accompanies the deoxygenation of haemoglobin.

Buffer mechanisms in the kidney

The kidneys play an important role in both the regeneration of bicarbonate buffer and in excretion of acids produced in cells during metabolism.

1. Renal bicarbonate reabsorption (Fig. 5.3)

- *H^+ secretion* into the tubular lumen occurs by active transport and is coupled to sodium reabsorption. For each H^+ secreted, one Na^+ and one HCO_3^- are reabsorbed.
- *HCO_3^- reabsorption*. Most of the H^+ secreted into the tubular fluid reacts with HCO_3^- to form carbonic acid which breaks down to form CO_2 and water. The CO_2 diffuses back into the proximal tubular cells, where it is rehydrated to H_2CO_3, which then dissociates into HCO_3^- and H^+. The buffering of secreted H^+ by filtered HCO_3^- is not a mechanism for H^+ excretion, since the CO_2 formed in the lumen from secreted H^+ returns to the tubular cell to form another H^+ and no net secretion of H^+ occurs.

2. Ammonium secretion (NH_4^+)

- Ammonia (NH_3) is produced by the deamination of amino acids, mainly glutamine, to form glutamic acid, and the oxidative deamination of other amino acids to form keto-acids in the renal tubule cells. NH_3 diffuses into the tubular lumen, where it accepts H^+ to become ammonium (NH_4^+), which is then excreted. NH_3 secretion is an important mechanism in the renal response to chronic respiratory or metabolic acidosis.

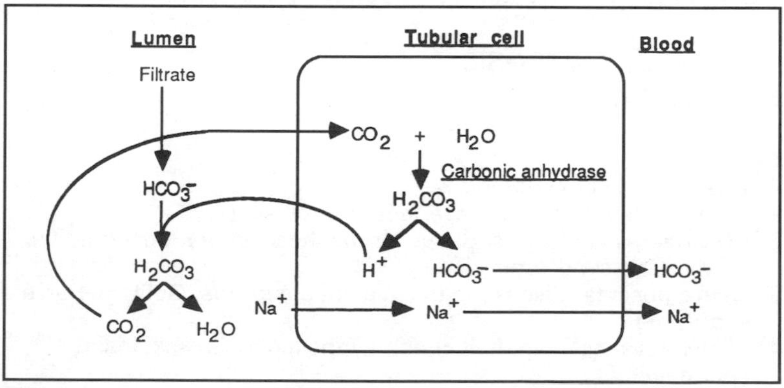

Fig. 5.3

3. Excretion of H^+ as dihydrogen phosphate

- The major titratable acid in the tubular fluid is phosphate. The titratable acidity measures that fraction of the acid excreted that did not combine with HCO_3^- or with NH_3.
- The exchange of H^+ for Na^+ converts monohydrogen phosphate into dihydrogen phosphate in the glomerular filtrate, which is excreted in the urine as titratable acid.
- Approximately 2/3rds of excess H^+ is excreted in the form of ammonium; the remaining 1/3rd of the excess acid is excreted as dihydrogen phosphate.

ACID–BASE DISTURBANCES

Table 5.3 Acid–base disturbances

Acid–base abnormality	*Primary disturbance*	*Effect*		*Base excess*	*Compensatory response*
		pH	*PO_2*		
Respiratory acidosis	↑ Pco_2	↓	↓		↑ $[HCO_3^-]$
Metabolic acidosis	↓ $[HCO_3^-]$	↓	N or ↑	–ve	↓ Pco_2
Respiratory alkalosis	↓ Pco_2	↑	N or ↑		↓ $[HCO_3^-]$
Metabolic alkalosis	↑ $[HCO_3^-]$	↑	N or ↑	+ve	↑ Pco_2

In general:

- Metabolic disturbances are compensated acutely by changes in ventilation, and chronically by appropriate renal responses.
- Respiratory disturbances are compensated by renal tubular secretion of H^+.
- A reduction in plasma $[HCO_3^-]$ may be due to metabolic acidosis or can indicate renal compensation for respiratory alkalosis.
- An elevated plasma $[HCO_3^-]$ can result from metabolic alkalosis or the secondary response to respiratory acidosis.

RESPIRATORY ACIDOSIS

This is often mixed.

Causes

Any cause of *hypoventilation*:

1. Obstructive airways disease (acute or chronic).
2. CNS depression, e.g. sedative drugs, head injury, encephalitis, Pickwickian syndrome.
3. Neuromuscular disease, e.g. myasthenia gravis, Guillain–Barré syndrome.
4. Skeletal disease, e.g. flail chest, kyphoscoliosis, ankylosing spondylitis.
5. Artificial ventilation.

Compensatory mechanisms

In acute respiratory failure (e.g. asthmatic attack or bronchopneumonia), rapid erythrocyte mechanisms are the major compensatory response. In chronic respiratory failure (e.g. emphysema) the renal tubular mechanism is the most important compensatory mechanism.

RESPIRATORY ALKALOSIS

Causes

Any cause of *hyperventilation*:

1. Psychogenic, e.g. hysteria, pain and anxiety.
2. Central, e.g. raised intracranial pressure, encephalitis, meningitis, cerebral haemorrhage.
3. Pulmonary, hypoxia (high altitude), pulmonary embolism, pneumonia, pulmonary oedema and pneumothorax.
4. Metabolic, e.g. hyperthyroidism, fever, metabolic acidosis, acute liver failure.
5. Drugs, e.g. early salicylate poisoning
6. Artificial ventilation.
7. Gram-negative septicaemia.

METABOLIC ACIDOSIS

Causes

Normal anion gap:

1. Intestinal loss of base, e.g. diarrhoea, fistulae, ureterosigmoidostomy (transplanation of ureters).
2. Renal loss of base, e.g. renal tubular acidosis (types 1 and 2), pyelonephritis.
3. Therapy with carbonic anhydrase inhibitors, e.g. acetozolamide, ammonium chloride and, rarely with hyperalimentation.

Conditions that cause a metabolic acidosis without an increase in unmeasured anions are associated with a high serum chloride.

Increased anion gap due to an increased acid pool:

1. Overproduction of organic acid, e.g. diabetic and alcoholic ketoacidosis or lactic acidosis secondary to hypoxia.
2. Decreased ability to conserve/generate HCO_3^- and to excrete acid, e.g. acute or chronic renal failure.
3. Advanced salicylate poisoning, ingestion of ethanol, methanol or paraldehyde.
4. Inborn errors of metabolism, e.g. maple syrup urine disease.

METABOLIC ALKALOSIS

Causes

1. Excess oral intake of alkali or forced alkaline diuresis.
2. Excess acid loss, e.g. gastric aspiration or persistent

vomiting as in pyloric stenosis (hypochloraemic alkalosis, see below).
3. Diuretic therapy (thiazide/loop).
4. Renal tubular acidosis due to chloride deficiency, potassium deficiency, hyperaldosteronism, Cushing's syndrome, corticosteroid treatment, or Bartter's syndrome.

MIXED DISORDERS

Causes
1. Respiratory alkalosis and metabolic acidosis in: salicylate overdose, renal failure with sepsis and septicaemia.
2. Respiratory acidosis and metabolic acidosis in: respiratory distress syndrome, cardiac failure, shock, hypothermia, cardiac arrest, severe CNS depression (e.g. drug overdose) and severe pulmonary oedema, or uncontrolled diabetes in patients with chronic lung disease.
3. Respiratory acidosis and metabolic alkalosis in: chronic lung disease and diuretic therapy or treatment of acute or chronic lung disease with steroids.
4. Respiratory and metabolic alkalosis in: overventilation of chronic respiratory acidosis.

HYPERCHLORAEMIC ACIDOSIS

Often associated with hypokalaemia. Occurs when HCO_3^- is lost in a one-to-one exchange for chloride.

Causes
1. Ureterosigmoidostomy (transplantation of ureters into upper sigmoid colon). Urine which contains chloride enters the intestinal lumen, where cells reabsorb some of this chloride in exchange for bicarbonate, causing bicarbonate depletion.
2. Renal tubular acidosis.
3. Acetazolomide treatment.
4. Hyperventilation.

HYPOCHLORAEMIC ACIDOSIS

Causes
1. Loss of gastrointestinal fluids, e.g. vomiting and diarrhoea.
2. Overtreatment with diuretics.
3. Chronic respiratory acidosis.
4. Diabetic acidosis.
5. Adrenal insufficiency, i.e. Addison's disease.

METABOLIC EFFECTS OF PROLONGED VOMITING

Prolonged vomiting may be caused by, e.g. pyloric stenosis.

Causes
1. Continued vomiting of acid gastric fluid with no loss of alkaline duodenal fluid.
2. Hypovolaemia and metabolic alkalosis due to HCl and K^+ loss.
3. Renal/HCO_3^- excretion inhibited by *hypochloraemic alkalosis*, hypokalaemia and reduced glomerular filtration rate.
4. Paradoxical aciduria.
5. Compensatory hypoventilation.

LACTIC ACIDOSIS

This is defined as a level >5 mmol/l. Normal plasma lactate (resting) = <1 mmol/l.

Causes
Increased generation of lactate:
1. Cardiac arrest due to decreased tissue perfusion.
2. Large tumour masses (leukaemia, lymphoma).
3. Cyanide and carbon monoxide poisoning.

Decreased utilization of lactate:
1. Phenformin and metformin in toxication.
2. Diabetes mellitus.
3. Alcoholism.
4. Hepatic failure due to decreased hepatic perfusion.

RENAL PHYSIOLOGY

FUNCTIONS OF THE KIDNEY

GLOMERULAR FILTRATION

Involves passage through three layers:
1. capillary endothelium lining the glomerulus.
2. glomerular basement membrane
3. epithelial layer of Bowman's capsule.

Depends on:

1. The balance of Starling forces where:
   Net filtration pressure across the glomerular membrane = (glomerular capillary hydrostatic pressure – hydrostatic pressure in Bowman's capsule) – colloid osmotic pressure of blood.
2. Permeability of glomerular capillary wall.
3. Total capillary area and number of glomeruli.
4. Glomerular capillary plasma flow.
   - The glomerular filtrate is an ultrafiltrate of plasma, with an identical composition except for a few proteins (0.03%).

Glomerular filtration rate (GFR)

- Total volume of plasma per unit time leaving the capillaries and entering the Bowman's capsule.
- GFR is approximately 180 l per day, or 120 ml/min.

Renal clearance

- Volume of plasma from which all of a given substance is removed per minute by the kidneys.

Measurement

- The measurement of clearance involves a comparison of the rate of urinary excretion (urine volume × urinary concentration) with the plasma concentration.
- Various substances can be used for measuring the GFR by determining its clearance. The properties of these include:
  1. Biologically inert, i.e. not metabolized.
  2. Freely filtered from the plasma at the glomerulus, i.e. not plasma protein bound.
  3. Neither reabsorbed nor secreted by the tubules.
  4. Concentration in plasma remains constant throughout the period of urine collection.

If the substance is neither excreted nor reabsorbed, i.e. all of the plasma filtered has been cleared of the substance, e.g. inulin, then Clearance = GFR

$$\text{Clearance} = \frac{\text{Amount excreted/min}}{\text{Plasma concentration of substance x}}$$

$$\text{GFR} = \frac{U_x V}{P_x}$$

where U_x = urine concentration (mmol/l)
V = urine volume (ml/min)
P_x = plasma concentration (mmol/l)
GFR = ml/min

- If Clearance > GFR, then there must be net secretion, as with para-amino hippuric acid (PAH).
- If Clearance < GFR, then there must be net reabsorption, as with urea.
- The 24-hour renal clearance of endogenous creatinine is often used clinically as an estimate of GFR (small amount of creatinine excreted). It declines with age, due to a decline in renal function and reduction in muscle mass. The plasma creatinine remains constant throughout life.

Renal blood flow (RBF)

- RBF = 1200 ml/min of whole blood (i.e. approximately 25% of the cardiac output).

- GFR and renal blood flow remain approximately constant, within a BP range of 80–180 mmHg, through the mechanism of autoregulation mediated by changes in the afferent arteriolar resistance.

Renal plasma flow (RPF)

- RPF is commonly measured using para-amino hippuric acid (PAH), by determining the amount of PAH in the urine per unit time, divided by the difference in its concentration in renal arterial or venous blood.
- RPF = 660 ml/min. Approximately 120 ml/min of the 660 ml/min is filtered at the glomerulus as ultrafiltrate, 65% is reabsorbed in the proximal tubule, 14% in the loops of Henlé, 15% in the distal tubules and 6% in the collecting ducts. Average urine output = 1.2 ml/min, i.e. only 1% of 120 ml/min of ultrafiltrate filtered at the glomerulus.

PROXIMAL TUBULE FUNCTION

1. *Iso-osmotic reabsorption* of 2/3rds of the glomerular filtrate.
2. *Active reabsorption* of sodium, potassium, glucose, galactose, fructose, amino acids, calcium, uric acid and vitamin C. Na^+ reabsorption can be coupled to the transport of other solutes by either co-transport with glucose, amino acids, bicarbonate and phosphate or exchange with, for example, H^+.
3. *Passive reabsorption* of urea and water due to the osmotic gradient generated by solute reabsorption.
4. *Active secretion* of organic acids, e.g. PAH, diuretics, salicylates, penicillins and probenicid.

Renal transport maximum (Tm) is the maximum amount of a given solute that can be transported (reabsorbed or secreted) per minute by the renal tubules. When the filtered load exceeds the transport maximum, the excess is not reabsorbed but excreted. Substances that have a Tm include phosphate, HPO_4^{2-}, SO_4^{2-}, glucose, many amino acids and uric acid.

LOOP OF HENLÉ FUNCTION

A *counter current multiplier system* exists between the ascending loop of Henlé, the collecting ducts (counter current multipliers), the vasa recta, which represent the vasculature of the juxtaglomerular nephrons (counter current exchangers) and the interstitial tissues. This establishes an interstitial concentration gradient, whereby osmotic pressure of the interstitial tissue of the kidney increases from cortex to medulla. In the presence of a normally functioning antidiuretic hormone (ADH) feedback mechanism, this permits maximum reabsorption of water and concentration of urine. In the absence of ADH, the kidney forms a dilute urine.

Mechanism

- Blood entering the outer medulla in the vasa recta receives NaCl from the descending loop of Henlé and so the interstitium becomes more concentrated.
- The tubular fluid in the descending limb loses water and so becomes more concentrated.
- The fluid in the ascending limb of the loop of Henlé loses NaCl, and so is hypotonic as it enters the distal convoluted tubule.
- The filtrate in the distal tubule and collecting ducts loses both water and urea (ADH increases permeability to water), so tubular urine becomes more concentrated again.

Summary
Fluid entering loop – isotonic
Fluid at tip of loop – hypertonic
Fluid leaving loop – hypotonic

DISTAL TUBULE/COLLECTING DUCT FUNCTION

1. *Reabsorption* of approximately 5% of sodium and 3% of bicarbonate. Variable water reabsorption in the collecting ducts, depending on the presence of ADH. Reabsorption is not iso-osmotic.
2. *Tubular secretion* (active or passive) of ammonium and H^+, and K^+ is under the influence of aldosterone. Also important for eliminating unwanted metabolic products and drugs. Both the distal convoluted tubule and collecting ducts are subject to the actions of aldosterone.

ENDOCRINE FUNCTION OF THE KIDNEY

1. Synthesis of erythropoetin under stimulus of hypoxia and anaemia.
2. 1,25-dihydroxycholecalciferol (vitamin D)
3. Renin
4. Prostaglandins A_2, E_2 and bradykinin.

RENAL TRANSPORT OF SODIUM

- 99% of filtered sodium load is reabsorbed (60% in proximal tubule, 25% in loop of Henlé, 10% in distal tubule/collecting ducts where 2% is under the control of aldosterone).

Reabsorbed by three principal mechanisms:
1. In proximal tubule by Na^+/H^+ exchange. Intracellular H^+ is provided by HCO_3^- absorption and carbonic anhydrase action.
2. In the thick ascending limb, Na^+ is absorbed by $Na^+/Cl^-/2K^+$ co-transport. The transport protein is inhibited by frusemide, and so prevents urine concentration by the loop of Henlé.

3. In the distal tubule, Na^+ is absorbed through an epithelial Na^+ channel which is electrically coupled to a K^+ channel. This dual channel mechanism results in net Na^+ absorption, coupled to net K^+ excretion. This mechanism is regulated by aldosterone.

REGULATION OF SODIUM BALANCE

1. Glomerular filtration rate
2. Aldosterone via the renin–angiotensin system
3. ? Atrial natriuretic peptide (see page 178).

ALDOSTERONE

- C-21 mineralocorticoid hormone secreted by the zona glomerulosa of the adrenal cortex.
- Normal plasma range = 0.9–3 μmol/l (on salt-restricted diet) and 0.1–0.4 μmol/l (on high salt diet)

Action

Promotion of sodium and chloride reabsorption in the distal tubules and collecting ducts, and excretion of K^+ and H^+. Similar exchange mechanism in the sweat glands, ileum and colon.

Control of secretion

1. Via the renin–angiotensin system (see Fig. 5.4); cAMP-mediated and independent of ACTH.
2. ACTH enhances aldosterone production by stimulating steroidogenesis. Negligible role.
3. Plasma K^+ and Na^+ in the absence of changes in plasma volume: a 10% increase in plasma [K^+] and a 10% decrease in plasma [Na^+] (effect often overridden by changes in the circulating volume), can stimulate the synthesis and release of aldosterone by a direct action on the zona glomerulosa.
   (i) Changes in ECF volume are detected by pressure receptors in the afferent arteriole; a fall in [Na^+] or rise in [K^+] is detected by receptors at the macula densa.
   (ii) Renin is secreted into the bloodstream, where it combines with the substrate, angiotensinogen, synthesized by the liver, to form angiotensin I. This is converted in the lung by angiotensin-converting enzyme (ACE), produced by pulmonary epithelial cells, to the physiologically active octapeptide (angiotensin II). This exhibits a negative feedback on its own production by inhibiting renin secretion.

Actions of angiotensin II
1. Potent arterial and venous vasoconstrictor.
2. Increases synthesis and release of aldosterone and ADH centrally.
3. Increases thirst by a central mechanism.
4. Increases level of prostaglandins.

Losartan is a non-competitive antagonist of the angiotensin II receptors AT1 and AT2. It is 30 000 times more selective for the AT1 than the AT2 receptor. It is now licensed for the treatment of essential hypertension. Unlike angiotensin-converting enzyme (ACE) inhibitors, it has no action on bradykinins, or substance P, i.e. no dry cough as associated with ACE inhibitors.

Causes of increased renin release:
A decrease in the effective circulating blood volume, Na^+ depletion, catecholamines, oral contraceptives, chronic disorders associated with oedema (cirrhosis, congestive heart failure and nephrotic syndrome) and standing.

Causes of decreased renin release:
1. Angiotensin II, ADH, hypernatraemia and hyperkalaemia.
2. Indomethacin and β-blockers reduce renin secretion.
3. Angiotensin-converting enzyme inhibitors (ACEI) prevent conversion of angiotensin I to II.

Angiotensin-converting enzyme
1. Plays a key role in the renin–angiotensin and kallikrein-kinin systems by activating angiotensin I to angiotensin II. These two peptide hormones have opposite effects on vascular tone and on smooth muscle proliferation. It remains unclear whether ACE levels are a risk factor for ischaemic heart disease.
2. The ACE gene has been cloned and is located on chromosome 17. Polymorphism exists with three genotypes: II, ID and DD. A DD genotype may be associated with increased risk of myocardial infarction.

Causes of increased aldosterone secretion
1. Upright position and when ambulant.
2. High potassium/low sodium intake.
3. Loss of ECF, e.g. haemorrhage.
4. Surgery, anxiety.
5. Primary hyperaldosteronism (Conn's syndrome).
   Biochemical features of primary hyperaldosteronism:
   (i) elevated plasma (and urinary) aldosterone, with decreased levels of plasma renin and angiotensin
   (ii) hypertension due to Na^+ and water retention
   (iii) hypokalaemic alkalosis.
   (iv) decreased haematocrit due to expansion of plasma volume.
   (v) absence of peripheral oedema.

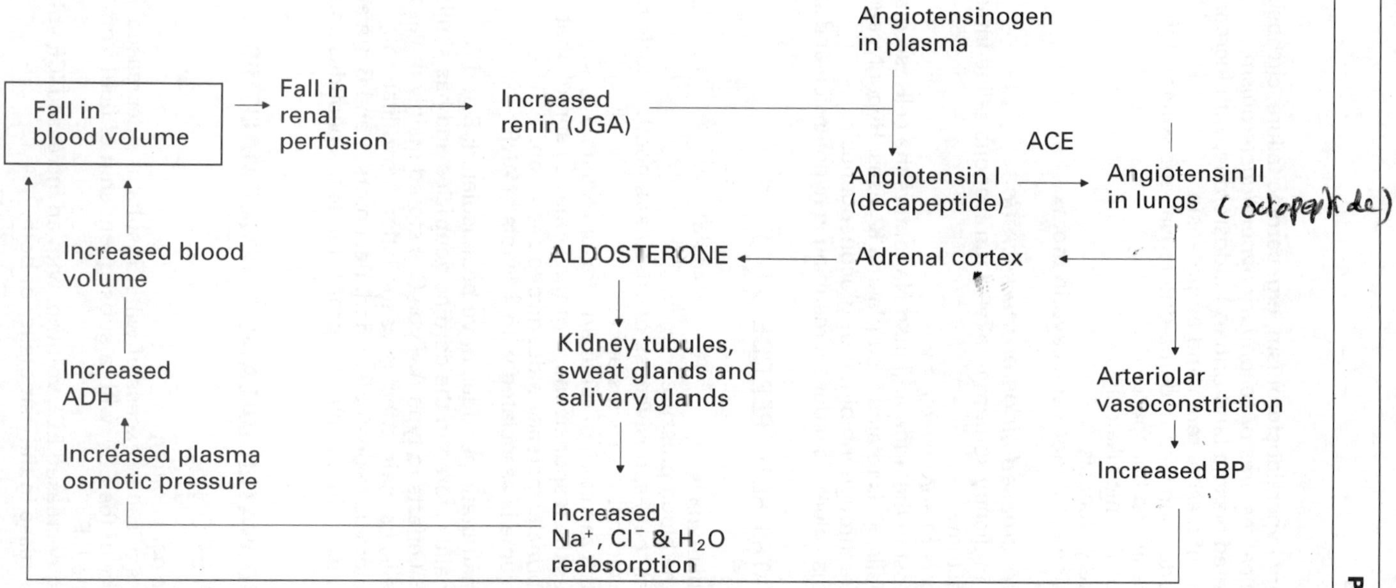

JGA, juxtaglomerular apparatus
ACE, angiotensin converting enzyme

Fig. 5.4 The renin–angiotensin system.

6. Secondary hyperaldosteronism, e.g. cardiac failure, cirrhosis.
   Biochemical features of secondary hyperaldosteronism:
   (i) elevated plasma (and urinary) aldosterone, with increased levels of plasma renin and angiotensin
   (ii) hypertension with oedema due to Na^+ and water retention in the interstitial space
   (iii) hypokalaemic alkalosis.
7. Renal artery stenosis
8. Constriction of inferior vena cava in thorax

Causes of decreased aldosterone secretion
1. Increase in dietary sodium intake or intravenous saline infusion
2. Adrenalectomy
   Main effects of adrenalectomy
   (i) Na^+ lost in the urine and also Na^+ enters the cells, so plasma Na^+ falls: K^+ is retained, so plasma K^+ rises. Hypoglycaemia occurs through inhibition of gluconeogenesis.
   (ii) Plasma volume is reduced, resulting in hypotension and shock.

ATRIAL NATRIURETIC PEPTIDE (ANP)

Actions
1. Marked natriuresis
2. Lowers the blood pressure
3. Decreases the responsiveness of vascular smooth muscle to many vasoconstrictor substances
4. Inhibits the secretion of renin and vasopressin
5. Decreases the responsiveness of the kidney to stimuli that would normally increase aldosterone secretion.
6. ↑ ECF volume is associated with ↑ levels of ANP.

Two other natriuretic peptides have been isolated: B and C. Type B is mainly stored in the cardiac ventricles and has similar physiological effects to type A. Type C is stored mainly in vascular epithelial cells. Its main effect is vasodilation (venodilation). Three receptors have been identified. Receptors A and B are active in signal transduction, while receptor C binds the peptides and terminates their effect.

SALT AND WATER BALANCE ABNORMALITIES

SALT DEPLETION

Hyposmotic dehydration.
1. A net loss of salt in excess of water results in a decreased osmolality of the ECF, with a subsequent shift of fluid from the ECF to the ICF.
2. Resulting decreased ECF volume, with an increased ICF volume and a decrease in the osmolality of both.

Causes: Addison's disease (renal loss of salt).

WATER DEPLETION

Hyperosmotic dehydration.

1. Main effect is a decreased ECF volume, with a fluid shift from the ICF to the ECF compartments.
2. Both the ECF and ICF volumes are decreased, and the osmolality of both is increased.
3. Resulting decreased GFR with associated release of aldosterone and ADH (i.e. renal tubular reabsorption of Na^+ and Cl^- increased).

Causes: decreased intake of water, diabetes insipidus, lithium.

WATER EXCESS

Hypo-osmotic overhydration.

1. Water enters the plasma, causing a decreased ECF osmolality, and hence a shift of fluid from the ECF to the ICF compartments.
2. Increase in the ECF and ICF volumes with a decrease in the osmolality of both compartments.

Causes: excessive intake of water, syndrome of inappropriate ADH secretion (SIADH).

SODIUM EXCESS

Hyperosmotic overhydration.

1. Sodium retention is usually accompanied by an equivalent retention of water and chloride.
2. The rise in plasma osmolality causes a shift of water from ICF to ECF. The ECF volume is increased and is borne by the interstitial fluid (oedema), whilst the ICF volume is decreased.
3. ADH release is inhibited, and the osmolality of both compartments is increased.

Causes: administration of large amounts of hypertonic fluid.

Causes of hypernatraemia

Normal extracellular sodium: water ratio is 140 mmol/l. Hypernatraemia occurs when the extracellular sodium: water ratio is greater than normal.

1. Sodium excess (i.e. increased total body sodium)
   - Excess IV saline, especially postoperatively.
   - Primary hyperaldosteronism, e.g. steroid therapy, Cushing's or Conn's syndrome.
2. Water depletion (i.e. low total body sodium)
   - Reduced water intake, e.g. coma, heat stroke, confusion in the elderly.
   - Extrarenal, e.g. fever, thyrotoxicosis, burns, diarrhoea and fistula.

- Renal, e.g. osmotic diuresis (some patients with hyperosmolar non-ketotic diabetic coma, postobstructive uropathy), diabetes insipidus (cranial/nephrogenic).

Causes of hyponatraemia

True hyponatraemia occurs when the extracellular sodium: water ratio is less than normal.

1. Water loading
   - (i) *Hypertonic hyponatraemia* – with sodium retention (i.e. increased total body sodium and water)
     - secondary hyperaldosteronism, e.g. congestive cardiac failure, nephrotic syndrome, liver cirrhosis
     - reduced GFR, e.g. acute/chronic renal failure.
   - (ii) *Hypotonic hyponatraemia* – without sodium retention
     - acute water overload, e.g. excess IV fluids, esp. dextrose in postoperative period (spot urine $[Na^+]$ <20 mmol/l)
     - psychogenic polydipsia
     - inappropriate ADH secretion, e.g. chlorpropamide, thiazide diuretics, carbamazepine, phenytoin, cytotoxic agents (cyclophosphamide, vincristine), TB, lung carcinoma, abscesses and other neoplasms.
2. Sodium depletion (i.e. decreased total body sodium)
   - (i) Renal loss (spot urine $[Na^+]$ >20 mmol/l) e.g. diuretics; osmotic diuresis due to diabetes, ketonuria, renal tubular damage (diuretic phase of acute renal failure), renal tubular acidosis, and Addison's disease
   - (ii) Extrarenal loss (spot urine $[Na^+]$ <20 mmol/l) e.g. sweating, extensive dermatitis, burns, vomiting, diarrhoea, fistulae, paralytic ileus and pancreatitis.

Other causes

Pseudohyponatraemia, e.g. hyperlipidaemia, sampling from IV infusion arm.

RENAL TRANSPORT OF OTHER SOLUTES

Potassium secretion

- 7% of filtered potassium load is excreted. Almost all potassium is actively reabsorbed in the proximal tubule.
- Passive secretion of potassium occurs in the distal tubule in exchange for sodium, promoted by aldosterone. Hydrogen and potassium ions compete for this exchange.
- Metabolic acidosis is associated with cellular K^+ efflux, a decreased K^+ secretion and hyperkalaemia. The converse is true with metabolic alkalosis.

Causes of hypokalaemia (See page 277)

1. Increased renal loss, e.g. diuretics, renal tubular acidosis, Fanconi syndrome, renal failure (diuretic phase of acute renal

failure/chronic pyelonephritis), diabetic ketoacidosis, Cushing's syndrome and steroid excess, hyperaldosteronism (primary and secondary).
2. Increased gastrointestinal loss, e.g. diarrhoea and vomiting, laxative abuse, carbenoloxone ingestion, intestinal fistulae, chronic mucous secreting neoplasms.
3. Other causes include insulin therapy, catabolic states, IV therapy with inadequate K^+ supplements, insulinoma, metabolic or respiratory alkalosis, familial periodic paralysis, drugs, e.g. carbenicillin, phenothiazines, amphotericin B and degraded tetracycline.

Causes of hyperkalaemia
1. Acute renal failure and advanced chronic renal failure.
2. Potassium-sparing diuretics.
3. Metabolic or respiratory acidosis.
4. Haemolysis (e.g. incompatible blood transfusion), tissue necrosis (e.g. major trauma and burns), severe starvation (e.g. anorexia nervosa), hypoaldosteronism.

Hydrogen secretion and bicarbonate reabsorption
- Hydrogen ion secretion (acidification) takes place throughout the entire length of nephron, except the loop of Henlé (85% in the proximal tubule, 10% in the distal tubules and 5% in the collecting ducts), in exchange for sodium.
- Three major mechanisms of hydrogen ion excretion (see pages 166–168).

Chloride transport
Cl^- moves passively in association with Na^+ except in the ascending limb of the loop of Henlé, where it is actively transported. Plasma chloride level varies inversely with that of plasma bicarbonate because these anions exchange for each other across cell membranes. Depression of plasma chloride will result in an alkalosis caused by the increase in plasma bicarbonate following the release of HCO_3^- from cells.

Sugars and amino acids
- Completely reabsorbed in proximal tubule via active, carrier-mediated mechanism. Sodium-dependent.
- Glucose reabsorption is saturatable: i.e. when blood glucose reaches 10 mmol/l, glycosuria occurs.

Urea
- 87% of filtered urea is reabsorbed; 50% is passively reabsorbed in the proximal tubule.
- Only one-fifth of the remaining urea entering the collecting duct leaves in the urine; the remainder is returned in the blood stream.

Causes of changes in plasma urea and creatinine:
Normal ratio of urea to creatinine, 10:1

1. Plasma urea and creatinine are raised in parallel
   - Chronic renal failure; established acute renal failure
2. ↑ urea > ↑ creatinine
   - Prerenal uraemia, e.g. sodium and water depletion, cardiac failure, gastrointestinal haemorrhage and trauma.
   - High protein intake (oral or IV) in presence of renal disease.
   - Protein catabolism, e.g. starvation, postoperative states, corticosteroid therapy, tetracycline therapy in the presence of renal disease.
   - Drugs via impairment of renal function, e.g. potent diuretics, indomethacin.
3. ↑ *creatinine* > ↑ *urea*
   - Rhabdomyolysis
4. ↓ *urea* > ↓ *creatinine*
   - Pregnancy; low protein diet; acute liver failure; high fluid intake.

RENAL TRANSPORT OF WATER

Water is reabsorbed passively along osmotic gradients set up by active transport of solutes, mainly Na^+, Cl^- and urea. 80% of filtered water is reabsorbed isosmotically in the proximal tubule. 10–15% is reabsorbed in the loop of Henlé, distal tubule and partly in the collecting ducts, in the presence of ADH.

CONTROL OF WATER EXCRETION

Counter current exchange together with multiplication is essential for the concentration of urine, and can only occur in the presence of ADH.

ANTIDIURETIC HORMONE (ADH, OR VASOPRESSIN)

- Synthesized in the cell bodies of the supraoptic and paraventricular nuclei of the hypothalamus.
- Transported along nerve axons and released from posterior pituitary. The neurophysins are the physiologic carrier proteins for the intraneuronal transport of ADH.
- Nonapeptide: the biologically active form is arginine vasopressin.

Control of secretion

- Release can occur in response to an increase in *osmolality* (via stimulation of osmoreceptors located in the anterior hypothalamus) and a decreased *fluid volume* (via a decrease in the tension or stretch of the volume receptors located in the left atrium, vena cavae, great pulmonary veins, carotid sinus and aortic arch).

Actions (Fig. 5.5)

- Acts via cyclic AMP on the distal tubules and collecting ducts.
- In absence of ADH, the distal tubule and collecting duct are fairly impermeable to water (8% is reabsorbed in distal convoluted tubules and collecting ducts, 12% is lost in the urine) and the urine is hypotonic.
- With maximal ADH effect, the walls of the collecting duct are permeable to water (19% is reabsorbed in distal convoluted tubule and collecting ducts, 1% is lost in the urine) and the urine is hypertonic.

Causes of ADH excess: syndrome of inappropriate ADH secretion (SIADH)

1. Increased pituitary ADH
   - hypoadrenalism, stress
   - drugs, e.g. nicotine, barbiturates, clofibrate, vincristine
   - lung disease, e.g. pneumonia, TB, pleural effusion, positive pressure ventilation

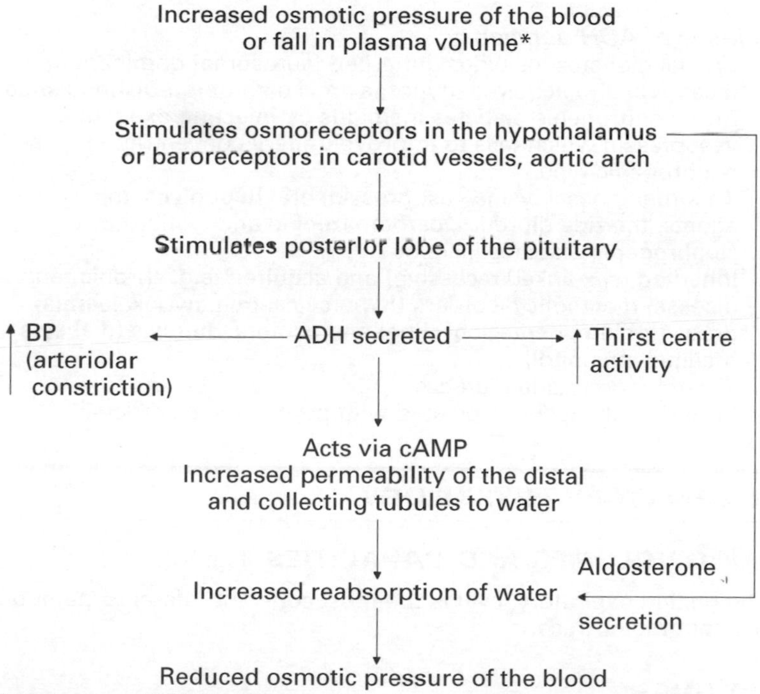
Increased osmotic pressure of the blood or fall in plasma volume*
Stimulates osmoreceptors in the hypothalamus or baroreceptors in carotid vessels, aortic arch
Stimulates posterior lobe of the pituitary
↑ BP (arteriolar constriction)
ADH secreted
↑ Thirst centre activity
Acts via cAMP
Increased permeability of the distal and collecting tubules to water
Increased reabsorption of water
Aldosterone secretion
Reduced osmotic pressure of the blood

*ADH release by fall in blood volume may override osmotic changes tending to inhibit release.

Fig. 5.5

- intracranial disease, e.g. head injury, stroke, cerebral tumours and encephalitis
- systemic disease, e.g. acute intermittent porphyria

2. Increased sensitivity to ADH, e.g. chlorpropamide, carbamazepine
3. Ectopic source of ADH, e.g. bronchogenic carcinoma

Criteria for diagnosis of inappropriate ADH syndrome
(Hypo-osmotic overhydration; page 179). Water retention occurs with an expansion of the ECF volume.
Oedema does not occur because aldosterone secretion is suppressed, which in turn causes increased urinary sodium excretion.

1. Hyponatraemia and low plasma osmolality: <270 mosmol/l.
2. Urine sodium output inappropriately high at 50 mmol/day.
3. Urine osmolality inappropriately high relative to serum osmolality: 350–400 mosmol/l.
4. No evidence of hypovolaemia.
5. Increasing plasma osmolality in response to a restricted intake of water.

Causes of ADH deficiency

1. Cranial diabetes insipidus: inherited (autosomal dominant or recessive) and acquired (hypothalamic disorders). Distinguished from nephrogenic diabetes insipidus by injecting exogenous vasopressin which fails to improve urinary concentration in the nephrogenic type.
   Treatment: nasal lysine vasopressin, oral hypoglycaemic agents, thiazide diuretics, carbamazepine and clofibrate
2. Nephrogenic diabetes insipidus
   Inherited (sex-linked recessive) and acquired, e.g. chronic renal disease, metabolic disorders (hypercalcaemia, hypokalaemia), drugs (lithium, demeclocycline) and osmotic diuresis (diabetes mellitus, mannitol)
   Treatment: thiazide diuretics
3. Primary polydipsia associated with psychiatric disorders.

RESPIRATORY PHYSIOLOGY

LUNG VOLUMES AND CAPACITIES (Fig. 5.6)

The resting expiratory level is the most constant reference point on the spirometer trace.

VOLUMES

Tidal volume (TV): 500 ml in males; 340 ml in females
Volume inspired or expired with each breath at rest.

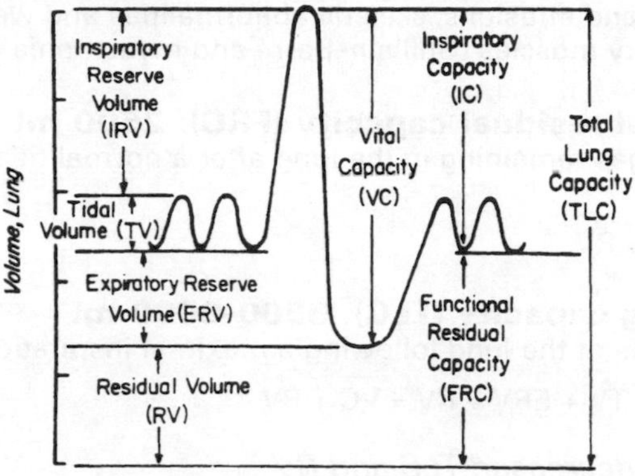

Fig. 5.6

Inspiratory reserve volume (IRV): 3000 ml
Maximum volume of air that can be inspired at the end of a normal tidal inspiration.

Expiratory reserve volume (ERV): 1000 ml
The maximum volume of air that can be forcibly expired after a normal tidal expiration.

Residual volume (RV): 1500 ml
Volume of air remaining after maximal voluntary expiration. Cannot be measured by spirometry. 25% of total lung capacity and increases with age.

RV = FRC (see below) – ERV

CAPACITIES

Inspiratory capacity (IC): 3500 ml
Maximum volume of air that can be inspired at the end of a normal tidal expiration.

IC = TV + IRV

Vital capacity (VC): 4500 ml in males; 3500 ml in females
Maximum volume of air that can be expired after a maximal inspiration. Values increase with size and decrease with age. Approx. 80% of total lung capacity.

VC = IC + ERV

Causes of decreased VC
1. Severe obstructive airways disease
2. Decreased lung volume, e.g. pulmonary fibrosis, infiltration,

oedema and effusions, skeletal abnormalities and weak respiratory muscles (Guillain–Barré and myasthenia gravis).

Functional residual capacity (FRC): 2500 ml

Volume of gas remaining in the lung after a normal tidal expiration.

FRC = ERV + RV

Total lung capacity (TLC): 5500–6000 ml

Total volume of the lung following a maximal inspiration.

TLC = IRV + TV + ERV + RV = VC + RV

Causes of decreased TLC and RV

1. 'Stiff lungs': i.e. reduced lung compliance, e.g. pulmonary fibrosis, pneumoconiosis, pulmonary infiltration and pulmonary oedema.
2. Chest wall disease, e.g. deformity of thoracic spine, respiratory muscle weakness (myopathies, neuropathies and myasthenia gravis).

Causes of increased TLC and RV

1. Increased lung compliance, e.g. emphysema.
2. Airways obstruction and gas trapping, e.g. chronic bronchitis, emphysema and asthma. (↑ in RV > ↑ in TLC)

Forced vital capacity (FVC) (See Note below)

The vital capacity when the expiration is performed as rapidly as possible.

Forced expiratory volume in one second (FEV) (See Note below)

Volume expired during 1st second of FVC. It is relatively independent of expiratory effort because of the dynamic collapse of the airways and the fact that expiratory flow is determined by the elastic recoil pressure of the lung and the resistance of airways proximal to the collapsing lung. Normally greater than 80% of the FVC.
Patients with restrictive lung disease have a reduced VC and TLC due to decreased lung compliance. $FEV_1/FVC > 80\%$.
Patients with obstructive lung disease have a large TLC and a reduced VC, because their RV is increased. $FEV_1/FVC < 80\%$.

Peak flow (See Note)

Maximum expiratory flow rate achieved during a forced expiration.

Note: These are spirometric measures. Spirometry cannot be used to calculate the RV, FRC and TLC. Helium dilution or total body plethysmography may be used.

Minute ventilation (or minute volume)

This is the volume of gas expired per minute
= Tidal volume × respirations/min = 500 × 12
= 6 l/min at rest.
May increase 20–30-fold on exercise.

Alveolar ventilation

This equals the minute ventilation minus the ventilation of the dead space, i.e. it represents the part of the minute ventilation that reaches the gas exchanging part of the airways. Approximately 5.25 l/min.

Dead space ventilation

Anatomical (150 ml)

Portion of tidal volume that remains in the non-exchanging parts of the airways, e.g. mouth, pharynx, trachea and bronchi up to terminal bronchioles.

Physiological

Identical to anatomical dead space in health. May be measured using the Bohr equation. In disease, physiological dead space may exceed anatomical dead space due to disorders of ventilation/ perfusion mismatch.

PULMONARY DYNAMICS

WORK OF BREATHING

1. Elastic resistance: reciprocal of compliance. Elastic recoil of lungs and thorax due to tissue elasticity and surface tension, due to the presence of pulmonary surfactant (see Note), in the lung alveoli.
   In patients with restrictive lung disease, low compliance must overcome large elastic forces during inspiration.
2. Non-elastic resistance: airways resistance (see below) and tissue resistance of lungs and thorax.

Note: *Pulmonary surfactant* is a lecithin-based material which decreases the surface tension at low lung volumes so increasing compliance. At high lung volumes it increases surface tension, decreasing compliance and facilitating expiration. Surfactant prevents alveolar collapse at end-expiratory alveolar pressures that would otherwise lead to atelectasis.

COMPLIANCE

- Change in volume produced by a unit change of pressure difference across the lungs. It is an index of lung distensibility.
- Normal value = 0.2 l/cmH_2O. Measured with an oesophageal

catheter, which provides an estimate of the change in pleural pressure that occurs during tidal breathing.

- Static compliance reflects the elastic recoil of the lungs and expansibility of the thoracic cage.
- Dynamic compliance (i.e. compliance during respiration) is influenced by airways obstruction. Compliance is greater for expiration than inspiration due to the viscous properties of the lungs.
- Compliance is non-linear. It is greatest at mid-lung volumes and decreases at its extremes.
- *Hysteresis* is the variation of pressure depending on volume.

Causes of decreased compliance
Pulmonary oedema, interstitial fibrosis, pneumonectomy and kyphosis.

Causes of increased compliance
Emphysema and age.

AIRWAYS RESISTANCE (Raw)

- Equals the transairway pressure gradient divided by the flow rate.
- Factors which affect Raw:
  1. Flow rate and airway radius: Raw depends largely on the small peripheral airways (20%).
  2. Lung volume: increases in lung volume cause a reduction in airway resistance by dilatation of the airways.
  3. Phase of respiration: resistance greater on expiration than inspiration (hence expiratory wheeze in asthma).
  4. Autonomic effects: increased sympathetic activity results in bronchodilation: increased parasympathetic activity results in bronchoconstriction.
  5. Elastic recoil: decreased elastic recoil seen in the elderly and in patients with emphysema.
  6. Local P_{CO_2}: a decrease in P_{CO_2} in expired air causes local bronchoconstriction: this mechanism is important in adjusting regional balance between ventilation and perfusion in the lungs.

Causes of increased Raw: include chronic bronchitis, emphysema, upper airways obstruction.

INTRAPLEURAL PRESSURE

(Quiet ventilation.)

- Equals the pressure in the pleural space minus the barometric pressure. Pleural pressure is less negative at the base than at the apex.
- Varies from – 4 cmH_2O in inspiration to 1 cmH_2O in expiration.

RESPIRATORY CYCLE

During inspiration, the pressure gradient from the extrathoracic to the intrathoracic veins increases and right ventricular filling and output increases. However, pulmonary venous return is decreased by the reduction in intrathoracic pressure. This produces a decrease in left ventricular stroke volume and cardiac output.

PULMONARY GAS EXCHANGE AND BLOOD GAS TRANSPORT (See pages 262–263)

PARTIAL PRESSURES OF GASES IN RESPIRATION (Fig. 5.7)

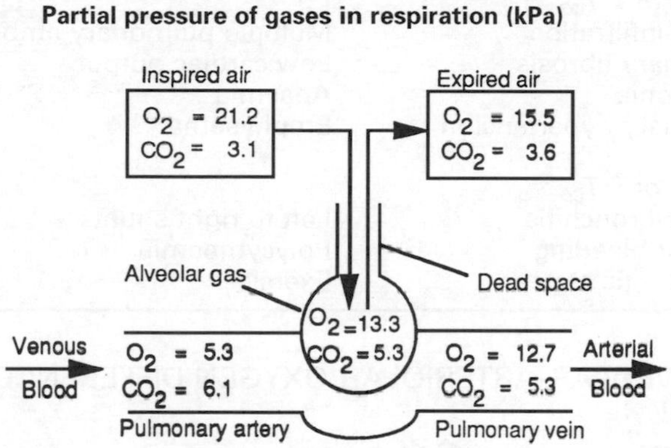

Fig. 5.7

BLOOD–GAS BARRIER

Consists of:
1. Layer of pulmonary surfactant
2. Alveolar epithelium
3. Epithelium basement membrane
4. Interstitium
5. Endothelium basement membrane
6. Capillary endothelium
7. Plasma
8. Red cell membrane
9. Intracellular fluid.

DIFFUSING CAPACITY OF THE LUNG OR TRANSFER FACTOR (T_{CO} measured in mmol/min/kPa)

- The rate at which a gas will diffuse from the alveoli into the blood.

- It is influenced by the rate of diffusion through three barriers:
  1. alveolar–capillary wall, major determinant
  2. plasma
  3. cytoplasm of the erythrocyte.
- Carbon monoxide is the only gas that is used to measure the diffusing capacity, where T_{CO} normally measures 25–30 ml CO/min/mmHg. The diffusing capacity for carbon dioxide is about 20-fold this value, because of greater solubility in tissue fluids.

BOX 5.1 CHANGES IN DIFFUSING CAPACITY

Causes of ↓ T_{CO}

Diffuse infiltration	Multiple pulmonary emboli
Pulmonary fibrosis	Low cardiac output
Pneumonia	Anaemia
Pulmonary hypertension	Emphysema

Causes of ↑ T_{CO}

Asthma/bronchitis	Left to right shunts
Alveolar bleeding	Polycythaemia
Hyperkinetic states	Exercise

THE ALVEOLAR–ARTERIOLAR OXYGEN DIFFERENCE ($P(A - a)O_2$)

- The difference between the partial pressure of oxygen in the alveoli and the arterial partial pressure of oxygen.
- It is the best single indicator of the gas-exchange properties of the respiratory system, and is increased by any process that interferes with the diffusion of gas across the alveolar–capillary barrier, such as interstitial lung disease. It can be used to follow the progress of lung disease; an increasing gradient indicates a deterioration in lung disease.
- The mean alveolar PO_2 (PAO_2) is calculated using the alveolar gas equation.
  $PAO_2 = PIO_2 - (PaCO_2/R) + F$ where PIO_2 is the partial pressure of inspired O_2, $PACO_2$ is the partial pressure of alveolar CO_2, R is the respiratory quotient which represents the balance between O_2 consumption and O_2 production. It normally varies between 0.7 and 1.0.
  F is a correction factor.
  PaO_2 is obtained from arterial blood gas analysis.
- The $P(A - a)O_2$ should normally not exceed 15–20 mmHg. This difference is due to physiologic shunts such as the bronchial and coronary circulations and to V–Q inequalities (see below), which exist in the lung as a function of gravity.

PULMONARY CIRCULATION

Mean pulmonary arterial pressure is 12–15 mmHg, and left atrial pressure is normally about 5 mmHg. Therefore the pressure gradient across the pulmonary circulation is 7–10 mmHg. The vascular resistance of the lung is approximately one-tenth that of the systemic circulation.

VENTILATION/PERFUSION RATIO (V/Q)

- Important in determining alveolar gas exchange. V = volume of air entering alveoli = 4 l/min Q = blood flow through lungs = 5 l/min V/Q = 0.8
- The distribution of ventilation is determined by the pleural pressure gradient and airway closure. In erect subjects, ventilation increases *slowly* from lung apex to base (due to the diaphragm pulling the alveoli open at the bases).
- Pulmonary blood flow (perfusion) varies in different parts of the lungs because of the low pressure head, the distensibility of the vessels, and the hydrostatic effects of gravity. Perfusion increases *rapidly* from lung apex to base (mainly due to the effect of gravity).

Therefore, V/Q ratio falls from 3.3 at apex to 0.63 at base.

Causes of V/Q imbalance

- A *low* V/Q ratio indicates right to left shunting of deoxygenated blood, i.e. wasted perfusion.
- A *high* V/Q ratio indicates a large physiological dead space, i.e. wasted ventilation and is associated with CO_2 retention and a high arterial $P\text{CO}_2$. Examples include hyaline membrane disease of the newborn, pneumothorax, bronchopneumonia and pulmonary oedema.
- Blockage of both ventilation and perfusion to one portion of a lung would maintain a constant V/Q ratio, e.g. surgical removal of a lung or a portion of a lung.

CONTROL OF BREATHING

- Coordinated activity between central regulatory centres, central and peripheral chemoreceptors, pulmonary receptors and the respiratory muscles.
- $P\text{CO}_2$ is the most important variable in the regulation of ventilation, through its effect on pH. Maximal increase in CO_2 can increase alveolar ventilation 10-fold.
- $P\text{O}_2$ and [H^+] play a less important role. Maximal increase in [H^+] can increase ventilation 5-fold and maximal decrease in $P\text{O}_2$ can increase it by about one and two-thirds.
- *Central regulatory centres* control rate and depth of respiration
  1. Medullary respiratory centre

2. Apneustic centre (lower pons)
3. Pneumotaxic centre (upper pons).

- *Central chemoreceptors* respond to changes in $[H^+]$, i.e. an increase in $[H^+]$ in brain ECF stimulates ventilation.
- *Peripheral chemoreceptors* respond to changes in the P_{O_2}, P_{CO_2} and H^+ concentrations of arterial blood. The carotid body chemoreceptors respond to decreases in arterial P_{O_2}, high P_{CO_2}, reduced flow and low pH. The aortic body chemoreceptors respond to increased level of P_{CO_2} and low P_{O_2}.
- *Pulmonary receptors*
  1. Pulmonary stretch receptors are responsible for the Hering–Bruer reflex (distension of the lung results in a slowing of the respiratory rate) via the vagi. Vagotomy abolishes this reflex.
  2. Irritant receptors are stimulated by an increase in any noxious agent (e.g. histamine, bradykinin), resulting in bronchoconstriction.
  3. J (juxtacapillary) receptors are stimulated by stretching of the pulmonary microvasculature.

RESPONSE TO CHRONIC HYPOXIA

For example, acclimatization to high altitude.
At high altitude (>3000 m), the partial pressure of O_2 in inspired air is reduced. Acute and chronic adaptation to hypoxia occur.

ACUTE ADAPTATION

- Increased minute ventilation (in response to hypoxia and raised CO_2 levels) by about 65%, which reduces the CO_2 level and causes an alkalosis. This is slowly corrected by renal excretion of HCO_3^-.
- Increased cardiac output and heart rate which returns to normal after two weeks at high altitude.
- Hypocapnia.
- Increased red cell 2,3,diphosphoglycerate (2,3,DPG) production stimulated by hypoxia. Causes decreased oxygen affinity for haemoglobin which facilitates O_2 release to the tissues, i.e. oxygen dissociation curve shifted to the right.

CHRONIC ADAPTATION

- Further increase in ventilation by about 400%.
- Polycythaemia: erythropoetin production stimulated by hypoxia, with an increase in haemoglobin concentration and haematocrit (from 40–45% to 60–65%).
- Circulatory blood volume increases by up to 50–90%.
- Pulmonary hypertension due to pulmonary vasoconstriction caused by chronic hypoxia.

CARDIAC PHYSIOLOGY

CONDUCTING SYSTEM OF THE HEART

VENTRICULAR MUSCLE

- The resting membrane potential of cardiac cells is about −90 mV.
- A typical action potential may be divided into 4 phases:
  Phase 0: Membrane depolarization. Rapid increase in permeability to sodium.
  Phase 1: Rapid repolarization: rapid decrease in permeability to sodium, small increase in permeability to potassium.
  Phase 2: Slow repolarization: plateau effect due to: (i) absence of large rapid increase in permeability to K^+; (ii) increase in Ca^{2+} permeability. Unique feature of cardiac action potential.
  Phase 3: Rapid repolarization: gradual increase in potassium permeability and inactivation of slow inward Ca^{2+} channels.

PACEMAKER CELLS

For example, sinoatrial node.
- Slow upstroke action potential, mediated by calcium channels.
- Smaller magnitude of action potential.
- No fast sodium channels.
- Spontaneously depolarizes during diastole (phase 4 depolarization).

CARDIAC CYCLE

A cardiac cycle showing the relationship between left ventricular pressure, heart sounds, venous pulse and ECG is shown in Figure 5.8.

PHASES OF THE CARDIAC CYCLE

1. *Atrial contraction*
   The pressure in the ventricles at the end of atrial contraction is termed the ventricular end-diastolic pressure and sets the preload for the next ventricular contraction.
2. *Isovolumetric contraction*
   Pressure in the ventricular cavities rises due to the onset of ventricular contraction. This reverses the pressure gradient across the atrioventricular (AV) valves and causes closure of the AV valve. Following closure, the ventricular volume remains constant until the ventricular pressure exceeds that in the arteries, when ventricular ejection begins.
3. *Rapid ejection*
   Almost 70% of the stroke volume is ejected in the first third of systole.

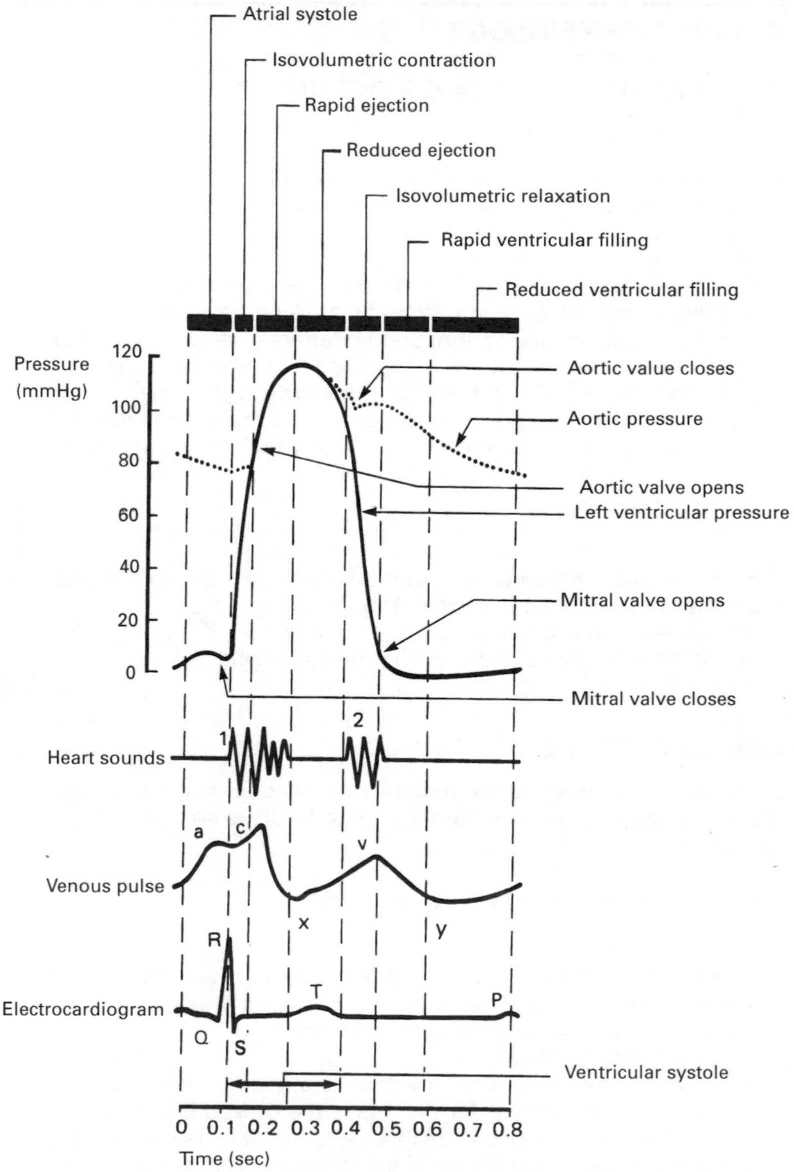
Atrial systole
Isovolumetric contraction
Rapid ejection
Reduced ejection
Isovolumetric relaxation
Rapid ventricular filling
Reduced ventricular filling
Pressure (mmHg)
120
100
80
60
40
20
0
Aortic value closes
Aortic pressure
Aortic valve opens
Left ventricular pressure
Mitral valve opens
Mitral valve closes
1
2
Heart sounds
a
c
v
x
y
Venous pulse
R
T
P
Q
S
Electrocardiogram
Ventricular systole
0 0.1 0.2 0.3 0.4 0.5 0.6 0.7 0.8
Time (sec)

Fig. 5.8

4. *Reduced ejection*
During the latter two-thirds of systole, the ejection rate declines with the ventricular and arterial pressures.
5. *Isovolumetric relaxation*
This phase extends from the closure of the semilunar valves and ends as ventricular pressure falls below atrial pressure and the AV valves reopen.
6. *Rapid ventricular filling*
During ventricular systole, venous filling continues and the atrial pressure reaches its peak just as the AV valves reopen. Once open, the pressure in both the atrial and ventricular cavities falls as ventricular relaxation continues.
7. *Reduced ventricular filling*
During the later stages of diastole, the atrial and ventricular pressures rise slowly as blood returns to the heart.

INTRACARDIAC PRESSURES

Table 5.4 Normal intracardiac pressures and oxygen saturation

Chamber	*Pressure (mmHg)*	*Oxygen saturation (%)*
Right atrium	3	65–75
Right ventricle	20/4	
Pulmonary artery	20/12 15 (mean)	
Pulmonary capillary wedge	8 (mean)	96–98
Left atrium	8	
Left ventricle	150/8	
Aorta	130/75 100 (mean)	

HEART SOUNDS (see Fig. 5.8)

1. First heart sound is due to closure of the AV (mitral and tricuspid) valves. Louder sound if PR interval is abnormally long or short, as valve leaflets close from a more widely separated position, e.g. mitral stenosis, hyperdynamic circulation, tachycardia. Normally split in tricuspid area on inspiration.
2. Second heart sound is high in frequency and is due to closure of the semilunar (aortic and pulmonary) valves. Physiological splitting of the second heart sound (A_2–P_2 interval; see Note). Fixed splitting occurs due to pressure or volume load on the right ventricle such as in an atrioseptal defect or pulmonary hypertension. Paradoxical splitting occurs whenever left ventricular systole is delayed or prolonged, such as in left

bundle branch block, aortic stenosis and occasionally systemic hypertension.

3. Third heart sound is due to rapid filling of the left ventricle. Best heard in children.
4. Fourth heart sound is due to ventricular distension caused by a forceful atrial contraction. Not heard in normal individuals.

Note: During expiration the A_2–P_2 interval is about 0.02 seconds, and during inspiration about 0.05 seconds. This is because during inspiration the ventricular ejection period is prolonged due to increased stroke volume secondary to increased venous return.

Effect of respiration on murmurs

- Respiration increases stroke volume of right ventricle and therefore increases the intensity of tricuspid stenosis, pulmonary stenosis and tricuspid incompetence.
- Respiration increases vascular volume of lungs and decreases stroke volume of left ventricle, therefore decreasing intensity of murmurs of mitral stenosis and incompetence, and aortic stenosis and incompetence.

Effect of drugs on murmurs

Vasodilators will decrease arteriolar resistance and increase systolic ejection murmurs and regurgitant murmurs at all valves. Drugs increasing arteriolar resistance will have the opposite effect.

ECG intervals (Table 5.5)

Table 5.5 ECG intervals (see also Fig. 5.8)

ECG intervals	*Time (sec)*	*Event*
PR interval	0.12–0.2	Atrial depolarization and conduction through AV node
QRS duration	0.08–0.1	Ventricular depolarization
QT interval	0.4–0.43	Ventricular depolarization plus ventricular repolarization

VENOUS PRESSURE CHANGES (Fig. 5.8)

- **a wave**: due to atrial systole.
  Disappears in atrial fibrillation; cannon waves are present in complete heart block. Giant 'a' waves are present in pulmonary hypertension, severe pulmonary and tricuspid stenosis.
- **c wave**: due to bulging of the AV valve during ventricular contraction. Synchronous with the pulse wave in the carotid artery.
- **v wave**: due to rise in atrial pressure before the AV valve opens during diastole.

- **x descent**: due to drawing away of the AV valve from the atrium during ventricular systole.
- **y descent**: due to fall in atrial pressure as blood rushes into ventricle when the AV valve opens. Deep 'y' descent occurs with any condition causing a high jugular venous pressure (JVP), such as constrictive pericarditis. A slow 'y' descent is seen with tricuspid stenosis.

CARDIAC PERFORMANCE

VENTRICULAR END-DIASTOLIC VOLUME (VEDV)

- The volume of blood in the ventricular cavity just prior to the first heart sound, i.e. at the end of atrial contraction. The normal LVEDV is about 120 ml.
- Influenced by the ventricular filling pressure, compliance and heart rate.
  RV filling pressure = central venous pressure (CVP)
  LV filling pressure = pulmonary wedge pressure

Central venous pressure

- Normal pressure = –2 cm H_2O to +12 cm H_2O
- Varies with cardiac cycle, respiration and position of patient

Causes of ↓ CVP
Non-cardiogenic shock.

Causes of ↑ CVP
Heart failure
Positive end-expiratory pressure ventilation and Valsalva manoeuvre impedes venous return
Expansion of blood volume.

VENTRICULAR END-SYSTOLIC VOLUME

- The volume of blood remaining in the ventricle at the end of ejection.
- The normal left ventricular end-systolic volume is 40 ml.

STROKE VOLUME (SV)

- The volume of blood ejected with each beat.
- Equal to the difference between the ventricular end-diastolic and end-systolic volumes.
- Approximately 70–80 ml.

EJECTION FRACTION

- Ratio of stroke volume to end diastolic volume (SV/EDV)
- Normal range 50–70%
- Useful index of overall left ventricular function (measured by gated blood pool scanning and 2-D echocardiography).
- Stroke volume and ejection fraction increase with contractility.

CARDIAC OUTPUT (CO)

- Volume of blood expelled from one side of the heart per minute.
- Determined by the heart rate (HR) and stroke volume (SV).

$$CO = HR \times SV$$

$$\frac{72 \times 70 \text{ ml}}{1000} = \text{5 l/min in average resting man; 20\% less in women.}$$

- May increase 4–5 times on strenuous exertion. Varies with body surface area.
- The cardiac index is the cardiac output per square metre of body surface and averages about 3.2 l.

Measurement of cardiac output

Techniques used:

1. *Fick method*

   Principle:

   Amount of oxygen delivered to the tissues must equal the oxygen uptake by the lungs, plus the oxygen delivered to the lungs in the pulmonary artery.

$$CO = \frac{\text{oxygen consumption rate by the body (ml/min)}}{\text{arterial oxygen content} - \text{venous oxygen content}}$$

$$= \frac{250 \text{ ml } O_2\text{/min}}{190 \text{ ml } O_2\text{/l blood} - 140 \text{ ml } O_2\text{/l blood}}$$

$$= 5 \text{ l/min}$$

2. *Dye dilution*

   Principle:

   If a known amount of indicator dye is mixed into an unknown volume of blood, and its concentration is measured, the volume of blood can be calculated from the factor by which the indicator has been diluted. The flow of blood can be measured if the mean concentration of the indicator is determined for the time required for that indicator to pass a given site.
3. *Thermodilution*

   Principle:

   Cold saline injected at the proximal end of a catheter in the right ventricle, mixes with blood in the right ventricle and the temperature change is measured by a distal thermistor downstream in the pulmonary artery.

Factors modifying cardiac output

- Heart rate
  1. Intrinsic rhythmicity
  2. Extrinsic factors: e.g. autonomic nervous system
- Stroke volume
  1. Contractility
  2. Preload
  3. Afterload.

Contractility

The force which the heart muscle generates as it contracts. Influenced by inotropic factors:

Causes of an increase in contractility i.e. positive inotropic factors.

1. Sympathetic nerve stimulation and catecholamines
2. Increase in extracellular [Ca^+]
3. Decrease in extracellular [Na^+]
4. Drugs, e.g. digoxin, glucagon, L-thyroxine.

Causes of a decrease in contractility, i.e. negative inotropic factors.

1. Drugs, e.g. β-blockers, anaesthetic agents, antiarrhythmic drugs
2. Heart failure
3. Hypoxia, hypercapnia and acidosis.

Preload

- The ventricular end-diastolic volume or pressure.
- The relationship between the preload (left ventricular end-diastolic volume) and stroke volume is described by the *Frank–Starling law*, which states that the force developed in a muscle fibre depends on the degree to which the fibre is stretched.
- Applied to cardiac dynamics, the initial fibre length is equivalent to the left ventricular end-diastolic volume (LVEDV).
- Ventricular function curves illustrating the Frank–Starling law are shown in Figure 5.9.
  —The LVEDV increases with venous return. Exercise, overtransfusion and sympathetic venoconstriction increase venous return, while haemorrhage, diuretics and venodilatation decrease venous return.
  —The LVEDV fails to increase normally with decreasing contractility.

Afterload

I.e. total peripheral resistance

- Tension or force in the ventricular wall during ventricular ejection.
- Determined by:
  1. aortic pressure

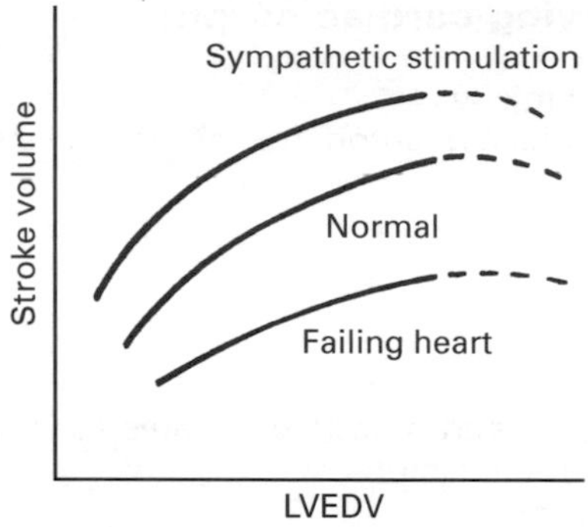

Fig. 5.9

2. aortic valve resistance
3. ventricular cavity size.

- At constant preload and contractility, the stroke volume is inversely related to the afterload, i.e. decreasing the peripheral resistance with a vasodilator increases the stroke volume.

BLOOD PRESSURE

- BP = Cardiac output × peripheral resistance
- Pulse pressure = Systolic pressure – diastolic pressure
- Mean arterial pressure = Diastolic pressure + 1/3rd of the pulse pressure

Control

1. Autonomic nervous system via baroreceptors in aortic arch via vagus and carotid sinus and medullary and hypothalamic cardiorespiratory centres.
2. Renin–angiotensin system

Main determinants of blood pressure

1. Heart rate: increase in heart rate increases arterial pressure by reducing time for diastolic run-off to the periphery. This increases the mean arterial volume and so the diastolic blood pressure.
2. Peripheral resistance: an increase in peripheral resistance raises the diastolic arterial volume by reducing peripheral run-off.
3. Stroke volume: an increase in stroke volume at a constant heart rate increases mean arterial volume and pressure and pulse pressure.
4. Aortic elasticity: an increase produces a greater pulse pressure (↑ in systolic and ↓ in diastolic pressures).

PERIPHERAL RESISTANCE (PR)

- Resistance to flow of blood through arterioles.

$$PR = \frac{\text{Mean arterial pressure}}{\text{Cardiac output}} = \frac{100}{5 \text{ l/min}} = 20 \text{ mmHg/l/min}$$

- *Control* of peripheral resistance is exerted by controlling vessel calibre. Arteriolar vasoconstriction causes an increase in peripheral resistance. Venous vasoconstriction causes an increase in stroke volume and cardiac output.

Factors affecting the calibre of the arterioles

Constriction	**Dilatation**
Increased sympathetic activity	Decreased sympathetic activity
Circulating catecholamines	Increased P_{CO_2}, decreased pH and P_{O_2}
Circulating angiotensin II	Lactic acid, histamine and prostaglandins
Locally released serotonin	
Decreased local temperature	Increased local temperature

THE CIRCULATION

VESSELS, FUNCTIONS AND DISTRIBUTION OF BLOOD (Table 5.6)

Table 5.6 Circulation

Vessel	*Function*	*% distribution of total blood volume*
Artery, Arteriole	Damping/resistance	12
Capillary	Exchange	7
Venule, Vein	Capacitance	50

CIRCULATION THROUGH SPECIAL AREAS

Cerebral circulation

- Cerebral blood flow = 0.75 l/min
- Depends on:
  1. Perfusion pressure (i.e. the arterial–venous pressure difference at the brain level).
  2. Cerebral vascular resistance, which is a function of intracranial pressure, the calibre of cerebral arterioles and blood viscosity. The vascular diameter is regulated by local factors, e.g. a local increase in P_{CO_2} or a local decrease in P_{O_2} or pH causes vasodilatation.

- Considerable degree of autoregulation to maintain an overall constant cerebral blood flow. Cerebral blood flow is not reduced until BP falls to <60 mmHg or exceeds 150 mmHg.

The *Cushing reflex* is a systemic vasoconstriction in response to an increase in the systemic blood pressure and CSF pressure, in order to maintain blood flow to the brain.

Coronary circulation

- Coronary blood flow = 200 ml/min at rest
- Depends on:
  1. pressure in the aorta
  2. length of diastole.
- In the left ventricle, ventricular pressure is slightly greater than aortic pressure during systole, but much less than the aortic pressure during diastole. Therefore coronary flow to the left ventricle only occurs during diastole.
- In the right ventricle and atria, aortic pressure is greater than right ventricular and atrial pressure during systole and diastole, therefore coronary flow to these parts continues throughout the cardiac cycle.
- Oxygen consumption = 7.9 ml/min/100 g.

CIRCULATORY ADAPTATIONS

1. Postural changes from supine to upright position
   ↓ venous return and ↓ CVP → ↓ stroke volume → ↓ cardiac output → ↓ BP.
   Compensatory ↑ heart rate and ↑ peripheral resistance. (Heart rate decreases on reversal of movement.)
2. Severe haemorrhage
   ↓ BP → vasoconstriction → ↓ in renal blood flow
   ↑ heart rate (4-fold) → ↑ stroke volume (1.5-fold) and ↑ cardiac output.
3. Exercise
   ↑ heart rate (4-fold) and stroke volume (2-fold)
   ↑ cardiac output (up to 30 l/min) which is redistributed to working muscles
   ↑ O_2 consumption (up to 20-fold) in blood to skeletal muscles and coronary circulation
   Peripheral vasoconstriction → ↑ systemic arterial pressure
   Pulmonary vessel dilatation → ↓ pulmonary vascular resistance
4. Altitude (see page 192).
5. Valsalva manoeuvre (or positive end-expiratory pressure)
   Increase in intrapulmonary and intrathoracic pressures, so that venous return impeded (Fig. 5.10).
   ↓ heart rate, stroke volume, and BP
   On release – ↑ in peripheral volume → overshoot of BP and ↓ HR.

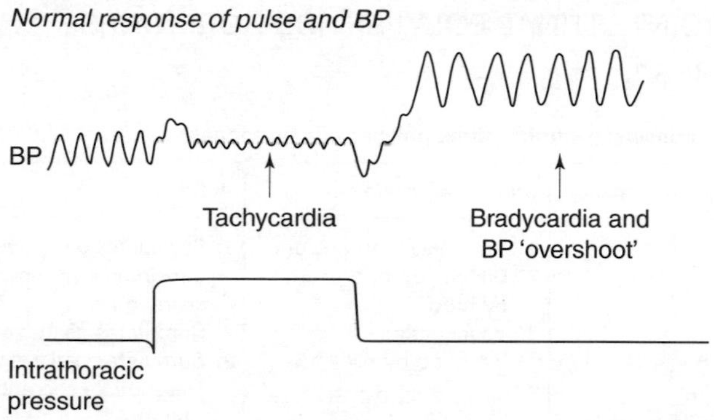

Fig. 5.10

GASTROINTESTINAL PHYSIOLOGY

STOMACH

GASTRIC JUICE

- Approximately 3 l/day
  1. Parietal (oxyntic) cells produce hydrochloric acid, Na^+, Ca^{2+}, Mg^{2+} and intrinsic factor.
  2. Surface mucosal cells produce mucus and bicarbonate.
  3. Chief (peptic) cells secrete pepsinogen, the inactive precursor of pepsin.

CONTROL OF GASTRIC SECRETION

Stimulation of gastric acid secretion

1. Neural: vagal stimulation increases both pepsin and acid output directly, as well as indirectly by causing secretion of gastrin. Vagotomy reduces basal acid secretion, and secretion in response to histamine or pentagastrin.
2. Hormonal: gastrin.
3. Histamine: via interaction with H_2 receptors on oxyntic cells. Blockage of histamine H_2 receptors by drugs such as cimetidine inhibits both the gastrin-induced and vagally mediated acid secretion.

Inhibition of gastric acid secretion

1. Higher centres, e.g. nausea, and fear through activation of the sympathetic nervous system.
2. Low gastric juice pH.
3. Small intestinal peptides, e.g. cholecystokinin–pancreozymin (CCK-PZ), secretin, and gastric inhibitory peptide (GIP).

GASTROINTESTINAL POLYPEPTIDE HORMONES

See Table 5.7.

Table 5.7 Principal gastrointestinal polypeptide hormones

Hormone and location	*Stimulus for release*	*Actions*
Gastrin G cells in gastric antrum	1. Aminoacids in antrum 2. Distension of antrum by food 3. Vagal action Inhibited by pH <1.5	1. Stimulates gastric acid, pepsin and intrinsic factor secretion 2. Stimulates gastric emptying 3. Stimulates pancreatic bicarbonate secretion and secretin
Secretin Duodenum and jejunum	1. Intraluminal acid (vagus has no direct action on secretin secretion)	1. Stimulates pancreatic bicarbonate secretion 2. Inhibits gastric acid and pepsin secretion 3. Delays gastric emptying
Cholecystokinin–pancreozymin (CCK-PZ) Duodenum and jejunum	1. Intraluminal fat, amino acids, peptides and certain cations e.g. Ca^{2+} and Mg^{2+}	1. Stimulates pancreatic enzyme and bicarbonate secretion 2. Stimulates gall bladder contraction (and relaxation of the sphincter of Oddi) 3. Inhibition of gastric emptying and motility of the small intestine
Gastric inhibitory peptide (GIP) Duodenum and jejunum		1. Inhibits gastric acid secretion and motility 2. Stimulates postprandial insulin secretion
Motilin Duodenum and jejunum		1. Stimulates gastric and intestinal motility
Pancreatic polypeptide (PP)* Pancreas		1. Inhibits pancreatic enzyme secretion 2. Relaxes gall bladder
Vasoactive intestinal peptide (VIP)* Small intestine		1. Inhibits gastric acid and pepsin secretion 2. Stimulates pancreatic and intestinal secretion

*Neurocrine system: VIP, substance P, and endorphins.

GASTRIC EMPTYING

See Table 5.8.

Table 5.8 Factors affecting gastric emptying

Increased	*Reduced*
Distension of stomach and antrum	Fatty acids
Gastrin	Hyperosmolar solution (e.g. amino acids and polypeptides)
Cold	Acid in duodenum
Emotion	Secretin, CCK-PZ Heat and emotion

PANCREAS

PANCREATIC JUICE

- Alkaline fluid (pH 8.0) containing electrolytes and digestive enzymes in the form of their proenzymes.
- 1200–1500 ml/day.
- Neutralizes gastric juice together with bile and duodenal juice and so creates the optimal pH for intestinal enzymes.
- Acinar cells produce a secretion rich in enzymes and electrolytes for the digestion of carbohydrates, proteins, fats and nucleic acids.
- The principal enzymes are: maltase, amylase, lipases, nucleases, and the proenzymes are trypsinogen, chymotrypsinogens, proaminopeptidase and procarboxypeptidases.
- Ductule cells produce water and electrolytes.

Control of pancreatic juice secretion

1. Gastric: food in the stomach stimulates the vagus, resulting in gastrin and acid release. Gastrin stimulates enzyme secretion by the acinar cells.
2. Intestinal: peptides, aminoacids, fatty acids and H^+ in the duodenum cause release of:
   (i) secretin which stimulates a secretion, rich in bicarbonate, by the acinar cells.
   (ii) cholecystokinin–pancreozymin (CCK-PZ) which stimulates the acinar cells to increase enzyme secretion.

BILIARY SYSTEM

250–1100 ml of bile are secreted daily by the liver. Bile is stored in the gall bladder and released into the duodenum through contraction of the gall bladder stimulated by CCK.

COMPOSITION OF BILE

Bile acids
Phospholipids
Cholesterol
Bile pigments (bilirubin and biliverdin)
Protein

Bile acids

- *Primary bile acids:* Cholic acid and chenodeoxycholic acid. Formed in the liver from cholesterol by the addition of hydroxyl and carboxyl groups.
- *Secondary bile acids:* Deoxycholic acid and lithocholic acids. Formed from the primary bile salts through the action of intestinal bacterial enzymes.

Functions of bile acids

1. Solubilize cholesterol by incorporation into micelles.
2. Aid emulsification of fats with phospholipids and fatty acids.
3. Aid absorption of fat-soluble vitamins.
4. Stimulate pancreatic secretion by releasing CCK-PZ.

HAEM AND BILIRUBIN CATABOLISM

- Worn out red blood cells are phagocytosed by reticuloendothelial cells in the spleen. The free haemoglobin released is bound to haptoglobin. This complex is transported in the bloodstream to the liver where hepatic reticuloendothelial cells split off the haemoglobin portion, converting it to its haem and globin moeties.
- The globin is hydrolysed into its component amino acids, which are added to the hepatic pool for reuse.
- Bilirubin is formed from the catabolism of the haem moeity and is transported to the liver bound to albumin. The iron released from haem in this process is stored in the liver for reuse.
- Bilirubin is conjugated with glucuronic acid catalysed by glucuronyl transferase to form water-soluble bilirubin diglucuronide which is excreted in bile. Bacterial metabolism of bilirubin in the bowel leads to the formation of urobilinogen, some of which undergoes an enterohepatic circulation and may be found in the urine.

Enterohepatic circulation (EHC)

In the intestine, both primary and secondary bile acids are deconjugated, reabsorbed in the terminal ileum and returned to the liver by the portal vein bound to serum albumin, where they are excreted. Recirculation occurs about six times a day.
EHC may be interrupted by:
1. drugs: chelating agents, e.g. cholestyramine

2. ileal disease causing impaired reabsorption
3. bacterial overgrowth causing increased deconjugation.

Control of biliary secretion

1. Neural: parasympathetic stimulation increases bile secretion; sympathetic stimulation decreases bile secretion.
2. Hormonal: gastrin and secretin increase the volume and bicarbonate concentration of bile. CCK increases bile output.

Bile pigment changes (Table 5.9)

Table 5.9 Summary of urinary and faecal bile pigment changes

	Obstructive	*Hepatocellular failure with no obstruction*	*Haemolytic*
Urinary bilirubin	↑	Normal or ↑	None
Urinary urobilinogen	↓	Normal or ↑	↑
Faecal stercobilinogen	↓	Normal	↑

SMALL INTESTINE

INTESTINAL JUICE

Approximately 2 l/day

1. Brünner's glands produce an alkaline secretion (with mucus).
2. Paneth cells at the base of the crypts of Lieberkühn produce a watery secretion.
3. Villus enterocytes (columnar cells) secrete digestive enzymes, and this is the principal site of absorption.

Digestive enzymes (Table 5.10)

Table 5.10 Digestive enzymes and products

Digestive enzymes	*Substrate*	*Products*
Several peptidases	Polypeptides	Peptides
Amylase	Starch	Glucose, maltose and maltotriose
Lactase	Lactose	Glucose and galactose
Sucrase	Sucrose	Glucose and fructose
Maltase	Maltose	Glucose
Isomaltose	Isomaltose	Maltose and glucose
Lipases	Fats	Free fatty acids and monoglycerides
Enterokinase	Trypsinogen	Trypsin

Control of secretion

Stimulation of secretion

1. Vagal stimulation.
2. Intestinal hormones, especially CCK-PZ and secretin.
3. Brünner's glands are inhibited by sympathetic stimulation.

Disorders of secretion

Causes of increased gastrin levels

1. Gastrinoma, antral G-cell hyperplasia.
2. Retained and isolated antrum.
3. Zollinger–Ellison syndrome with intractable peptic ulcers and high gastric acid.
4. Vagotomy.
5. Achlorhydria, e.g. pernicious anaemia and gastric ulcer.
6. Short bowel syndrome.
7. Renal failure.
8. H_2 blockers and omeprazole.

Causes of decreased gastrin levels

1. Fasting states
2. Diseases causing hyperacidity, e.g. duodenal ulcer.

Causes of high VIP levels

VIPoma, resulting in the Werner–Morrison syndrome or WDHA syndrome (**W**atery **D**iarrhoea, **H**ypokalaemia and **A**chlorhydria).

Causes of high glucagon level

Glucagonoma (tumour of A cells in pancreatic islets) resulting in a necrolytic migratory erythema, diabetes, weight loss, anaemia and stomatitis.

Causes of a high somatostatin level

Somatostatinoma (flush, diabetes and hypochlorhydria).

SMALL INTESTINE MOTILITY (Table 5.11)

Table 5.11 Factors affecting small intestine motility.

Increased	*Decreased*
Parasympathetic activity	Sympathetic activity
Cholinergic agents	Adrenergic agents
Gastrin, CCK-PZ, motilin	Secretin
Prostaglandins	
Serotonin	

DIGESTION AND ABSORPTION IN THE SMALL INTESTINE:
(pages 233, 245, 255)

- Mainly occurs in the duodenum and upper jejunum, e.g. sugars, amino acids, salts, folic acid, and vitamins B and C via a passive transport system (monosaccharides and amino acids require carrier protein).
- Fatty acids, monoglycerides, cholesterol and fat-soluble vitamins A, D, E and K are released from micelles and are passively absorbed across the cell membrane.
- Little absorption takes place in the ileum except vitamin B_{12} and bile salts.
- Movement of water across the gastrointestinal mucosa is by passive diffusion and follows the transport of osmotically active solutes, e.g. Na^+, glucose, chloride and amino acids.

COLON

FUNCTIONS

1. Active absorption of Na^+ and Cl^- and passive absorption following the osmotic gradient established by Na^+ and Cl^- absorption.
2. Secretion of mucus, K^+, and HCO_3^-.

LARGE INTESTINE MOTILITY (Table 5.12)

Table 5.12 Factors affecting large intestine motility

Increased	*Decreased*
Parasympathetic activity	Sympathetic activity
Cholinergic agents	Anticholinergic agents
Distension (gastrocolic reflex)	Inflammation
Emotion	Emotion
CCK-PZ	
Laxatives	

ENDOCRINE PHYSIOLOGY

CLASSIFICATION OF HORMONES (see Table 5.13)

MECHANISMS OF HORMONE ACTION

On cell membrane

1. Via cyclic adenosine 3′,5′-monophosphate (cAMP) as a 'second messenger', e.g. most polypeptide hormones (ACTH, ADH, TSH,

Table 5.13 Hormone classification

Polypeptide	*Steroid*	*Amine*
Most hypothalamic hormones	Hormones of adrenal cortex, gonads and fetoplacental unit	Thyroid hormones Catecholamines
Hormones of anterior and posterior pituitary		
Hormones of the pancreas and GI tract		
Growth factors		

LH, PTH and glucagon), many biogenic amines and some prostaglandins.
—The first messenger is the hormone that binds to the membrane receptor and leads to the activation of the membrane-bound enzyme adenyl cyclase, which converts adenosine triphosphate to cyclic AMP (cAMP).
—cAMP exerts biologic activity via the phosphorylation of cAMP-dependent protein kinases, which can lead to the activation (e.g. via phosphorylase kinase, or phosphorylase) or the inactivation (e.g. via glycogen synthetase) of the substrate.

2. By membrane control of permeability (not via cyclic AMP). e.g. insulin-induced increased entry of glucose into cells. Other peptide hormones that may change membrane permeability include GH, ACTH, ADH and PTH.

In cytosol

Via a hormone–receptor complex, e.g. mainly steroid hormones, T3, T4 and somatomedin.

- Binding of free hormone to specific cytosol receptor proteins in target cells. The hormone–receptor complex then migrates to the nucleus, where the usual effect is to increase mRNA synthesis.

HYPOTHALAMIC REGULATORY HORMONES (see Table 5.14)

- Neurons from the supraoptic and paraventricular nuclei of the hypothalamus send axons to the posterior pituitary (neurohypophysis).
- The portal hypophyseal vessels form a vascular connection between the median eminence of the ventral hypothalamus and the anterior pituitary.

Table 5.14 Hypothalamic regulatory hormones

Hypothalamic hormone	*Pituitary hormone released*
Releasing hormones:	
Thyrotrophin-releasing hormone (TRH)	Thyroid-stimulating hormone (TSH) and prolactin Follicle-stimulating hormone (FSH) in men
Growth hormone-releasing hormone (GHRH)	Growth hormone (GH) Insulin, glucagon and gastrin release
Prolactin-releasing hormone (PRH)	Prolactin
Corticotrophin-releasing hormone (CRH)	ACTH
Gonadotrophin-releasing hormone (GnRH)	Luteinizing and follicle-stimulating hormone (LH and FSH)
Inhibiting hormones:	*Suppresses release of*:
Prolactin-inhibiting factor or dopamine (PIF)	Prolactin, luteotrophin
Growth hormone-inhibiting hormone or somatostatin	GH, TSH, FSH

ANTERIOR PITUITARY HORMONES

HISTOLOGY (Fig. 5.11)

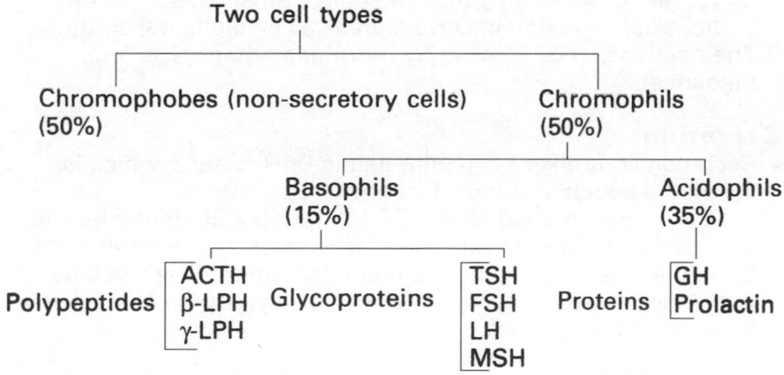

Fig. 5.11

ADRENOCORTICOTROPHIC HORMONE (ACTH)

Structure (Fig. 5.12)

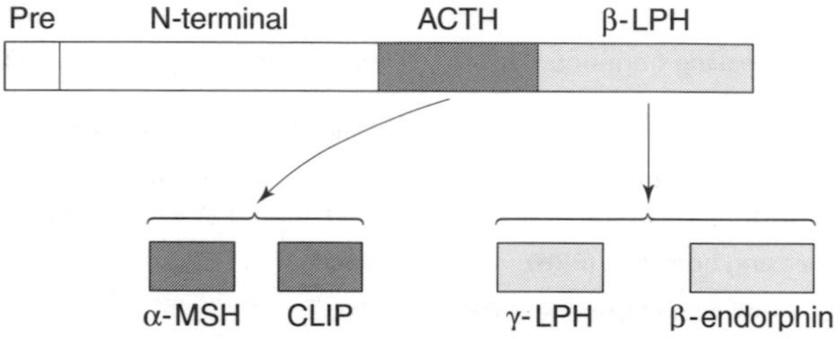

Fig. 5.12

Single-chain polypeptide (39 amino acids: first 24 essential for biological activity). ACTH, β-lipotrophin (β-LPH) and pro-γ-melanocyte-stimulating hormone (pro-γ-MSH) originate from a common precursor molecule, pro-opiocortin, which is synthesized in the hypothalamus and broken down in the anterior pituitary.

ACTH-related peptides

- These include β-LPH, γ-LPH, corticotrophin-like intermediate peptide (CLIP), endorphins (α β γ), met-enkephalin and leu-enkephalin (Fig. 5.12).
- Endogenous opiates: endorphins and enkephalins bind to morphine (opiate) receptors. They have an analgesic action and possibly function in certain areas as synaptic transmitters. Their action can be blocked by morphine antagonists (e.g. naloxone).

Secretion

- Secretion controlled by hypothalamic CRH release, which is subject to negative feedback control from cortisol.
- Striking circadian rhythm in ACTH output by pituitary which in turn causes a diurnal secretion of cortisol by the adrenal cortex. Lowest levels occur at midnight and maximum levels at 8.00 a.m. Loss of rhythm occurs in Cushing's syndrome, depression, heart failure and stress.

Stimuli for release

Stress, e.g. hypoglycaemia, surgery, exercise, fever

Actions

Acts via cAMP.

1. ↑ secretion of cortisol by the adrenal cortex
2. ↑ adrenal blood flow
3. ↑ cholesterol concentration → cortisol
4. ↑ protein synthesis in the adrenal cortex.

THYROID-STIMULATING HORMONE (TSH)

Structure

- Glycoprotein 209 amino acids and two subunits: α and β.
- α-Subunit common to LH, FSH and human chorionic gonadotrophin (HCG); β-subunit confers biological specificity and immunological properties.

Secretion

- Secreted in response to hypothalamic TRH, and subject to negative feedback that depends on plasma thyroid hormones (free T4 and T3) acting at hypothalamic and pituitary levels.
- Circadian rhythm.

Actions

1. Stimulates growth of the thyroid gland and increased iodine uptake.
2. Synthesis and release of T3 and T4 hormones.

LUTEINIZING HORMONE (LH) AND FOLLICLE-STIMULATING HORMONE (FSH)

Structure

Glycoproteins and each consists of two subunits: α subunit is common to FSH, LH and TSH and β-subunit is hormone-specific.

Secretion

- Secreted in response to gonadotrophin-releasing hormone (GnRH), and subject to feedback control from both oestrogen and androgen effects.
- **FSH** is elevated in early proliferative (follicular) phase. A fall occurs preceding ovulation; with a further brief rise at ovulation. Levels fall again in secretory (luteal) phase.
- **LH**: pattern of secretion similar to FSH.
- **Both** peak at mid-ovulatory cycle. LH peak higher than FSH. Triggered by rise in plasma oestradiol.

High levels of FSH and LH in:
Postmenopausal women
Primary gonadal failure
Kleinfelter syndrome

Low levels in:
Hypopituitarism

Actions

- **FSH** via FSH receptor on Sertoli cell.
  1. Females: controls the development and maturation of the Graffian follicle.

2. Males: influences growth of seminiferous tubules and spermatogenesis. Induces responsiveness to LH.

- **LH** via LH receptor on Leydig cells.
  1. Females: controls development of corpus luteum and secretion of progesterone.
  2. Males: increases production of testosterone by the Leydig cells.

MELANOCYTE-STIMULATING HORMONE (γ-MSH)

Structure

- Pro-opiocortin contains three components with MSH activity α-MSH (in ACTH component); β-MSH (in LPH component); α-MSH.
- Formed by enzyme degradation of pro-opiocortin and its ACTH and LPH components. Function unclear.

GROWTH HORMONE (GH, SOMATOTROPIN)

Structure

- Most abundant hormone in the pituitary
- Structurally similar to prolactin and placental lactogen.

Secretion

- Under hypothalamic control through GHRF and GHRIF (somatostatin).
- Somatomedins exhibit negative feedback control of GH secretion.
- Basal secretion low during the day with increased secretion during the first few hours of sleep.

Stimuli for release

Stress (emotion, fever and surgery)
Vigorous exercise
Insulin-induced hypoglycaemia
↑ circulating amino acids, e.g. protein meal, arginine infusion
Sleep
Glucagon
Bromocriptine

Stimuli for inhibition of release

Fatty acids
Somatostatin
Hyperglycaemia
↑ cortisol

Somatomedins

- Family of small peptides synthesized in the liver and other sites in response to growth hormone.
- Responsible for overall body growth in addition to other growth factors which affect individual tissues or organs.

- Primary somatomedins include insulin-like polypeptides (IGF-I and IGF-II). Other growth factors include nerve growth factor, epidermal growth factor, ovarian growth factor, fibroblast growth factor and thymosin. They also have insulin-like actions on carbohydrate and fat metabolism.

Actions
Mostly mediated by the somatomedins.
1. Raises blood sugar
2. Stimulates lipolysis.
3. Stimulates protein synthesis and cell proliferation: promotes positive nitrogen balance.
4. Stimulates growth of bone, cartilage and connective tissue.

PROLACTIN (PRL; LUTEOTROPIC HORMONE, LTH)

Structure
Single-chain polypeptide of 198 amino acids. Similar in structure to GH.

Secretion
- Under inhibitory control of PIF synthesized in the hypothalamus.
- Dopamine is physiologically the most important prolactin inhibiting factor (PIF).
- Secreted intermittently in pulses lasting about 90 min. Secretion highest at night and falls during the morning.

Stimuli for release

PRH, TRH
Exercise
Sleep (circadian rhythm)
Stress, e.g. surgery, myocardial infarction
Pregnancy/oestrogens / SSRI
Suckling/lactation
Puberty in girls

Pathological causes

Hypothalamic/pituitary diseases
Hypothyroidism
Renal failure
Drugs, e.g. L-dopa and dopamine agonists (bromocriptine)

Causes of decreased secretion

Reversal of above factors
PIF, i.e. dopamine
Drugs, e.g. L-dopa and dopamine agonists (bromocriptine)

Actions
1. Milk synthesis: induces and maintains lactation post-partum.
2. Responsible for inhibitory effect on ovaries and normal breast development.

POSTERIOR PITUITARY HORMONES

Produces two important hormones.
1. **Vasopressin (antidiuretic hormone, ADH)**
2. **Oxytocin**

Both synthesized in paraventricular and supraoptic nuclei, and transported via the hypothalamoneurohypophyseal tracts to the posterior pituitary. Secretion is through stimulation of cholinergic nerve fibres.

ADH

See pages 182–184.

OXYTOCIN

Structure
Nonapeptide

Secretion
Stimuli for release
1. Milk-ejection reflex
2. Coital reflex
3. Labour (2nd stage).

Actions
1. Uterine contraction
2. Milk ejection due to contraction of myoepithelial cells

ADRENAL CORTEX

STRUCTURE OF STEROID HORMONES

Basic structure for all steroid hormones is the cyclopentanoperhydrophenanthrene nucleus (Fig. 5.13)
Oestrogens: C_{18} steroids
Androgens: C_{19} steroids
Glucocorticoids, Mineralocorticoids, Progestogens } C_{21} steroids

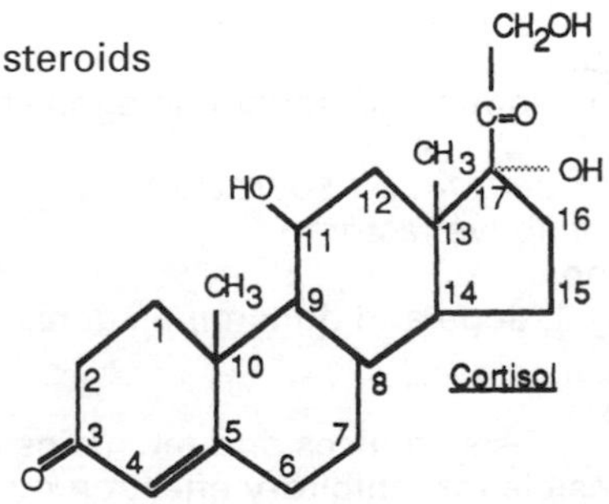

Fig. 5.13

Secretion

Table 5.15 Secretion of steroid hormones

Site of production	*Hormone*
Zona glomerulosa	Mineralocorticoids — aldosterone — deoxycorticosterone — corticosterone (also a glucocorticoid)
Zona fasiculata	Glucocorticoids (cortisol) Androgens (dehydroepiandrosterone, androstenedione, testosterone)
Zona reticularis	Oestrogens (oestradiol) Progestogens

BIOSYNTHESIS OF ADRENAL STEROIDS

- Occurs in adrenal cortex, testis and ovary.
- The rate-limiting step in the biosynthesis of adrenal steroids is the mitochondrial conversion of cholesterol to pregnenolone (Fig. 5.14).
- About 75% of plasma cortisol is bound to cortisol-binding globulin; 15% is bound to plasma albumin and 10% is unbound, which represents the physiologically active steroid.

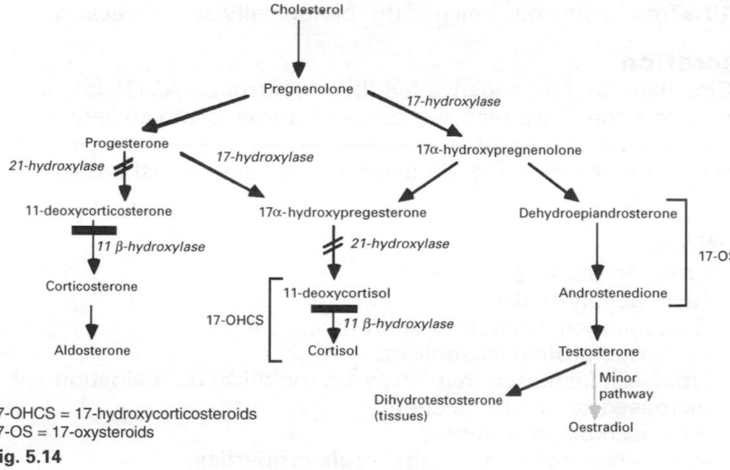

17-OHCS = 17-hydroxycorticosteroids
17-OS = 17-oxysteroids

Fig. 5.14

Urinary metabolites
1. Urinary free cortisol.
2. Urinary 17-hydroxycorticosteroids (17-OHCS). Increased levels with Cushing's disease and pregnancy.
3. Urinary 17-oxysteroids (17-OS)/17-ketosteroids (17-KS). Group of metabolites formed mainly from androgens, (adrenal, testicular or ovarian in origin). Increased levels with Cushing's syndrome, congenital adrenal hyperplasia, polycystic ovaries and some testicular tumours.

DISORDERS OF SECRETION

Congential adrenal hyperplasia

11β-hydroxylase defect: autosomal recessive
- Principal steroids excreted are androgens and 11-deoxycortisol metabolites.
- Clinical features include hypertension with virilization.

21-hydroxylase defect: autosomal recessive
- Increased excretion of androgens: 17-ketosteroid and 21-deoxysteroids in the blood and urine.
- Two types:
  1. Severe, with salt-losing syndrome in infancy.
  2. Mild, with virilism in female and pseudoprecocious puberty in male.

GLUCOCORTICOIDS

- Cortisol and corticosterone (secreted at 1/10th amount of cortisol).
- Bound to corticosteroid-binding globulin (CBG) or transcortin; 10% free in plasma, which is the biologically active fraction.

Secretion
- Circadian rhythm: negative feedback control on ACTH, but can be overridden by stress, e.g. severe trauma, acute anxiety, infections and surgery.
- Highest in the morning (around 8.00 am) and lowest around midnight.

Actions
Anti-insulin actions
1. Glycogenolysis (liver).
2. Gluconeogenesis from protein (liver).
3. Increased protein catabolism.
4. Lipolysis, increased free fatty acid mobilization, oxidation and increased ketone production.
5. Increased plasma glucose.
6. Anti-inflammatory and antiallergic properties.
7. Increased resistance to stress.
8. Some mineralocorticoid action.

9. Decreased lymphocytes and eosinophils; increased neutrophils, platelets and red blood cells.
10. Decreased protein matrix in bone. Increased urinary calcium.
11. Increased secretion of hydrochloric acid and pepsin.

MINERALOCORTICOIDS

Aldosterone

See pages 175–178.

SEX HORMONES

Androgens: testosterone, androstenedione, and dehydroepiandosterone
Oestrogens: oestradiol
Progesterone

ADRENAL MEDULLA

Consists of chromaffin cells which are derived from the primitive neuroectoderm, and have a common origin with ganglion cells of sympathetic nervous system.

CATECHOLAMINES

- Adrenal cells contain two catecholamines: noradrenaline (20%) and adrenaline (80%).
- Bound to ATP and protein and stored as membrane-bound granules, called chromaffin granules.

Synthesis and metabolism of catecholamines (Fig. 5.15)

- The plasma half-life of the catecholamines is 1–3 minutes.
- Sympathetic nerve endings take up the catecholamines from the circulation, which leads to non-enzymatic inactivation by intraneuronal storage and to enzymatic inactivation in the synaptic cleft.
- These transmitters are destroyed by the enzymes, monoamine oxidase (MAO) and catechol-o-methyltransferase (COMT).

Stimuli for release

Stress, Fear, Hypoglycaemia } → Hypothalamus → Adrenal medulla (via greater splanchnic nerves)

Actions

(See page 268)
Mediated principally by adrenaline.

1. Increased glycogenolysis (liver, muscle)
2. Increased gluconeogenesis
3. Increased lipolysis (fat cells).

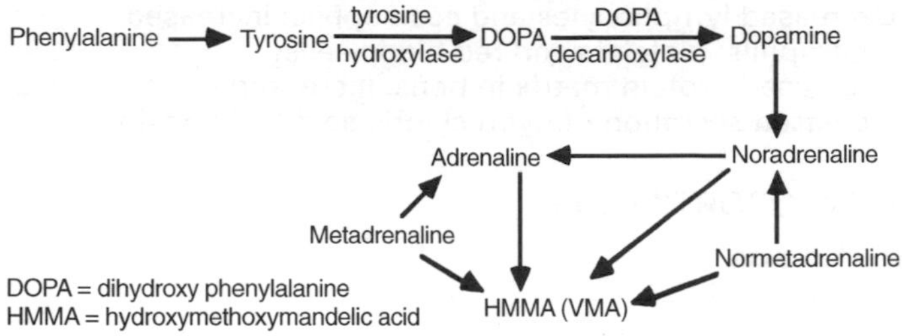

Fig. 5.15

THYROID

- Consists of colloid-filled follicles (acini) containing the thyroid hormones stored as thyroglobulin, surrounded by a layer of cubical epithelial cells.
- Parafollicular (C) cells are also found between the acini. Secrete calcitonin, which prevents calcium mobilization from bone and so lowers the calcium level in the blood.

THYROID HORMONE

Structure

Thyroid hormone secreted in two forms:

1. *Thyroxine (T_4)*: 90% of active thyroid hormone. Mainly protein bound: 75% to thyroxine-binding globulin (TBG), 15% to thyroxine-binding prealbumin (TBPA) and 10% to albumin. 0.05% exists as the free hormone which is the physiologically active form.
2. *Tri-iodothyronine (T_3)*: 0.5% exists as the free hormone. Five times as potent as T_4, with a shorter half-life and less strongly bound. T_3 is active hormone at tissue level. Approximately 1/3rd of T_4 is converted to T_3 in tissues.

Thyroid hormone biosynthesis (Fig. 5.16)

Secretion

Under control of TSH. Free thyroid hormone mediates negative feedback control of TSH, and acts directly on the anterior pituitary to decrease cell response to TRH.

Actions

1. Increases metabolic rate: increases O_2 consumption and metabolic rate of almost all metabolically active tissues.
2. Essential for skeletal growth and sexual maturation.
3. Essential for brain development and function.
4. Stimulates glucose absorption from the intestinal tract.
5. Lowers blood glucose.
6. Converts carotene to vitamin A.

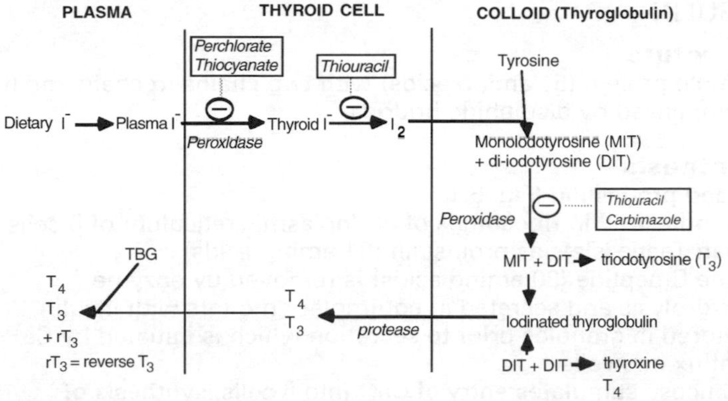

Fig. 5.16

7. Lowers circulating cholesterol level.
8. Potentiates the action of catecholamines on the heart (due to up-regulation of β-receptors).

Causes of increased serum thyroid-binding globulin
1. Pregnancy
2. Oestrogen therapy/oral contraceptive pill
3. Drugs, e.g. phenothiazines, clofibrate
4. Myxoedema.

Causes of decreased serum thyroid-binding globulin
1. Hypoproteinaemia, e.g. nephrotic syndrome
2. Acromegaly
3. Glucocorticoids, androgens and anabolic steroids
4. Thyrotoxicosis.

Causes of reduced TBG binding
1. Renal failure
2. Drug displacement by, e.g. salicylates, phenytoin, phenylbutazone.

PANCREAS

THE ISLET CELLS (Fig. 5.17)

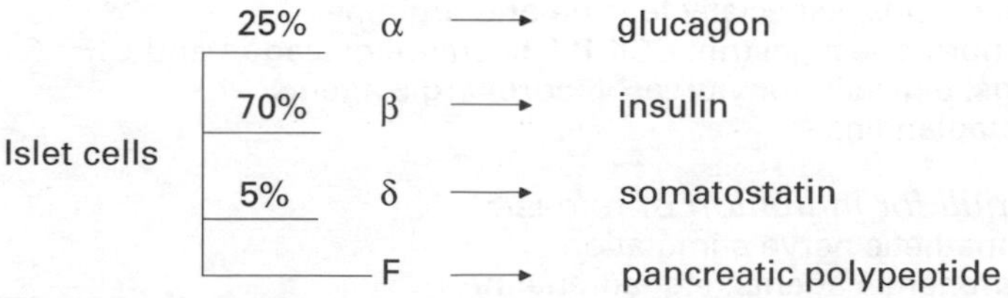

Fig. 5.17

INSULIN

Structure
Soluble protein (51 amino acids) with two chains (α chain and β chain) linked by disulphide bridges.

Synthesis
Folded pro-insulin (Fig. 5.18)
- Synthesized in ribosomes of endoplasmic reticulum of β-cells of pancreatic islets as proinsulin (81 amino acids).
- The C-peptide (30 amino acids) is removed by enzyme hydrolysis and secreted in equimolar amounts with insulin.
- Stored in granules prior to secretion which is initiated by Ca^{2+} influx into cells.
- Glucose stimulates entry of Ca^{2+} into β cells, synthesis of proinsulin and secretion of insulin, C-peptide and small amounts of proinsulin.
- 80% of insulin is degraded in the liver and kidneys.

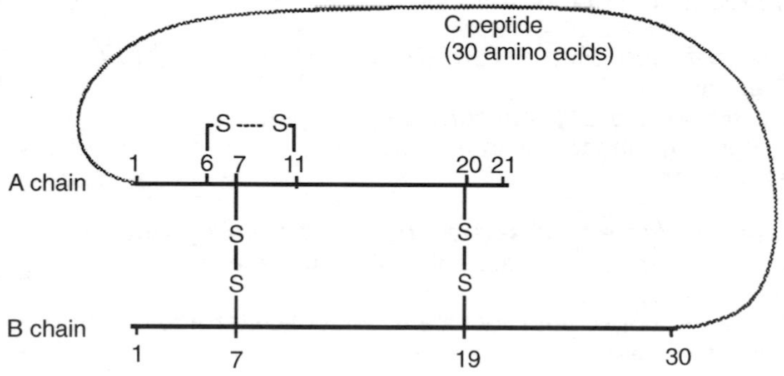

Fig. 5.18

Secretion
Stimuli for release
Glucose
Fatty acids and ketone bodies
Vagal nerve stimulation
Amino acids, especially leucine and arginine
Gut hormones: gastrin, CCK-PZ, secretin, glucagon and GIP
Drugs, e.g. sulphonylureas, β-adrenergic agents
Prostaglandins.

Stimuli for inhibition of release
Sympathetic nerve stimulation
α-Adrenergic agents, e.g. adrenaline
β-Blockers

Dopamine
Serotonin
Somatostatin

Insulin antagonists: include cortisol, adrenalin, glucagon, growth hormone, oestrogens and T_4.

Actions (see page 268)

Adipose tissue
Increased glucose entry
Increased fatty acid synthesis and lipid storage
Inhibition of lipolysis
Activation of lipoprotein lipase and hormone-sensitive lipase

Muscle
Increased glucose uptake
Increased glycogen synthesis
Increased amino acid uptake
Increased protein synthesis
Decreased protein catabolism.

Liver
Increased glucose uptake
Increased glycogen synthesis
Inhibition of gluconeogenesis
Increased lipogenesis
Inhibition of ketogenesis.

Effect of insulin on glucose transport
- Glucose influx increased by 15–20-fold by insulin.
- Transport is by means of facilitated diffusion carrier mechanism down a concentration gradient (*not* active transport), since intracellular glucose concentration is lower than extracellular.
- Insulin has no effect on glucose transport in brain, renal tubules, intestinal mucosa and red blood cells.

GLUCAGON

Structure
- Polypeptide (29 amino acids). Secreted by α cells of the pancreatic islets.
- Glucagon, secretin, VIP and GIP have some homologous amino acid sequences.
- Rapidly degraded in the tissues (especially in the liver and kidney) and by kallikrein in plasma.

Secretion
Stimuli for release
Amino acids
β-Adrenergic stimulation

Fasting, hypoglycaemia
Exercise
Gastrin, CCK and cortisol

Stimuli for inhibition of release
Glucose
Somatostatin
Free fatty acids
Ketones
Insulin

Actions (see page 268)
1. Glycogenolytic, gluconeogenic, lipolytic, ketogenic.
2. Stimulates secretion of GH, insulin and somatostatin.
3. Reduces intestinal motility and gastric acid secretion.

SOMATOSTATIN

- Synthesized as a large precursor molecule, and then cleaved to produce a prohormone, which undergoes further modification to produce the biologically active products, somatostatin 14 and 28.
- Somatostatin inhibits the release of thyrotropin from the pituitary gland and growth hormone release.
- It also acts as a neurotransmitter in other areas of brain, and has a wide range of inhibiting effects on the gastrointestinal tract.
- Octreotide is a structural analogue of somatostatin and has been used in treatment of acromegaly, thyrotropin-secreting adenomas and non-secreting pituitary adenomas.

PHYSIOLOGICAL RESPONSE OF MOTHER TO PREGNANCY

1. Cardiovascular changes
↑ CO, HR and SV
↑ blood flow to many tissues and organs
Compression of vena cava in supine position → ↓ VR, CO and BP (supine hypotensive syndrome).

2. Respiratory changes
↑ minute volume by 30–50%
↑ oxygen consumption by 20–30%
↑ basal metabolic rate
↓ lung volumes (cf: for restrictive lung disease).

3. Renal
↑ renal blood flow by 25%
↑ GFR by 50%
↑ clearance of urea, uric acid and creatinine (glucose and amino acids may be lost in urine).

4. Blood

↑ red cell mass and plasma volume
↓ plasma [Hb], [iron]: ↑ plasma [transferrin] and total iron-binding capacity
↓ [plasma protein]
↑ β-globulin and fibrinogen.

5. Endocrine

↑ placental hormone production
↑ plasma throxine and TBG

6. Nutrition

↑ 15% calorie requirement
↑ 50% protein requirement
↑ requirement for folate, calcium, phosphorus, Mg^{2+}, iron, vitamins A and C, zinc and iodine.

6. Biochemistry and clinical chemistry

CHAPTER CONTENTS

PART I: METABOLIC PATHWAYS

OVERVIEW OF MAJOR METABOLIC PATHWAYS AND CYCLES (Summarized in Fig. 6.1)

INTERRELATIONSHIP OF CARBOHYDRATE, FAT AND PROTEIN METABOLISM (Fig. 6.1)

Amino acids and lipids feed into the pathways of carbohydrate metabolism and the citric acid cycle, where they are degraded to hydrogen and carbon dioxide. The hydrogen ions are then oxidized to water by enzymes of the electron transport chain, and adenosine triphosphate (ATP) is generated.

TRICARBOXYLIC ACID (TCA) – CITRIC ACID CYCLE (Fig. 6.1)

- Final common pathway for the oxidation of carbohydrate, fat and some amino acids to CO_2 and H_2O.
- Takes place in the mitochondria.
- Oxaloacetate and acetyl-CoA condense to form citrate, which is then converted to oxaloacetate by a series of nine reactions. The net result is the conversion of the acetyl residues to two molecules of CO_2 and eight hydrogen atoms per turn of cycle, which enter the electron transport chain with the generation of two ATP molecules and oxaloacetate.
- Regulated by the availability of acetyl-CoA, oxaloacetate, NADH and FAD^+. The control enzymes are pyruvate dehydrogenase, citrate synthase, isocitrate dehydrogenase and α-ketoglutarate dehydrogenase.

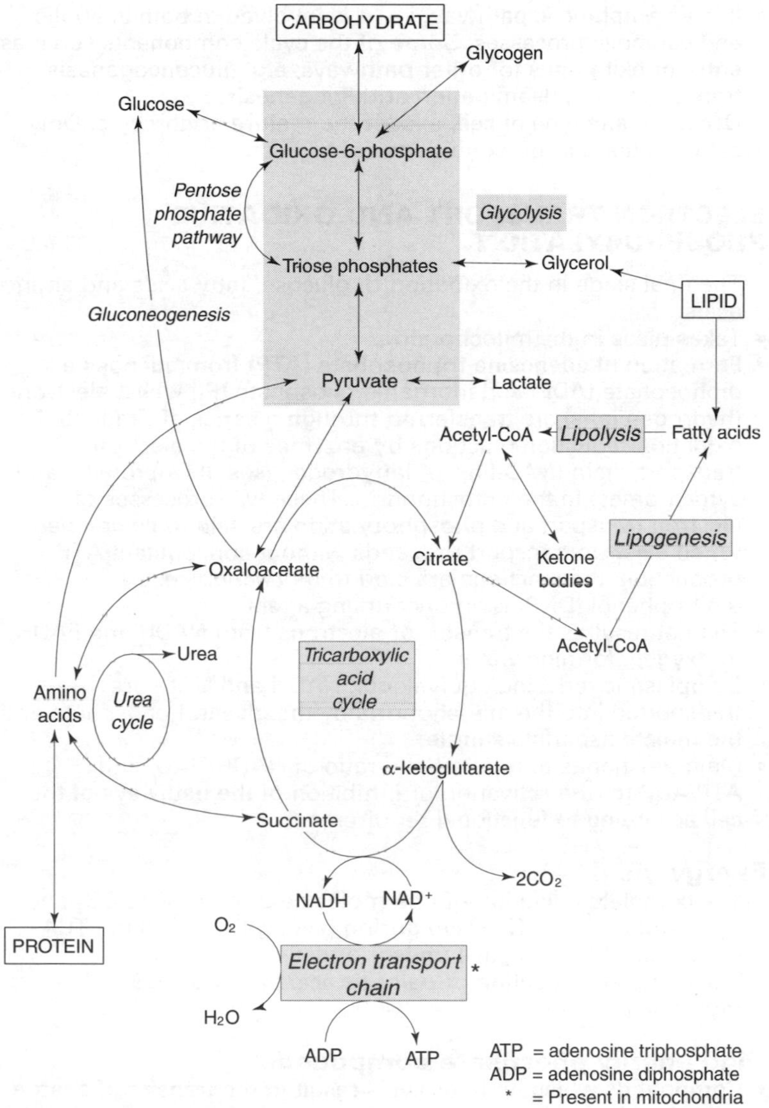
CARBOHYDRATE
Glycogen
Glucose
Glucose-6-phosphate
Pentose phosphate pathway
Glycolysis
Triose phosphates
Glycerol
LIPID
Gluconeogenesis
Pyruvate
Lactate
Acetyl-CoA
Lipolysis
Fatty acids
Lipogenesis
Oxaloacetate
Citrate
Ketone bodies
Acetyl-CoA
Urea
Amino acids
Urea cycle
Tricarboxylic acid cycle
α-ketoglutarate
Succinate
2CO2
NADH
NAD+
O2
Electron transport chain *
H2O
PROTEIN
ADP
ATP
ATP = adenosine triphosphate
ADP = adenosine diphosphate
* = Present in mitochondria

Fig. 6.1

- It is an amphibolic pathway, i.e. it is involved in both anabolic and catabolic processes. Some of the cycle components serve as entry or exit points for other pathways, e.g. gluconeogenesis, transamination, deamination and lipogenesis.
- Occurs in any type of cell, except the mature erythrocyte. Only active under aerobic conditions.

ELECTRON TRANSPORT AND OXIDATIVE PHOSPHORYLATION

- The final stage in the oxidation of glucose, fatty acids and amino acids.
- Takes place in the mitochondria.
- Formation of adenosine triphosphate (ATP) from adenosine diphosphate (ADP) and inorganic phosphate (Pi) whilst electrons (hydrogen ions) are transferred through a series of sequential oxidation-reduction reactions by enzymes of the electron transport chain (NAD-linked dehydrogenases, flavoproteins and cytochromes) in the mitochondria. These two processes of electron transport and phosphorylation are said to be *coupled*. When electron transport proceeds without concomitant ATP production, the reactions are said to be *uncoupled*; 2,4-dinitrophenol (DNP) is an uncoupling agent.
- The net result is the transfer of electrons from NADH and $FADH_2$ to oxygen, forming water.
- Cytoplasmic reducing equivalents, NADH and NAD^+ are transported into the mitochondria by the glycerol-phosphate and the malate-aspartate shuttle.
- Main function is to regulate the ratio of NADH/NAD^+ and ATP/ADP for the activation or inhibition of the pathways of the cell according to functional requirements.

Energy yield

- The complete oxidation of one molecule of *glucose* to CO_2 and H_2O produces 38 ATP. (Two during glycolysis, two in the TCA cycle and 34 by oxidative phosphorylation).
- The complete oxidation of *palmitic acid* produces 129 ATP molecules.

High energy phosphate compounds

- Compounds which on hydrolysis result in the transfer of a large quantity of energy.
- Most important is adenosine triphosphate (ATP). On hydrolysis to adenosine diphosphate (ADP) it liberates energy directly to processes as muscle contraction, active transport and the synthesis of many chemical compounds.
- Other high energy phosphate compounds include creatine phosphate, guanosine triphosphate (GTP), uridine triphosphate (UTP) and cytidine triphosphate (CTP).

CELL COMPARTMENTS AND ORGANELLES

Nucleus: gene expression
Cytoplasm: metabolism and protein synthesis
Mitochondria: energy production. Has its own genome.
Golgi apparatus: protein processing
Endoplasmic reticulum: protein modification
Lysosome: protein degradation
Peroxisome: oxidation reactions

CELL CYCLE

The sequence of events leading to cell reproduction (Fig. 6.2).

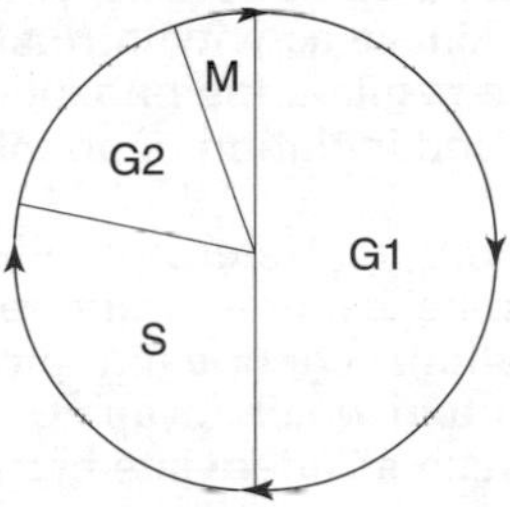

- G1 (6–12 hours); RNA and protein is synthesized; there is no DNA replication
- S (6–8 hours); period of DNA replication
- G2 (3–4 hours); during this period the cell has two complete diploid sets of chromosomes
- M (1 hour); mitosis, the period of actual cell division

Fig. 6.2

CELL SIGNALLING

Drugs, hormones, growth factors, metabolites and physical stimuli such as photons of light interact with cell receptors to stimulate second messenger systems to produce changes in the state of cells.
Ligand-gated ion channels, e.g. nicotinic acetylcholine (ACh) receptor. Binding of ACh results in a conformational change in the receptor and the rapid influx of sodium ions and depolarization of the cell membrane.
Voltage-gated ion channels, e.g. skeletal muscle sodium channel respond to changes in local membrane potentials.

Ion channel-associated diseases

Voltage-gated channels

- Long QT syndrome: mutation in potassium channel genes.
- Myotonia congenita: skeletal muscle chloride channel.

- Hyperkalaemic periodic paralysis: skeletal muscle sodium channel.
- Hypokalaemic periodic paralysis: skeletal muscle calcium channel.

Ligand-gated channels
- Cystic fibrosis: ATP-gated chloride channel
- Nocturnal frontal lobe epilepsy: neuronal nicotinic acetylcholine receptor
- Startle disease: glycine receptor

Membrane receptors
- Tyrosine kinase receptors, e.g. insulin receptor. Binding of ligand induces dimerization and autophosphorylation at a tyrosine residue. The tyrosine kinase activity intrinsic to the receptor is then activated and the result is the phosphorylation of cytoplasmic proteins and initiation of an intracellular cascade of second messengers.
- G-protein-coupled receptors. Heterotrimeric G-proteins are associated with seven-helical membrane receptors. On ligand binding the conformational change in the receptor leads to the activation of the G-protein which swaps GDP for GTP. Second messenger systems such as adenylate cyclase are then activated. G-proteins can be inhibitory or facilitatory.

Nuclear hormone superfamily: corticosteroids, vitamin D, retinoic acid, sex steroids. The lipophilic hormone crosses the plasma membrane and binds to intracellular receptors. The complex then travels to the nucleus where the receptor acts as a transcription factor by binding to recognition elements in the 5′ end of genes.

SECOND MESSENGER SYSTEMS

Activation or inhibition of adenylate cyclase (Fig. 6.3)

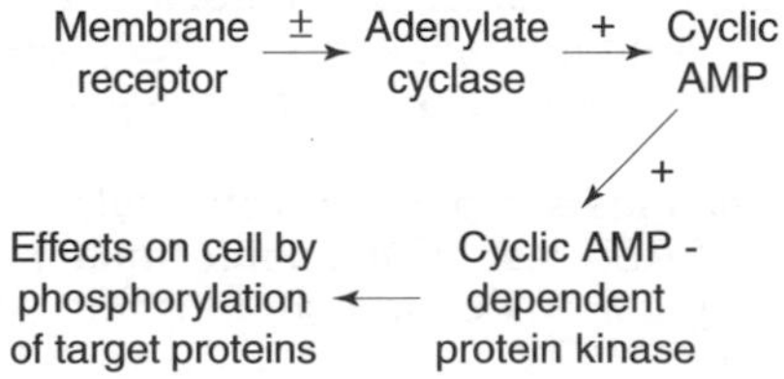

Fig. 6.3

Phospholipase activation

Both protein kinase C and inositol triphosphate act as second messengers in important cellular pathways.

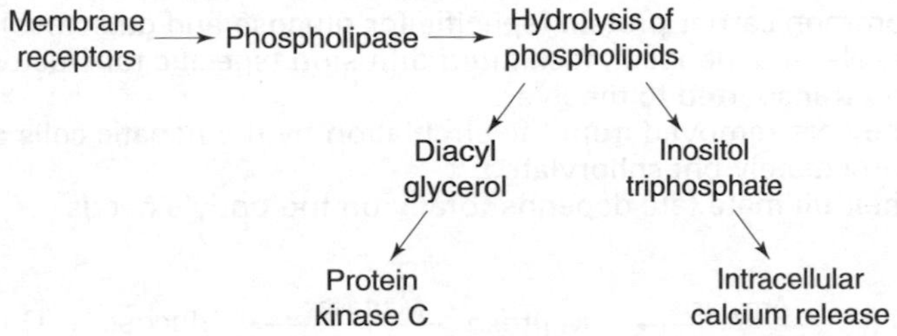

Fig. 6.4

CARBOHYDRATES AND METABOLISM

TYPES OF CARBOHYDRATE

Dietary carbohydrate consists mainly of starch, amylose, and amylopectin (polysaccharides), cellulose, sucrose, lactose and maltose (disaccharides), with small amounts of free glucose and fructose (monosaccharides). Most of the monosaccharides occurring in the body are D-isomers.
Complex carbohydrates include:

1. Glycoproteins: proteins which have oligosaccharides covalently attached to the protein chain, e.g. most membrane and plasma proteins. Sugars found in glycoproteins include glucose, galactose, mannose, galactosamine, arabinose, N-acetyl neuraminic acid or sialic acid.
2. Glycolipids: lipids containing a covalently attached oligosaccharide, e.g. many cell surface antigens.
3. Proteoglycans: complex molecules composed of a core protein with covalently attached glycosaminoglycans, e.g. chondroitin sulphate, hyaluronate and dermatan sulphate.
4. Glycosaminoglycans (GAGs): linear polysaccharides generally composed of alternating hexosamine and either uronic acid and/or galactose. Usually found as constituents of proteoglycans. The sugars found include N-acetylglucosamine, galactosamine, glucuronic acid and iduronic acids.

DIGESTION OF THREE MAIN CARBOHYDRATES

1. Carbohydrates are partially hydrolysed by salivary and pancreatic α-amylase to limit dextrans and oligosaccharides, maltose and maltotriose.

2. These are then hydrolysed by disaccharidases on the intestinal mucosal membrane to monosaccharides (glucose, fructose and galactose) (Fig. 6.5).
3. In the small intestine, the monosaccharides are absorbed either by an active cellular process, coupled to Na^+ transport using a common carrier protein (specific for glucose and galactose) or via Na^+ independent, facilitated diffusion (specific for fructose) and transported to the liver.
4. They are removed from the circulation by the hepatic cells and immediately phosphorylated.
5. Their ultimate fate depends totally on the body's needs.

Starch $\xrightarrow{\text{Amylase}}$ Maltose $\xrightarrow{\text{Maltase}}$ Glucose + Glucose

Lactose $\xrightarrow{\text{Lactase}}$ Glucose + Galactose

Sucrose $\xrightarrow{\text{Sucrase}}$ Glucose + Fructose

Fig. 6.5

CARBOHYDRATE METABOLISM

Fate of glucose

Glucose may be:

- oxidized to give energy, or
- stored as glycogen (muscle), or
- converted to triglycerides, amino acids and proteins.

GLYCOLYTIC PATHWAY (EMBDEN–MEYERHOF) (Fig. 6.6)

- The oxidation of glucose to pyruvate with generation of ATP in muscle, fat and non-gluconeogenic tissue. The pathway also metabolizes glucose derived from glycogen, galactose and fructose.
- May also occur in the absence of oxygen (i.e. anaerobic), when pyruvate is converted to lactate.
- Takes place in the cytoplasm.
- The net yield is two moles of ATP and NADH per glucose molecule.

Control of glycolysis

Control of glycolysis is through three regulatory enzymes:

1. hexokinase (glucokinase in the liver)
2. phosphofructokinase
3. pyruvate kinase.

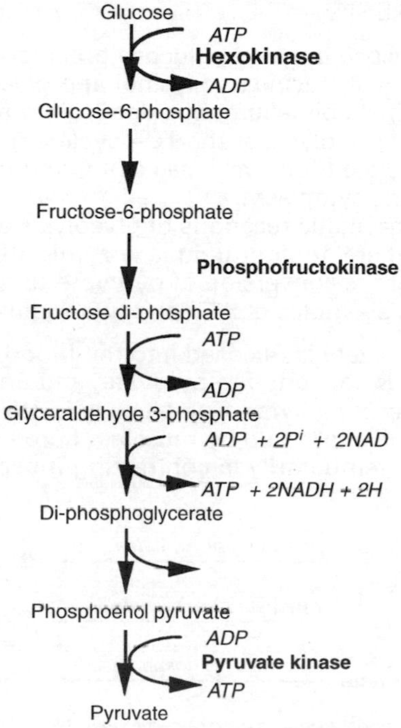

Fig. 6.6

Pyruvate kinase deficiency

Inadequate production of ATP reduces the activity of the Na^+/K^+-stimulated ATPase pump in the red blood cell. The cells swell and lyse resulting in a haemolytic anaemia.

Pyruvate is an intermediary product of glucose metabolism in the cytoplasm, that links together glycolysis, the TCA cycle, amino acid metabolism and fatty acid oxidation. It crosses the mitochondrial membrane and may:

1. React with coenzyme A to produce acetyl-CoA and NADH (*pyruvate dehydrogenase*), which can then enter the TCA cycle or lipid metabolism.
2. Condense with CO_2 to form oxaloacetate (*pyruvate carboxylase*).
3. Form alanine (*transamination*).
4. Be reconverted to glucose (*gluconeogenesis*).
5. Be reduced to lactate in the absence of oxygen (*lactate dehydrogenase*), with net synthesis of two molecules of ATP per molecule of glucose.

GLUCONEOGENESIS

- Synthesis of glucose from non-glucose precursors, especially amino acids (except leucine and lysine) and glycerol in the liver, kidney or intestinal epithelium, but also from any of the intermediates of glycolysis or the TCA cycle e.g. pyruvate, oxaloacetate, lactate (Cori cycle, see Note) and fructose.
- Takes place in the cytoplasm.
- Generally the enzymatic reactions of glycolysis are reversible, but in addition there are four unique enzymic steps (Fig. 6.7):
- The net result of the conversion of pyruvate to glucose is the consumption of six moles of ATP and two moles of NADH.

Note: Cori cycle. Lactate is released into the blood and travels to the liver, where it is converted to pyruvate, and finally to glucose, by the gluconeogenic pathway. The glucose is released into the circulation where it is taken up by muscle. Therefore, lactic acid production occurs temporarily in contracting muscles.

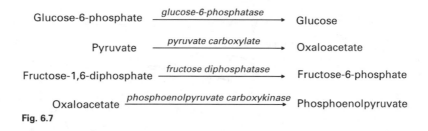

Glucose-6-phosphate $\xrightarrow{\textit{glucose-6-phosphatase}}$ Glucose

Pyruvate $\xrightarrow{\textit{pyruvate carboxylate}}$ Oxaloacetate

Fructose-1,6-diphosphate $\xrightarrow{\textit{fructose diphosphatase}}$ Fructose-6-phosphate

Oxaloacetate $\xrightarrow{\textit{phosphoenolpyruvate carboxykinase}}$ Phosphoenolpyruvate

Fig. 6.7

Functions

1. Important during starvation and interdigestive periods (especially at night) to maintain a steady blood glucose for brain cell metabolism. During fasting, protein is the most important glucose source.
2. During severe exercise, gluconeogenesis allows the use of lactate from anaerobic glycolysis and of glycerol from fat breakdown.
3. Allows the use of dietary protein in carbohydrate pathways after disposing of the amino acid nitrogen as urea.

LACTATE PRODUCTION

During strenuous muscular activity, glycogenolysis is stimulated and the resulting glucose-6-phosphate (G-6-P) is further metabolized by the glycolytic pathway and then by oxidation within the TCA cycle to supply the necessary energy. When the rate of glycolysis exceeds the availability of oxygen, glucose is converted to lactate by the muscle *anaerobic* glycolytic pathway.

$$\text{Glucose} \rightarrow 2\text{Lactate} + 2H^+$$

Pathological lactic acidosis

High blood lactate levels (>5 mmol) can be due to increased production (i.e. increased rate of anaerobic glycolysis, e.g. in severe illnesses) or decreased utilization (i.e. impairment of the TCA cycle or gluconeogenesis, e.g. phenformin) or both, as in tissue hypoxia.

Causes

See page 171.

PENTOSE PHOSPHATE PATHWAY OR HEXOSE MONOPHOSPHATE SHUNT (Fig. 6.8)

- Takes place in the cytoplasm. Occurs in muscle, liver, fat cells, thyroid, lactating mammary gland and erythrocytes.
- Consist of two branches, an oxidative and non-oxidative branch.
- The net result is the production of 12 NADPH, 6 CO_2 and one glyceraldehyde-3-phosphate molecule for each glucose-6-phosphate molecule passing through the pathway.

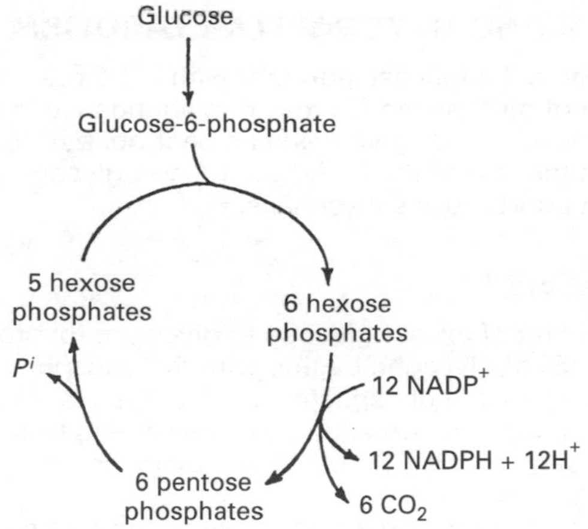

Fig. 6.8

Main functions

1. Provides reducing equivalents, e.g. reduced nicotinamide adenine dinucleotide phosphate (NADPH) for the reductive synthesis of fatty acids, cholesterol and other steroids, and for maintenance of glutathione in a reduced form inside erythrocytes. Two dehydrogenases are involved: *glucose-6-phosphate-dehydrogenase (G6PDH)* and *6-phosphogluconate dehydrogenase* (Fig. 6.9).

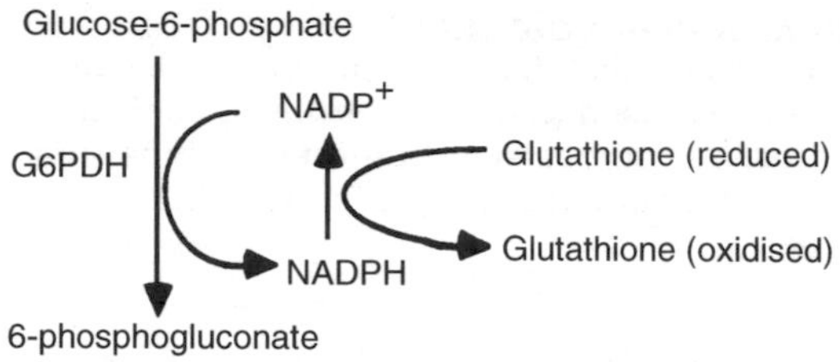

Fig. 6.9

2. Source of pentoses, e.g. ribose for nucleotide and nucleic acid synthesis.
3. Oxidizes glucose to CO_2.
4. Maintenance of integrity of red cell membrane as follows.
   (i) Production of NADPH which maintains glutathione in reduced state. The most important disease of the pathway is G6PDH deficiency.
   (ii) Glycolysis to produce 2 ATP which maintains Na^+ and K^+ distribution across the cell membrane.

GLYCOGEN AND GLYCOGEN METABOLISM

Glycogen is an α-1,4 glucose polymer with α-1,6 branches. It is the storage form of glucose, and is found in abundance in the liver, kidney and muscle. Liver glycogen can be mobilized for the release of glucose to the rest of the body, but muscle glycogen can only be used to support muscle glycolysis.

GLYCOGENESIS

- The conversion of excess glucose to glycogen for storage.
- The synthesis of glycogen begins with the phosphorylation of glucose to glucose-6-phosphate, which is then isomerized to glucose-1-phosphate and added to a glycogen primer, uridine diphosphoglucose (UDPG). Catalysed by *glycogen synthetase*, which exists in two forms:
  1. an active (D or dependent) form, since the enzyme is active in the absence of glucose-6-phosphate
  2. an inactive (L or independent) form, which is in active in the absence of glucose-6-phosphate.

GLYCOGENOLYSIS

- Glycogen is degraded in two distinct steps:
  1. *Phosphorylase* splits the α-1,4 linkage, releasing glucose-1-phosphate.
  2. A debranching enzyme then splits the α-1,6 bond producing free glucose.

- The glucose-1-phosphate can then be isomerized to glucose-6-phosphate and either enter glycolysis or be hydrolysed to free glucose.
- Phosphorylase b is the inactive form of the enzyme and is converted to the active form, phosphorylase a, by phosphorylation catalysed by phosphorylase b kinase.

Regulation of glycogen synthesis and degradation by cyclic AMP

Cyclic AMP (cyclic adenosine 3′,5′-monophosphate) activates a cAMP-dependent protein kinase, which in turn activates both phosphorylase b kinase and glycogen synthetase kinase. This results in glycogen breakdown with inhibition of glycogen synthesis. The enzymes that promote glycogenolysis are active in the phospho-forms and inactive in their dephospho-form. The reverse is true for glycogen synthetase.

Glycogenesis is promoted by glycogen synthetase.

Glycogenolysis is promoted by phosphorylase.

Adrenaline or glucagon activate glycogen degradation and inhibit glycogen synthesis.

Insulin activates glycogen synthesis and inhibits glycogen degradation (see page 268).

ABNORMAL STATES OF CARBOHYDRATE METABOLISM (Table 6.1)

INBORN ERRORS OF CARBOHYDRATE METABOLISM (see Table 6.1)

STARVATION AND KETOGENESIS

- During fasting, endogenous triglycerides in adipose tissue are reconverted to fatty acids and glycerol by lipolysis.
- Blood glucose levels are maintained initially by increased liver gluconogenesis using glycerol (which enters the pathway at the triose phosphate stage) and amino acids (mainly from muscle).
- This is supplemented by conversion of the fatty acids to acetyl coA, and also into ketone bodies, via β-hydroxy-3-methylglutaryl-coA (HMG-CoA). The ketone bodies include acetone, acetoacetate and β-hydroxybutyrate, and are used as a fuel by all cells except those of the brain.
- On prolonged starvation, brain cells can also adapt to using ketone bodies as a major source of fuel. The liver is the chief ketogenic organ.
- Ketosis occurs whenever the rate of hepatic ketone body production exceeds the rate of peripheral utilization as in severe diabetes, starvation, during anaesthesia and with a high fat, low carbohydrate diet.

Table 6.1 Inborn errors of carbohydrate metabolism (Fig. 6.10)

Disease	*Enzyme defect*	*Clinical features*	*Diagnosis*	*Treatment*
1. Glycogen storage diseases Incidence 1: 60 000 births		1. Recurrent hypoglycaemia 2. Hepatomegaly 3. Muscle weakness 4. Cardiac failure		
Type I von Gierke's	Glucose-6-phosphatase (G-6-P → glucose + P_i)	Usually presents in infancy, with features as above (plus metabolic acidosis, hyperlipidaemia, hyperuricaemia and ketosis)	Liver biopsy* and liver enzyme analysis	Frequent glucose feeds and restriction of fructose and galactose intake
Type II Pompe's	Lysosomal α-glucosidase (Glycogen → glucose)	Presents at or soon after birth, with features as above and cardiorespiratory failure	Muscle/liver biopsy* and enzyme analysis on muscle, fibroblasts or amniotic cells	Supportive only
Type III Cori's limit dextrinosis and *Type IV* Andersen's	Debranching and branching enzyme (Limit dextran → glucose)	Types III and IV have a presentation similar to Type I, but milder	Muscle/liver biopsy* and leucocyte enzyme levels	
Type V McArdle's	Muscle phosphorylase (Glycogen → G-1-P)	Presents in adult life with muscle cramps on exercise, myoglobinuria, muscle weakness and wasting but *no* hypoglycaemia	Muscle biopsy*, histochemistry or enzyme analysis. No normal rise in blood lactate after exertion	

Table 6.1 *(cont.)*

Disease	*Enzyme defect*	*Clinical features*	*Diagnosis*	*Treatment*
2. Galactosaemia Incidence 1 : 60 000 births	Galactose-1-phosphate-uridyl transferase (Galactose → glucose)	Presents at commencement of milk feeds with failure to thrive, vomiting, diarrhoea and jaundice. Also hepatomegaly, ascites, cataracts and mental retardation	Urine contains galactose (Clinitest +ve, Clinistix –ve) Erythrocyte enzyme analysis (for prenatal and carrier state diagnosis)	Lactose-free diet
3. Fructose intolerance Incidence 1 : 20 000 births	Fructose-1-phosphate-aldolase (F-1-P → DHA-P + α-glycerophosphate)	Provoked by fructose-containing foods Nausea, vomiting, abdominal pain, hypoglycaemia, growth retardation hepatomegaly, liver failure and aminoaciduria	Dietary history (onset of symptoms with introduction of sucrose into the diet) Fructosaemia and fructosuria after sucrose ingestion Liver enzyme analysis	Sucrose/fructose-free diet
4. Benign/essential fructosuria Incidence 1 : 130 000 births	Fructokinase	Asymptomatic	Fructosaemia and fructosuria after ingestion	

*Excessive glycogen deposition

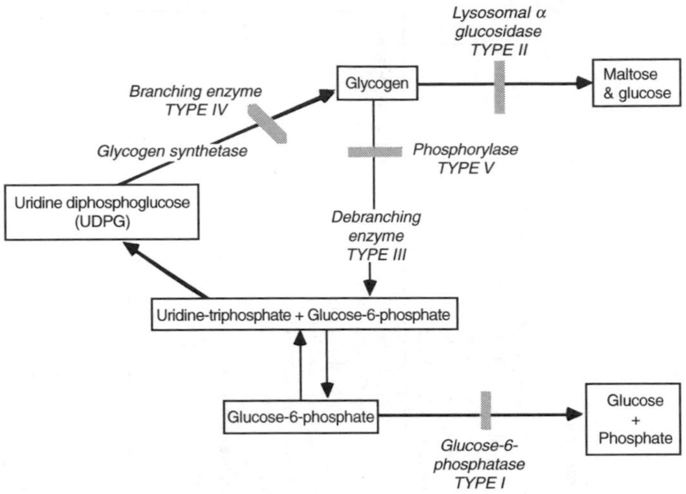

Fig. 6.10

DIABETIC KETOACIDOSIS

The mechanism of ketosis in diabetes is the same as that in fasting, but is more severe and occurs in the presence of hyperglycaemia. In prolonged fasting the supply of glucose to the cells is insufficient for normal glycolysis or lipolysis. With insulin deficiency, there is simply an impaired uptake of glucose into the cells, resulting in an intracellular glucose deficiency. Excessive lipolysis occurs, causing ketosis and acidosis.

SPONTANEOUS HYPOGLYCAEMIA

Causes

1. Glycogen storage diseases (Types I & III)
2. Galactosaemia
3. Fructose intolerance
4. Leucine sensitivity
5. Addison's disease } – due to inhibition of gluconeogenesis
6. Hypopituitarism }
7. Post-gastrectomy syndrome
8. β-Cell islet tumours
9. Alcoholic cirrhosis, due to inhibition of gluconeogenesis and glycogenolysis
10. Hypothyroidism

but not in:

1. Glycogen storage diseases (Types II and V)
2. Gaucher's disease
3. Glucose-6-phosphate dehydrogenase (G6PDH) deficiency.

LIPIDS AND METABOLISM

MAIN CLASSES OF LIPIDS

FATTY ACIDS

- Long, straight chain monocarboxylic acids with an even number of carbon atoms (usually between 16 and 24).
  $CH_3.CH_2.CH_2.CH_2.COOH$
- Classified as:
  Saturated fatty acids (i.e. no double bonds) e.g. palmitic (16 C) and stearic (18 C) acids or
  Unsaturated fatty acids (i.e. one or more double bonds) e.g. oleic, linoleic and arachidonic acids.
- Fatty acids may be esterified with glycerol to form glycerides, or they may be free fatty acids (FFA) or non-esterified free fatty acids (NEFA).
- *Essential fatty acids:* certain polyunsaturated fatty acids cannot be synthesized, e.g. linoleic and linolenic acids. They may function as:
  1. Precursors of prostaglandins (see Prostanoids, page 248).
  2. Confer on membrane phospholipids many of the properties associated with membrane function.

TRIGLYCERIDES

- Major dietary lipids of nutritional value. They are degraded in the small intestine by lipases into monoglycerides, fatty acids and glycerol.
- Esters of glycerol with three fatty acids.

$CH_2.O$ — FA
|
$CH_2.O$ — FA
|
$CH_2.O$ — FA

- Mostly resynthesized into triglycerides in mucosal cells, and transported via the lymphatic system as chylomicrons into the systemic circulation.
- Adipose tissue and liver are the major sites of endogenous triglyceride synthesis. Transported from the liver as VLDL.

PHOSPHOLIPIDS

Phosphoglycerides and sphingomyelin (Fig. 6.11).

- Triglycerides with one of the fatty acid residues replaced by a nitrogenous base, e.g. choline (phosphatidylcholine or lecithin), ethanolamine (phosphatidylethanolamine), serine or inositol (phosphatidylinositol), and linked to the glycerol via a phosphate residue.

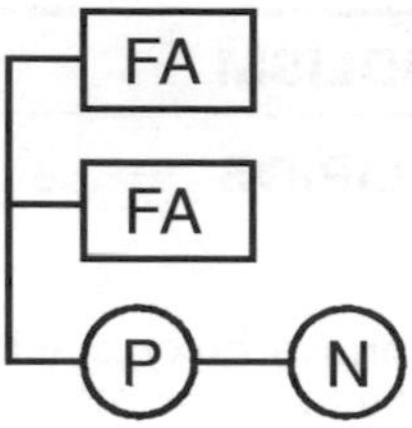

Fig. 6.11

- Mainly synthesized in the mucosa of the small intestine and in the liver.
- Important constituents of biological membranes and of the plasma lipoproteins.
- Includes the sphingolipid class which are characterized by the presence of the base sphingosine and comprise the ceramides, cerebrosides, sulphatides, gangliosides and sphingomyelin; all components of white matter in the central nervous system.

CHOLESTEROL (Fig. 6.12)

- Major constituent of the plasma membrane and of plasma lipoproteins. Widely distributed in all cells, but particularly nervous tissue.
- Two sources of cholesterol: *dietary cholesterol* (mostly triglycerides) ~ 70 g/day and *de novo synthesis* from acetate.

OTHERS

Other lipids of clinical significance include carotene, vitamins A, D, E and K.

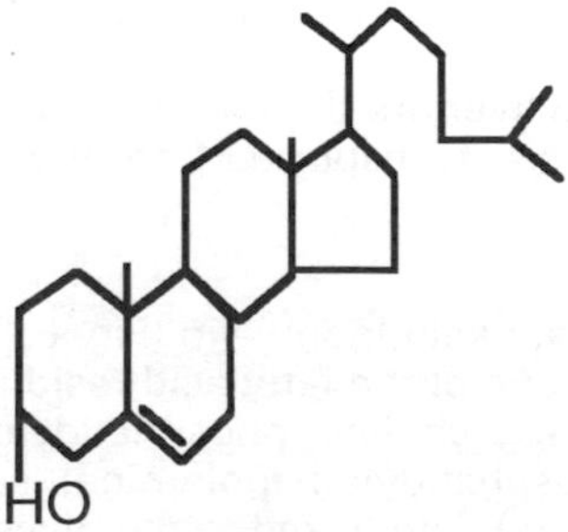

Fig. 6.12

DIGESTION OF FATS

- The entry of fats into the duodenum causes the release of pancreozymin-cholecystokinin, which in turn stimulates evacuation of the gall bladder.
- Hydrolysis of dietary triglycerides by pancreatic lipase takes place in the small intestine. The resulting free fatty acids, glycerol and monoglycerides are emulsified by bile salts and form micelles which are then absorbed along the brush border of mucosal cells.
- Small fatty acids enter the portal circulation bound to albumin. Larger ones are re-esterified within the mucosal cell into triglycerides which combine with lesser amounts of protein, phospholipid and cholesterol to create chylomicrons.
- Chylomicrons represent triglycerides and esters of cholesterol, with a coating of phospholipid, protein and cholesterol. These enter the lymphatic system and are transported via the thoracic duct to the bloodstream.
- The main sites for removal of chylomicrons are the muscle and liver. *Lipoprotein lipase*, an enzyme bound to the capillary endothelium of extrahepatic tissues, hydrolyses triglycerides in chylomicrons, and VLDL into free fatty acids and glycerol. After entering adipose tissue or muscle, these compounds are esterified and stored.
- The smaller remnant particles contain mainly cholesterol, and pass to the liver where they are metabolized further.

LIPID TRANSPORT: LIPOPROTEINS (Table 6.2 and Fig. 6.13)

- In plasma, free fatty acids (FFA) are bound to albumin. Other lipids (e.g. cholesterol, triglycerides and phospholipids) circulate with carrier apoproteins to form a series of soluble lipoprotein complexes. In general, the lipoproteins consist of a hydrophobic core of cholesterol and triglyceride esters surrounded by phospholipid and protein.
- Most endogenous cholesterol and triglycerides formed in the liver are transported from the liver as VLDL. In the peripheral tissues triglycerides are removed in the same way as chylomicrons. The smaller complex is further degraded via intermediate density lipoprotein (IDL) to form LDL, which is mainly composed of cholesterol. Most cells have surface receptors for LDL. LDL is bound and enters the cells by a process of receptor-mediated endocytosis, where the cholesterol is released and which in turn suppresses endogenous cholesterol synthesis.
- HDL carries the cholesterol formed peripherally from the peripheral tissues to the liver, to be excreted in the bile. An enzyme *lecithin-cholesterolacyl transferase (LCAT)* is associated

Table 6.2 Lipids and metabolism

	Chylomicrons (CM)	*Low density or β-lipoprotein (LDL)*	*Very low density or pre-β-lipoprotein (VLDL)*	*High density α-lipoprotein (HDL)*
Site of synthesis	Intestine	In blood and liver from VLDL	Liver and intestine	Liver and intestine
Function	Transport of dietary fat from the intestine to the liver and adipose tissue. The triglycerides are hydrolysed by lipoprotein lipase, and the cholesterol rich remnants are taken up by the liver	Transport of cholesterol to the tissues. LDL is removed by a receptor-mediated process	Transport of endogenous triglycerides from the liver. Degraded by lipoprotein lipase, resulting in the production of IDL*, then LDL	Transport of cholesterol from the plasma to the liver for excretion
Diameter (nm)	100–1000	25	50	10
Apoprotein†	A, B, C	B	B, C	A, C
% Triglyceride	85	10	50	10
% Cholesterol	4	50	20	15
% Protein	1	20	7	45

*IDL, intermediate density lipoprotein
†Nine apolipoproteins: Apo A-I, A-II, A-IV, B, C-I, C-II, C-III, D and E have been isolated and characterized.

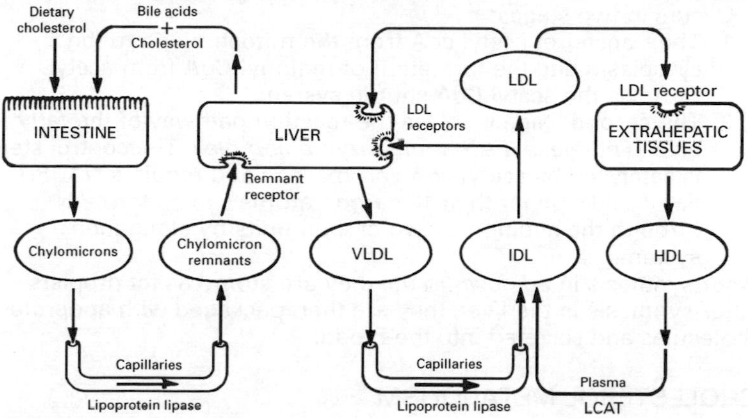

Fig. 6.13

with HDL and esterifies cholesterol. In LCAT deficiency, free unesterified cholesterol accumulates in the tissues.
HDL levels increase with: age, exercise, fish diet and alcohol.
HDL levels decrease with: progestin-type contraceptives, androgens, smoking, obesity and dietary carbohydrates.

LIPID METABOLISM

LIPOLYSIS

- Adipose tissue also contains an enzyme, *hormone-sensitive lipase (HSL)*, that hydrolyses triglycerides to produce fatty acids and glycerol. HSL is activated by catecholamines, ACTH, TSH and glucagon and inhibited by insulin, which stimulates glucose uptake for lipogenesis.
- The fatty acids released from adipose tissue are either bound to plasma albumin or circulate as free fatty acids (FFA) or non-esterified fatty acids (NEFA) and are taken up by the peripheral tissues for oxidation.
- *β-Oxidation of fatty acids:* is the process of degradation of fatty acids for energy and involves the removal of two carbon units at a time. It takes place in the mitochondria of the liver and muscle and results in the formation of acetyl coA and fatty acid residue.

LIPOGENESIS

- Synthesis of triglycerides from fatty acids, glycerophosphate and non-fat materials, especially carbohydrate.
- Occurs mainly in the liver, but also in the adipose tissue within the microsomes. Takes place in the cytoplasm.

- Occurs in two stages:
  1. The transfer of acetyl coA from the mitochondria to the cytoplasm and the formation of malonyl-CoA from acetyl-CoA, via the acetyl CoA shuttle system.
  2. The second stage involves the reaction pathway of the *fatty acid synthetase (FAS) multienzyme complex*. The control step is catalysed by acetyl-coA carboxylase and requires NADPH. Fatty acids longer than 16 carbon atoms can be formed through the addition of two carbon units by elongation systems.

After synthesis in *adipose tissue*, they are stored as fat droplets. After synthesis in the *liver*, they are then packaged with apoprotein molecules and secreted into the blood.

CHOLESTEROL METABOLISM

- *Hydroxymethyl-glutaryl-CoA reductase (HMGCoA reductase)* is a key enzyme that catalyses the reduction of β-hydroxy-β-methylglutaryl-coenzyme A (HMG-CoA) to mevalonate and regulates the activity of the pathway for cholesterol synthesis from acetate.
- The greater the dietary intake of cholesterol, the lower the rate of endogenous cholesterol biosynthesis in the liver and adrenal cortex. Synthesis in the peripheral tissues is regulated by the plasma LDL level. Diets high in fat or carbohydrate increase hepatic cholesterol synthesis.

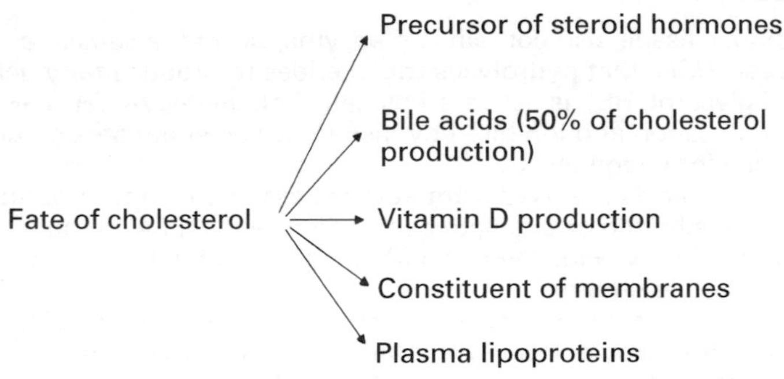

Fig. 6.14

PROSTANOID (EICOSANOID) METABOLISM

1. Prostaglandins (PGs)
   20-carbon unsaturated fatty acids containing a 5-carbon cyclopentane ring.
   Each *series* (A,B,E,F) has a different cyclopentane ring.
   Each *subset* ($_{1,2,3,4,}$) denotes the degree of unsaturation of hydrocarbon chain.

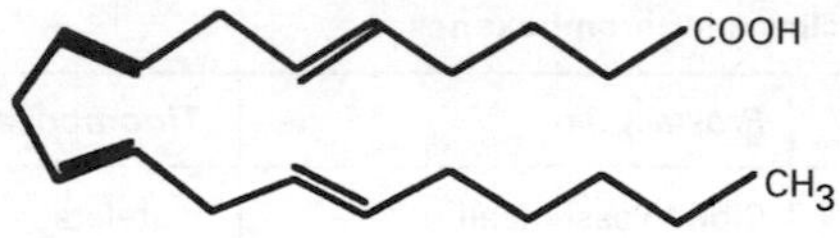

Fig. 6.15

2. Prostacyclin
3. Thromboxanes (TX)
4. Leucotrienes (LT).

PATHWAYS OF SYNTHESIS AND METABOLISM

Synthesized in almost any tissue. The lung is most important site for breakdown.

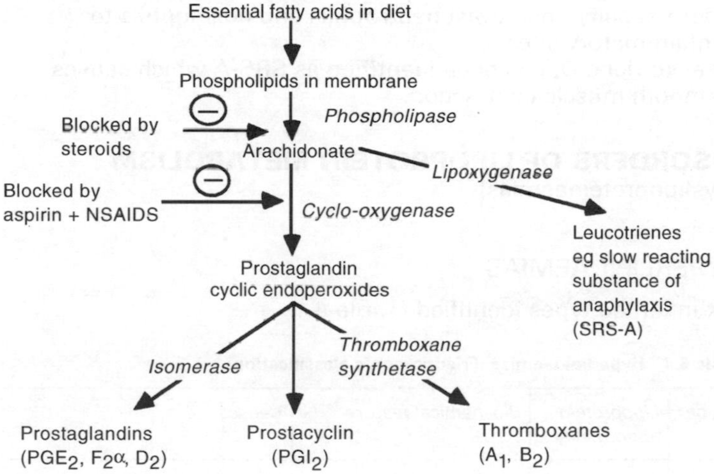

Fig. 6.16

PHARMACOLOGICAL EFFECTS

Variable effects on smooth muscle and blood vessels depending on the prostaglandin series.

COMPARISON OF PROSTACYCLINS AND THROMBOXANES (Table 6.3)

THE LEUKOTRIENES

- Synthesized by leucocytes. Mediators of inflammation and allergic reactions.

Table 6.3 Prostacyclins and thromboxanes

	Prostacyclin	*Thromboxanes*
Site of synthesis	Blood vessel wall	Platelets
Platelet aggregation	Inhibited	Stimulated
Coronary arteries	Relaxed (vasodilatation)	Constricted (vasoconstriction)
Blood pressure	Lowered	Raised
Smooth muscle	Relaxation PGE_1 and E_2 inhibits motility of non-pregnant uterus but increases contraction of pregnant uterus	Contraction

- Produce arteriolar and bronchoconstriction, increase vascular permeability and attract neutrophils and eosinophils to inflammatory sites.
- Leukotriene D_4 has been identified as SRS-A which causes smooth muscle contraction.

DISORDERS OF LIPOPROTEIN METABOLISM
(Dyslipoproteinaemias)

HYPERLIPIDAEMIAS

Six inherited types identified (Table 6.4).

Table 6.4 Hyperlipidaemias (Friedrickson's classification)

*Type**	*Lipoprotein abnormality*	*Biochemical feature*	*Causes*
I	↑Chylomicron	Marked hypertriglyceridaemia (↑ TG)	1° Usually familial (lipoprotein lipase deficiency: autosomal recessive)
IIa	↑ LDL	Hypercholesterolaemia with normal triglycerides (↑ CHOL)	1° Familial hypercholesterolaemia (absence or deficiency of normal receptor for LDL: autosomal dominant) 2° Hypothyroidism, obstructive jaundice, nephrotic syndrome, pregnancy, diabetes mellitus, obesity
IIb	↑LDL and VLDL	Familial combined hyperlipidaemia (1° ↑ TG + CHOL)	1° Usually familial

Table 6.4 *(cont.)*

*Type**	*Lipoprotein abnormality*	*Biochemical feature*	*Causes*
III	Abnormal β-lipoprotein	Combined hyperlipidaemia (2^0 ↑ TG + CHOL)	2^0 Diabetes mellitus, hypothyroidism, renal disease
IV	↑ VLDL and chylomicron	Familial hypertriglyceridaemia (1° ↑ TG ± ↑ CHOL)	1^0 Usually familial 2^0 Diabetes, hypothyroidism, obesity, liver disease, alcoholism, nephrotic syndrome, pancreatitis, pregnancy, oral contraceptives, steroids, anorexia nervosa and glycogen storage diseases
V	↑ VLDL and chylomicron	Equivalent of Type I and IV	

*In general: all types except Type I have an ↑ cholesterol and all types except Type II have ↑ triglycerides

SPHINGOLIPIDOSES AND MUCOPOLYSACCHARIDOSES

Disorders of sphingolipid and mucopolysaccharide metabolism are described in Tables 6.5 and 6.6.

HYPOLIPOPROTEINAEMIAS

1. Abetalipoproteinaemia
    - Rare, autosomal recessive. LDL deficiency due to complete absence of apoprotein B. Chylomicrons, VLDL, IDL and LDL are absent from the plasma.
    - Clinical features include: steatorrhoea, failure to thrive, ataxia, nystagmus, muscle weakness, abnormal red cell morphology (acanthocytosis) and low serum lipid concentrations.
2. Tangier disease (α-lipoprotein (HDL) deficiency)
    - Rare; autosomal recessive.
    - Reduced HDL, LDL and very low levels of apoA due to a high rate of catabolism.

APOLIPOPROTEINS

1. Apo A-I and apo A-II
    - Major components of HDL
2. Apo B
    - Structural protein for chylomicron remnants, VLDL, LDL.
3. Apo C-I, apo C-II, and apo E-III
    - Normally stored in HDL between meals, but transfer to triglyceride-rich lipoproteins after meals.

Table 6.5 Disorders of sphingolipid metabolism (sphingolipidoses)

Disease	*Defective enzyme*	*Clinical features/prognosis*	*Laboratory features/comments*
1. Tay-Sachs	Hexosaminidase A (Ganglioside $GM_1 \rightarrow GM_2$)	Presents at 6–9 months with mental retardation, spastic motor weakness and progressive optic atrophy (cherry red spot at the macula) No organomegaly or bony involvement Death aged 3–5 years	Reduced serum hexosaminidase activity Prenatal detection available, but 80% of cases represent first appearance of disease in families High frequency of heterozygotes in Ashkenazi Jews
2. Gaucher's	β-Glucosidase (Glucocerebroside → galactose)	Mental retardation with spasticity, marked hepatosplenomegaly and erosion of long bones in infants Death occurs within months in *infant* form, but almost normal lifespan in *adult* form	Cerebroside-filled Gaucher cells in marrow or liver biopsy Raised serum acid phosphatase High frequency in Ashkenazi Jews
3. Niemann–Pick	Sphingomyelinase (Sphingomyelin → ceramide + phosphorylcholine)	Mental retardation and hepatosplenomegaly May resemble Tay–Sachs with a cherry red spot at the macula Early death	Typical foam cells in marrow and liver biopsy
4. Metachromatic leucodystrophy	Arylsulphatase-A (catabolism of sulphides)	Mental retardation and demyelination in adults	Reduced enzyme activity in leucocytes

Table 6.6 Disorders of mucopolysaccharide metabolism (mucopolysaccharidoses*). Accumulation of glycosaminoglycans in fibroblasts and chrondrocytes.

Syndrome	*Defective enzyme*	*Clinical features/ prognosis*	*Laboratory features*	*Treatment*
1. **Hurler's** (best recognized form) 2. **Hunter's**	Iduronidase and iduronate sulphatase respectively (degradation of dermatan and heparan sulphate)	Both have similar clinical features with severe mental and growth retardation by end of first year, facial abnormalities ('gargoylism'), macroglossia, hepatosplenomegaly, heart disease, corneal opacities (Hurler's syndrome only) and conductive nerve deafness Death occurs in childhood	Dermatan sulphate and heparan sulphate in urine, tissues and amniotic fluid Presence of mucopolysaccharide inclusion bodies (Alder–Reilly bodies) in white blood cells	Plasma infusion/ enzyme replacement

*Other mucopolysaccharidoses include Sanfilippo's, Morquino's and Scheie's syndromes (mental retardation absent or slight).

4. Apo E-I, apo E-II, apo E-III, and apo E-IV
   - Enter plasma with nascent HDL produced in liver.
   - Transfer with cholesterol ester from HDL to triglyceride-rich lipoprotein remnants.

PROTEINS AND METABOLISM

AMINO ACIDS

- All the common amino acids (except for proline) have the same general structure: α-carbon bears a carboxy (COOH) and an amino (NH_2^-) group, but they differ with respect to their sidechain or 'R' groups.
- The 'R' groups confer their characteristic properties on each amino acid.

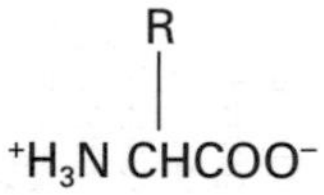

Table 6.7 The essential and non-essential amino acids

Essential (cannot be synthesized in the body, therefore must be present in the diet)	*Non-essential* (synthesized in the body from other pathway metabolites)
Isoleucine — aliphatic	**Alanine** — aliphatic non-polar
Leucine — non-polar	**Aspartic acid** — acidic side chain
Valine	**Hydroxyproline**
Phenylalanine	**Glutamic acid** — acidic side chain
Tyrosine — aromatic	**Glycine** — aliphatic non-polar
Tryptophan	**Cystine**
Methionine, **Cysteine** } sulphur-containing	**Proline** — imino acid **Serine** — hydroxy side chain
Arginine — basic	**Tyrosine**
Histidine — basic	**Cysteine**
Lysine — basic	**Hydroxylysine**
Threonine — hydroxy side chain	

BOX 6.1 ESSENTIAL AMINO ACIDS

Mnemonic for essential amino acids: **P.V.T. T.I.M. H.A.L.L.**

P — phenylalanine	T — tryptophan	H — histidine
V — valine	I — isoleucine	A — arginine
T — threonine	M — methionine	L — lysine
		L — leucine

PROTEINS

- Linear, unbranched polymers constructed from 20 different α-amino acids.
- The peptide bond is formed between the α-carboxyl group (C-terminal) of one amino acid and the α-amino group (N-terminal) of another.
- The *specific biological action* of the protein is determined by its primary, secondary, tertiary and quaternary structure.
  1º structure is the specific order of amino acids in the peptide chain.
  2º structure is the spatial relationships of neighbouring amino acid residues produced by twisting and turning, e.g. α-helix.
  3º structure is the spatial relationship of more distant residues produced by arrangement of the secondary structure into layers, crystals and fibres.
  4º structure is the spatial relationship between individual polypeptide chains, e.g. arrangement of subunits of haemoglobin.

BIOLOGICAL VALUE

- The *biological value* of a protein is determined by its content of essential amino acids.
- A *high* biological value protein supplies all the essential amino acids in optimal proportions, e.g. most animal proteins (meat and eggs).
- A *low* biological value protein is deficient in one or more essential amino acids, e.g. rice protein is deficient in lysine and threonine.

DIGESTION OF PROTEINS

- Pepsin hydrolyses protein in the stomach (pH optimum 2.5) to produce shorter peptide chains.
- Further breakdown into free amino acids occurs through the action of the pancreatic proteolytic enzymes (endopeptidases and carboxypeptidases) and the brush border enzymes (dipeptidases and aminopeptidases).
- The gastric and pancreatic proteases are secreted into the duodenum as zymogens, or inactive precursors, e.g. pepsinogen, trypsinogen and chymotrypsinogen.

- The small intestine absorbs these free amino acids by active transport. They then enter the hepatoportal venous system and are carried to the liver.

Intestinal transport mechanisms

- Several specific intestinal transport mechanisms exist for different classes of amino acids (e.g. small neutral, large neutral, basic and acidic amino acids and proline).

The transport is tightly coupled to the entry of Na^+ into the cell, with the energy derived from the Na^+ gradient.
For defects in the transport of amino acids see page 257.

PROTEIN METABOLISM

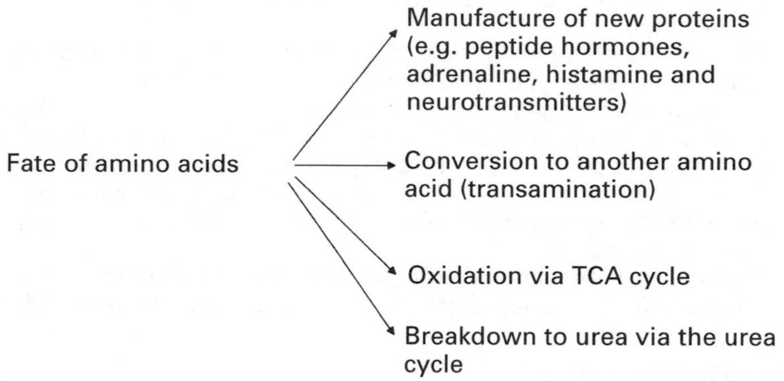

Fig. 6.17

PROTEIN CATABOLISM

- Breakdown of protein to free amino acids. Main site of catabolism is in the liver; the kidney is a secondary site.
- The metabolic pathways of amino acid degradation include transamination, oxidative deamination, direct deamination and the urea cycle. The carbon skeletons of the amino acids can be oxidized to make glucose in the process of gluconeogenesis.

Urea cycle

- Takes place in the liver and brain and involves the condensation of ornithine with carbomyl phosphate to form citrulline which then combines with aspartic acid to form arginosuccinate. Arginosuccinate is cleaved to arginine which is then hydrolysed to urea and ornithine.
- The first two reactions are rate-controlling, catalysed by: *carbamoyl phosphate synthetase* and *ornithine transcarbamoylase*, both located in the mitochondria.
- The remainder of the urea cycle takes place in the cytoplasm.

Nitrogen balance

Positive nitrogen balance exists if the total daily nitrogen losses in urine, skin and faeces are less than the total daily nitrogen intake, e.g. as in healthy, growing children or convalescing adults.
Negative nitrogen balance exists if nitrogen losses are greater than intake, e.g. in disease involving tissue wasting or in starvation.

AMINO ACID TRANSPORT DEFECTS (Table 6.8)

Generalized aminoaciduria

Causes

1. 'Overflow'
   Amino acid infusion, liver failure and inborn errors of metabolism, e.g. phenylketonuria, maple syrup urine, homocystinuria.
2. Renal causes
   (i) Specific transport defects, e.g. cystinuria, Hartnup's disease
   (ii) General tubular damage, e.g. Fanconi syndrome, heavy metal poisoning, drugs (neomycin), nutritional deficiencies (e.g. vitamins D and B_{12}), acute tubular necrosis, nephrotic syndrome and renal transplant rejection.

Specific transport defects

1. Cystinuria (not an inborn error of metabolism). Defective transport of the basic amino acids (*cystine, ornithine, arginine* and *lysine*) in the renal tubule and the gastrointestinal tract.

Clinical features

Cystine urinary calculi and crystals in the urine. The cyanide-nitroprusside urine test is positive in cystinuria and homocystinuria.
2. Hartnup's disease (not an inborn error of metabolism). Defective renal and intestinal transport of neutral amino acids, especially tryptophan.

Clinical features

Malabsorption, ataxia and pellagra rash.

Table 6.8 Inborn errors of amino acid metabolism (see Fig. 6.18)

Disease	*Site of metabolic block*	*Clinical features*	*Laboratory features*	*Treatment*
1. Phenylketonuria (PKU) Incidence 1: 12 000 births	Phenylalanine hydroxylase pathway (**1**)	Presents in early childhood with reduced pigmentation, eczema, mental retardation (IQ usually <20) and seizures	Raised blood phenylalanine at approx. 1 week after birth; phenylpyruvic acid in urine (phenistix +ve) Prenatal diagnosis available	Low phenylalanine diet. Early treatment important
2. Alkaptonuria Incidence 1: 300 000 births	Homogentisic acid oxidase pathway **(2)**	Deposition of homogentisic acid in cartilage and other tissues causing ochronosis, pigmentation of face, ears and sclera and arthritis Urine darkens on exposure to air		
3. Albinism Three types: 1. Oculocutaneous (autosomal recessive) 2. Ocular (X-linked) 3. Cutaneous (autosomal dominant)	Tyrosinase pathway **(3)**	White hair, photosensitive skin Prominent red reflex from unpigmented fundus. Strabismus, nystagmus, photophobia, and loss of visual acuity		
4. Homocystinuria Incidence 1: 160 000 births	Cystathione-β-synthetase (Homocysteine + serine → cystathionine)	Mental retardation, seizures, spastic paraplegia, osteoporosis, cataracts, and thromboembolic disease Some features similar to Marfan's syndrome, i.e. dislocation of lens (but downwards) arachnodactyly, high arched palate, lax ligaments, kyphoscoliosis; but no dissecting aneurysm	Elevated plasma methionine and urinary homocystine Prenatal diagnosis and carrier detection available	Dietary restriction of methionine with cystine supplementation
5. Maple syrup urine disease Incidence 1: 175 000 births	Branched chain ketoacid decarboxylase	Presents in 1st week of life, with mental deficiency, areflexia, dysphagia, metabolic acidosis and hypoglycaemia	Characteristic urine smell Leucocyte/fibroblast enzyme analysis	Reduced intake of branched chain aminoacids

General tubular damage

1. Fanconi syndrome

Causes

Cystinosis, galactosaemia, hereditary fructose intolerance, glycogen storage disease Type I, and Wilson's disease.

Clinical features

Generalized aminoaciduria, glycosuria, and hyperphosphaturia, rickets or osteomalacia, *also* acidosis, hypokalaemia, polyuria and hypouricaemia.

2. Cystinosis (compare with cystinuria and homocystinuria (page 258). Deposition of L-cystine crystals in the proximal renal tubule, reticuloendothelial tissue and cornea.

Clinical features

Fanconi syndrome, renal tubular acidosis, progressive renal failure and hepatosplenomegaly.

Inborn errors of amino acid metabolism (Table 6.8 and Fig. 6.18)

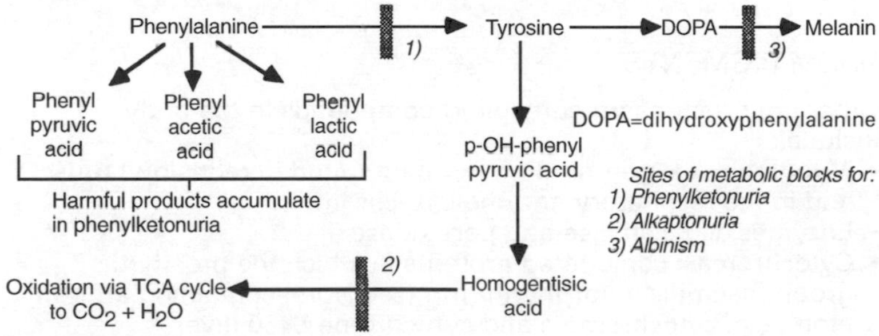

Fig. 6.18

SPECIALIZED PROTEINS

HAEMOGLOBIN

Structure (See also Table 6.9)

Table 6.9 Normal human haemoglobins

Haemoglobin	*% of normal adult haemoglobin*	*% of haemoglobin at birth*	*Globin structure*
A	97	10–50	$\alpha_2\beta_2$
A_2	2.5	Trace	$\alpha_2\delta_2$
F (fetal)	0.5	50–90	$\alpha_2\gamma_2$

- Mol. weight = 67 000
- Each haemoglobin molecule consists of a globin molecule and four haem groups (tetramer). Each haem group is a binding site for oxygen.
- *Haem part*: ferrous complex of protoporphyrin IX arranged in four pyrrole rings.
- *Globin part*: two pairs of polypeptide chains (α and β chains) are linked through histidine residues with one haem molecule. In both myoglobin and haemoglobin, the iron of the haem group is in the Fe^{2+} form. When in the ferric or Fe^{3+} form, the proteins are methaemoglobin and metmyoglobin.

Porphyrin and haem synthesis (Fig. 6.19)

Three main successive steps in the pathway:

1. Biosynthesis of δ-amino laevulinic acid (ALA) from the precursors, glycine and succinyl coA. The enzyme for this reaction, *δ-aminolaevulinate synthetase (ALA-S)* is the rate-controlling enzyme for porphyrin synthesis.
2. Two molecules of ALA condense to form porphobilinogen.
3. Conversion of porphobilinogen to the cyclic tetrapyrrole porphyrin ring and haem. Haem, the end-product of porphyrin synthesis inhibits ALA-synthetase.

HAEM PIGMENTS

Other important haem-containing compounds in the body include:

- Myoglobin: oxygen-binding pigment found in red (slow) muscle and in the respiratory enzyme cytochrome c.
- Enzymes, e.g. catalase and peroxidase
- Cytochromes: conjugated proteins in which the prosthetic group (haem) is a porphyrin ring (see Note) containing an iron atom, e.g. cytochrome c and cytochrome p450 (liver microsomes).

Note: Large, flat, heterocyclic ring structures made up of four pyrrole rings linked together by —C= bridges, and found in all aerobic cells.

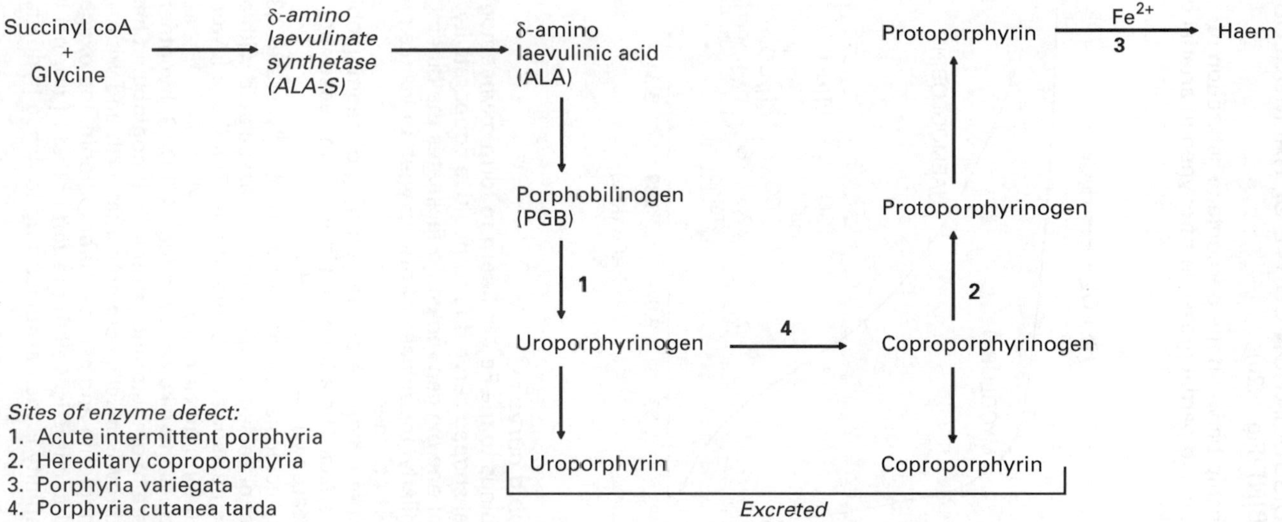

Sites of enzyme defect:
1. Acute intermittent porphyria
2. Hereditary coproporphyria
3. Porphyria variegata
4. Porphyria cutanea tarda

Fig. 6.19 Porphyrin and haem synthesis

OXYGEN DISSOCIATION CURVE OF HAEMOGLOBIN (AND MYOGLOBIN) (Fig. 6.20)

The relationship between the percentage saturation of haemoglobin and partial pressure of oxygen in arterial blood ($Pa\text{O}_2$).

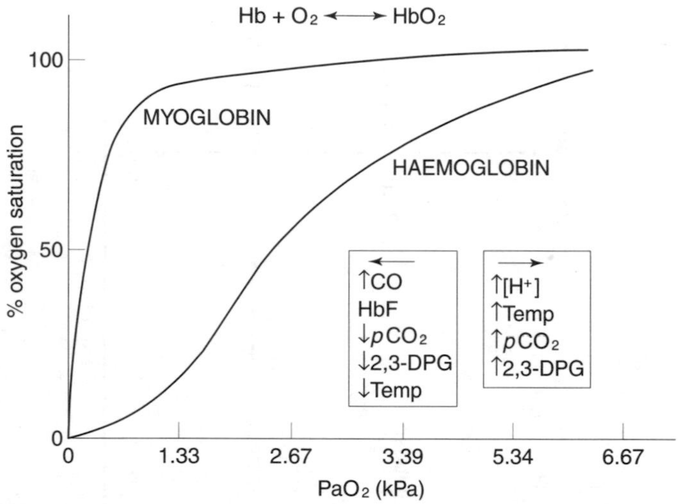

Fig. 6.20

Haemoglobin curve

- Oxygen binds to the Fe^{2+} in haem to form oxyhaemoglobin.
- Sigmoidal-shaped curve due to positive cooperativity, i.e. the binding of one oxygen molecule facilitates the binding of the next. Similarly, the release of one oxygen molecule promotes the release of others.
- The effect of pH on the oxygen binding of haemoglobin is called the *Bohr effect*. The affinity of Hb for O_2 increases at higher pH, and decreases with a fall in pH.
- High $P\text{CO}_2$, acidosis, raised 2,3-diphosphoglycerate (2,3-, DPG) (see Note) or raised temperature are associated with a shift in the oxygen dissociation curve to the *right* (i.e. a lower O_2 saturation for a given $Pa\text{O}_2$).
- Low $Pa\text{CO}_2$, acute alkalosis, reduced 2,3-DPG, hypothermia, certain rare haemoglobinopathies (haemoglobins Chesapeake and Heathrow), in cells containing fetal Hb and with methaemoglobin and carboxyhaemoglobin, the oxygen dissociation curve is well to the *left* of that of normal Hb, i.e. oxygen affinity is increased, leading to tissue hypoxia.

Myoglobin curve

- One oxygen molecule bound per haem molecule, i.e. the myoglobin molecule does not alter conformation on oxygenation, and shows no Bohr effect. Follows Michaelis–Menten kinetics and produces a hyperbolic curve.

Table 6.10 Summary of binding characteristics

Myoglobin	*Haemoglobin*
Monomer	Tetramer, 2α and 2β chains
Binds one O_2	Binds $4O_2$
Binding kinetics hyperbolic	Binding kinetics sigmoidal

Note: *2,3-diphosphoglycerate (2,3-DPG)* is synthesized in the red cells from metabolites of the glycolytic pathway. It binds to haemoglobin, stabilizing the deoxy form, and reduces the affinity of haemoglobin for oxygen, causing the release of oxygen. Production is stimulated by hypoxia, e.g. anaemia and altitude.

CARRIAGE OF GASES

Oxygen

1. Combined with haemoglobin in the red cell: 1 g of haemoglobin carries 1.39 ml of oxygen.
2. Dissolved in plasma: at 100 mmHg, 0.3 ml oxygen is dissolved in every 100 ml of blood.

Carbon dioxide

1. In plasma, mostly as bicarbonate, but also as carbonic acid and carbamino compounds with plasma proteins.
2. In red blood cells as carbaminohaemoglobin (30%) and bicarbonate (60%).
3. Dissolved in plasma (5%).

Carbon dioxide has 20 times the rate of diffusion of oxygen.
The capacity of blood and tissues for CO_2 is three times and 100 times respectively greater than for oxygen.
The CO_2 dissociation curve is relatively linear over a physiological range of oxygen tensions.

DISORDERS OF HAEM SYNTHESIS (Table 6.11)

Other causes of excessive porphyrin excretion

1. Lead poisoning

Inhibits several enzymes in haem synthesis.

Table 6.11 Disorders of haem synthesis

	Hepatic porphyrias	*Porphyria cutanea tarda (PCT)*	*Erythropoietic porphyrias**	
	Acute intermittent porphyria (AIP) Porphyria variegata (VP) Hereditary coproporphyria (HCP)		Congenital porphyria (Gunther's disease)	Erythropoietic porphyria
Cell affected	Liver	Erythrocyte and liver	Erythrocyte	Erythrocyte
Inheritance	Autosomal dominant Increased activity of liver ALA-S	No family history Usually secondary to chronic (especially alcoholic) liver disease	Autosomal recessive Rare	Autosomal dominant
Clinical features	1. GI: abdo pain, vomiting and constipation 2. CNS: peripheral neuropathy, confusion and psychosis 3. CVS: tachycardia and hypertension 4. Fragile skin with VP 5. Acute attacks precipitated by: drugs (see page 331), alcohol, hormonal change, diet and infection	1. Skin photosensitivity, hypertrichosis, skin pigmentation 2. Liver function test abnormal	Pink teeth, hypertrichosis and severe photosensitivity	Photosensitivity and hepatocellular damage
Accumulating materials	δ-Aminolaevulinic acid (ALA) and porphobilinogen (PBG)	Uroporphyrins	ALA and PBG excretion are normal. Uroporphyrin I and coproporphyrin	ALA and PBG excretion are normal. Protoporphyrin
Diagnosis	1. ↑ ALA and PBG in the urine and ↑ faecal porphyrins with VP and HCP 2. Urine turns deep red in sunlight†	Excess plasma, faecal and urinary uroporphyrins and coproporphyrins	Both compounds in erythrocytes, urine, and faeces (red urine)	↑ erythrocyte, urine and faecal protoporphyrin

*Acute attacks do not occur.
†Porphyrinogens, ALA and PBG are colourless, but oxidize to corresponding porphyrins which are dark red and fluoresce in UV light.

Clinical features
Intestinal colic, gingivitis, blue line on gums. Lead encephalopathy (mortality 25%), motor neuropathy. Haematological effects: anaemia (may be sideroblastic), basophilic stippling, reticulocytosis, increased serum iron, Large amounts of urinary coproporphyrin and ALA.

2. Liver disease
Increased urinary coproporphyrin, possibly due to decreased biliary excretion.

ABNORMAL DERIVATIVES OF HAEMOGLOBIN

Methaemoglobin
Form of oxidized Hb (Fe^{2+} replaced by Fe^{3+}), so that ability to act as an O_2 carrier is lost.

Causes of methaemoglobinaemia
1. Haemoglobinopathies, e.g. HbM, deficiency of NADH-methaemoglobin reductase.
2. Drugs: phenacetin, primaquine, sulphonamides, nitrites, nitrates (after conversion to nitrites in the gut), and various aniline dye derivates.

Carboxyhaemoglobin (HbCO)
- Haemoglobin can combine with carbon monoxide (CO) to form carboxyhaemoglobin.
- Affinity of haemoglobin for CO is 200 times that for O_2, so CO will displace O_2 from oxyhaemoglobin.

Glycosylated haemoglobin
- Glycosylation occurs as the result of binding between adult haemoglobin A and glucose during the 120-day life span of the red blood cell, and is an irreversible reaction.
- Normally about 6–9% of adult HbA is glycosylated and in the diabetic about 12–21%. Useful for providing a picture of the long-term state of diabetic control (over 2–3 months). Difficult to interpret in the presence of abnormalities of red blood cells.

DISORDERS OF GLOBIN SYNTHESIS

1. Haemoglobinopathies
Abnormal polypeptide chains are produced.

Sickle cell disease
- Substitution of valine for glutamic acid at 6th position on β chain. Abnormal HbS is produced, which is less soluble in the deoxygenated state.
- Homozygotes produce HbS with HbF and HbA_2. Heterozygotes produce 30–40% HbS and the rest HbA.
- World distribution of HbS: Central Africa, Mediterranean and India.

2. Thalassaemias

Polypeptide chains are normal in structure but are produced in decreased amounts.

1. β-thalassaemia

- Homozygotes (thalassaemia major) are characterized by ↓ β-chain production and ↑ HbA_2 and HbF production. Mild disease in heterozygotes (thalassaemia minor) with Hb A_2 ↑.
- World distribution: Middle East.

2. α-thalassaemia

↓ α chain production. Severe disease in homozygotes with death in utero, e.g. Hb-Barts of HbH, but insignificant disease in heterozygotes.

COLLAGEN

Structure and synthesis

- Collagen is formed by fibroblasts in connective tissues, osteoblasts in bone and chondroblasts in cartilage.
- Synthesized in an inactive form called procollagen which is then proteolytically processed outside the cell into tropocollagen. Three chains of tropocollagen twist around each other in a right-handed superhelix. Cleavage of the ends of tropocollagen forms collagen, which is held together by cross-links between hydroxylysine residues.
- Collagen has a unique distribution of amino acid residues with 33% glycine, 10% proline, 10% hydroxyproline and 1% hydroxylysine.
- Other examples of fibrous proteins are elastin and fibronectin.

Disorders of metabolism of collagen

1. Scurvy
2. Ehlers–Danlos syndrome type VI
   - Enzyme lysyl hydroxylase is deficient and collagen with a reduced hydroxylysine content is formed.
   - Clinical features include musculoskeletal deformities, especially hypermobility of the joints and poor wound healing.
3. Homocystinuria
4. Ehlers–Danlos syndrome type VIII
   - No proteolytic cleavage of the N-terminal peptide on procollagen.
   - Clinical features include hyperelastic skin which bruises easily and bilateral hip dislocation.

PURINE AND PYRIMIDINE METABOLISM

Physiologically important purines and pyrimidines

Purines: adenine, guanine, hypoxanthine and xanthine
Pyrimidines: cytosine, uracil and thymidine

SYNTHESIS

Most purines and pyrimidines are synthesized de novo from amino acids, especially in the liver, via complex pathways involving the incorporation of many molecules into the purine and pyrimidine structure or from the breakdown of ingested amino acids. The nucleotides of RNA and DNA are then synthesized.

CATABOLISM (Fig. 6.21)

- 90% of the purine and pyrimidine bases and nucleosides obtained from the breakdown of cellular polynucleotides are not catabolized, but salvaged and re-utilized. Minor amounts are excreted unchanged in the urine. The pyrimidines are catabolized to CO_2 and NH_3, and the purines are converted to uric acid.
- Two salvage pathways exist to regenerate AMP and GMP released from nucleosides.
  1. *Adenine phosphoribosyl transferase (APRT)* adds ribose phosphate from phosphoribosyl pyrophosphate (PRPP) to adenine to regenerate AMP.
  2. *Hypoxanthine guanine phosphoribosyl transferase (HGPRT)* catalyses the same reaction with guanine. In addition, adenosine may be deaminated to inosine, which then liberates its ribose forming hypoxanthine.
- Xanthine oxidase (XO) transforms hypoxanthine to xanthine and then into uric acid.

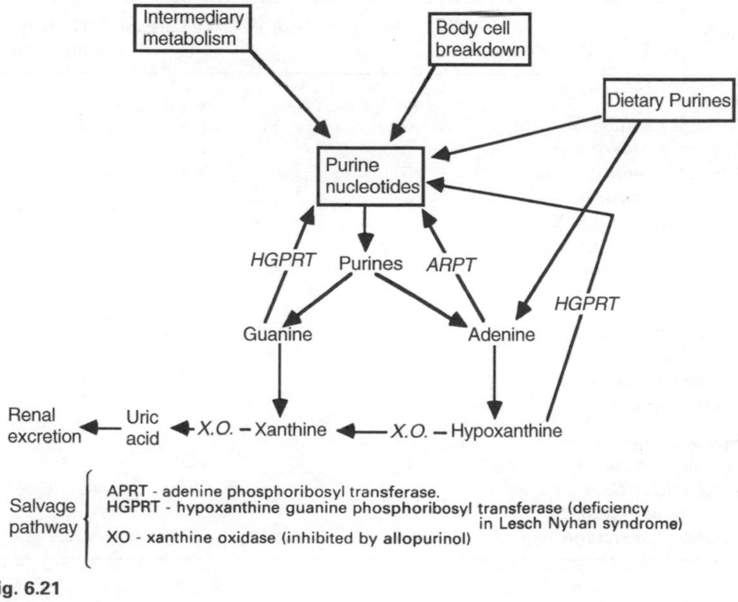

Fig. 6.21

DISORDERS OF PURINE AND PYRIMIDINE METABOLISM: HYPERURICAEMIA

Causes

1. *Increased purine synthesis*
Primary gout (25% of cases due to increased synthesis de novo) Lesch–Nyhan syndrome (HGPRT deficiency), Type I glycogen storage disease.

2. *Increased purine turnover*
Myeloproliferative and lymphoproliferative disorders, polycythaemia, severe exfoliative psoriasis, high purine diet.

3. *Decreased excretion of uric acid*
Primary gout (75% of cases), renal failure, increased levels of organic acids, e.g. exercise, alcohol, diabetic ketoacidosis, starvation, hyperparathyroidism and lead poisoning.

4. *Drugs*
Thiazide and loop diuretics, pyrizinamide, ethambutol, salicylate in low doses, cytotoxic agents and alcohol.

HORMONAL CONTROL OF METABOLISM

Table 6.12 The principal actions of insulin, glucagon, adrenaline, cortisol and growth hormone

Action	*Insulin*	*Glucagon*	*Adrenaline*	*Cortisol*	*Growth hormone*
Liver					
Glycogen synthesis	↑	↓	↓	↑	↑
Glycogen breakdown	↓	↑	↑		
Gluconeogenesis	↓	↑	↑	↑	
Glucose release	↓	↑	↑	↑	↑
Ketone body production	↓	↑	↑		
Amino acid catabolism	↓	↑		↑	
Fatty acid synthesis	↑	↓	↓		
Muscle					
Fatty acid utilization			↑		↑
Glycogen breakdown	↓		↑		
Glucose uptake	↑		↓	↓	↓
Protein synthesis	↑			↓	↑
Adipose tissue					
Glucose uptake	↑	↑			
Fatty acid release	↓		↑	↑	↑
Triglyceride synthesis	↓				↑
Triglyceride storage	↑				

PART II: CLINICAL CHEMISTRY

VITAMINS

Vitamlns: Organic molecules required for certain metabolic functions that must be supplied in very small amounts (<50 mg/day).

Coenzyme: Non-protein organic molecule that binds to an enzyme to aid in the transfer of small functional groups. When it binds tightly, it is considered to be a *prosthetic* group of an enzyme.

Cofactor: Differs from a coenzyme only because it is usually a metallic ion rather than an organic molecule, e.g. Fe^{2+} in the cytochromes, and Mg^{2+} for enzymes utilizing ATP.

See Tables 6.13 and 6.14.

Table 6.13 Water-soluble vitamins

Vitamin	*Source*	*Function*	*Deficiency state* and causes*	*Laboratory diagnosis*
Thiamine Vitamin B_1	Wholemeal flour, cereals (germinal layer), peas, beans and yeast	Coenzyme: thiamine pyrophosphate (TPP) for decarboxylation of α-ketoacids (pyruvate to acetyl-CoA) and transketolation reactions	1. 'Dry' beri-beri: (polyneuritis and weight loss) 2. 'Wet' beri-beri: (high output cardiac failure) 3. Wernicke–Korsakoff syndrome: *Causes:* Occurs in chronic alcoholics and when polished rice is the main food	↑ Blood pyruvate and ↓ Red cell transketolase activity ↓ Urinary thiamine excretion
Riboflavin Vitamin B_2	Meat, milk, wholemeal flour, fish and eggs	Coenzyme of flavoproteins, e.g. flavin adenine dinucleotide (FAD) and flavin mononucleotide (FMN) (act as reversible electron carriers) for oxidation-reduction reactions	1. Angular stomatitis and cheliosis 2. Seborrhoeic dermatitis 3. Vascularized cornea 4. Peripheral neuropathy	↓ Plasma glutathione reductase
Niacin, nicotinic acid, nicotinamide Vitamin B_3	Liver, wholemeal flour, and nuts Also synthesized from tryptophan in the body	Coenzyme, e.g. nicotinamide adenine dinucleotide (NAD), and NAD phosphate (NADP) (act as reversible electron carriers) for oxidation-reduction reactions, e.g. glycolysis and oxidative phosphorylation	1. Pellagra (*3Ds*: diarrhoea, dementia and dermatitis) 2. Neurological disease: (dementia and signs similar to those of subacute combined degeneration of the cord) *Causes* Alcoholism, malabsorption, Hartnup's disease and isoniazid therapy	↑ Urinary excretion of N′-methyl nicotinamide

Table 6.13 *(cont.)*

Vitamin	*Source*	*Function*	*Deficiency state* and causes*	*Laboratory diagnosis*
Pyridoxine Vitamin B_6	Very widespread	Coenzyme, e.g. pyridoxal phosphate (PP) for decarboxylation, transmination and deamination of amino acids	1. Glossitis and seborrhoea 2. Peripheral neuropathy and convulsions 3. Hypochromic anaemia *Causes:* Pregnancy, alcoholics, isoniazid or penicillamine therapy administration	↑ Urinary excretion of xanthurenate†
Panthothenic acid	Widespread, but mainly liver, eggs, meat and milk	Component of coenzyme A for the transport of acetyl and succinyl units	Lethargy and paraesthesia	
Biotin	Widespread Synthesized by intestinal bacteria	Coenzyme for carboxylation and decarboxylation reactions, e.g. malonyl-coA from acetyl-coA and oxaloacetate from pyruvate	Seborrhoeic dermatitis, paraesthesia and lethargy Induced by avidin (a protein in raw egg white), or by antibiotic therapy	

Table 6.13 *(cont.)*

Vitamin	*Source*	*Function*	*Deficiency state* and causes*	*Laboratory diagnosis*
Cyanocobalamin Vitamin B_{12}	Liver and all foods of animal origin Normal body stores take 3–5 years for depletion (Gastric intrinsic factor (IF) facilitates its absorption in the terminal ileum)	1. Coenzyme: (methylcobalamin, 5′-deoxyadenosyl cobalamin) in synthesis of nucleic acids and coenzymes 2. Transfer of methyl groups from N5-methyltetrahydrofolate to homocysteine, regenerating methionine Homocysteine | *Methylcobalamin* *(+ folic acid)* ↓ Methionine 3. One-carbon reaction in the conversion of methylmalonyl-coA to succinyl-coA Methylmalony-coA | *5′-deoxyadenyl cobalamin* ↓ Succinyl-coA 4. Stimulates erythropoiesis‡	1. Megaloblastic anaemia, leucopaenia and thrombocytopaenia 2. Peripheral neuropathy: 'glove and stocking' distribution 3. Subacute combined degeneration of the cord 4. Optic atrophy, tobacco amblyopia 5. Depression and psychosis *Causes:* (i) Dietary deficiency (ii) Malabsorption *Stomach* (lack of IF) e.g. pernicious anaemia, partial/total gastrectomy *Gut* e.g. Crohn's disease, ileal resection, jejunal diverticulae, blind loop syndrome and fish tapeworm	↑ AST and ALT Serum B_{12} Schilling test: see Table 6.15, page 276 ↑ Methylmalonic acid excretion in urine in deficiency states ↑ Levels of serum B_{12} in liver disease and myeloproliferative disorders

Table 6.13 *(cont.)*

Vitamin	*Source*	*Function*	*Deficiency state* and causes*	*Laboratory diagnosis*
Folic acid Contains: 1. Pteridine ring 2. Para-aminobenzoic acid (PABA) 3. Glutamate	Widespread in small amounts, especially green vegetables, fruits and liver; also, synthesized by gut bacteria	Coenzyme, e.g. tetrahydrofolic acid for reactions of 1-carbon units (e.g. conversion of homocysteine to methionine and conversion of serine to glycine) and for synthesis of purines and pyrimidines	Megaloblastic anaemia *Causes* (i) Dietary deficiency (especially in alcoholics and the elderly) (ii) Malabsorption, e.g. coeliac disease (most common), gastrectomy and Crohn's disease (iii) Excessive utilization, e.g. haematological disease (leukaemia, chronic haemolytic anaemia), malignancy, and inflammatory disease (rheumatoid arthritis, psoriasis) (iv) Drugs, e.g. phenytoin and methotrexate (v) Excessive loss e.g. chronic dialysis	↓ Serum and red cell folate ↑ Urinary excretion of forminoglutamate (FIGLU)
Vitamin C Ascorbic acid	Fresh fruit, vegetables and liver Destroyed by cooking (only primates and guinea pigs can synthesize vitamin C)	Antioxidant and coenzyme in oxidation reactions. Required for: 1. Collagen synthesis (hydroxylation of proline and lysine residues) 2. Steroid metabolism 3. Electron and cytochrome p450 function 4. Increased gastrointestinal absorption of iron 5. Hydroxylation of tyrosine, tryptophan and proline	Scurvy	↓ Plasma, leucocyte and urinary ascorbate

*Glossitis occurs in all five of the vitamin B deficiency states, in addition to iron deficiency anaemia.

†24-hour urinary excretion of xanthurenate is measured before and after a loading dose of 2 g of L-tryptophan. Increased levels are excreted in patients with pyridoxine deficiency.

‡Other substances essential to erythropoesis include: erythropoetin, vitamins B_1, B_2, B_{12} and C, folic acids, protein, iron and trace elements (Mn, Co), hormones including thyroxine, cortisol, androgen and prolactin.

Table 6.14 Fat-soluble vitamins

Vitamin	*Source*	*Function*	*Deficiency state*
Vitamin A* Provitamin = β-carotene Vitamin = retinol	Liver, dairy produce, fish oils and eggs	Maintenance of epithelial surfaces and integrity of cartilage Night vision (11-*cis*-retinal) 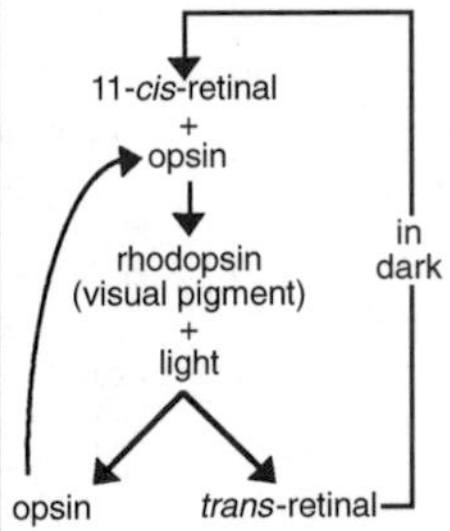 	Night blindness Xerophthalmia Follicular hyperkeratosis
Vitamin D Provitamins = ergosterol (plants) and 7-dehydrocholesterol (skin) Vitamins D_2 (ergocalciferol) and D_3 (cholecalciferol) *Synthesis* Provitamins converted to vitamins by UV light Cholecalciferol (vit. D_3) is hydroxylated first in the liver to produce 25-hydroxycholecalciferol (25-HCC) and next in the kidney to generate both 1,25-dihydroxycholecalciferol (1,25-DHCC)† and 24,25-dihydroxycholecalciferol	Dairy produce, fish liver oils and UV light	Regulates calcium and phosphate metabolism 1,25-DHCC acts directly on bone, muscle, kidney and intestine	Rickets in children and osteomalacia in adults. Tetany and muscle weakness *Causes* (i) Dietary vitamin D deficiency (ii) Chronic severe liver disease (iii) Malabsorption, e.g. bowel resection gastric surgery, intestinal bypass operations (iv) Chronic renal failure and renal tubular disease (v) Familial hypophosphataemic rickets and hypophosphatasia

Table 6.14 *(cont.)*

Vitamin	*Source*	*Function*	*Deficiency state*
Vitamin E Tocopherols	Widely distributed in small amounts, especially green vegetables and vegetable oils	Biological antioxidant	Areflexia, gait disturbance, gaze paresis and haemolytic anaemia *Causes* Abetalipoproteinaemia
Vitamin K K_1 = phylloquinone K_2 = menaquinone	Widely distributed in small amounts, e.g. green vegetables Synthesized by intestinal bacteria	Acts as a coenzyme Essential for activation of clotting factors by the liver (II, VII, IX and X)	1. Easy bruising due to impaired clotting 2. Fat malabsorption *Causes* (i) Prolonged obstructive jaundice (ii) Prematurity (iii) Gut sterilization (antibiotics) (iv) Drugs, e.g. antibiotics and anticoagulants

* Laboratory diagnosis of deficiency: plasma vitamin A level. †Production of 1,25-DHCC is stimulated by a low circulating phosphate concentration, a high circulating PTH, oestrogen, prolactin and growth hormone.

Table 6.15 Urinary B_{12} excretion in the Schilling test

Oral preparation	*Pernicious anaemia*	*Bacterial overgrowth*	*Ileal disease*
B_{12}	Low	Low	Low
B_{12} + intrinsic factor	Normal	Low	Low
B_{12} after antibiotic therapy	Low	Normal	Low

MINERALS

See also page 282, Table 6.18.

SODIUM

Factors affecting plasma sodium concentration

The intracellular fluid (ICF) Na^+ concentration is less than one-tenth of that in the extracellular fluid (ECF).

1. Aldosterone and the renin–angiotensin system.
2. Changes in glomerular filtration rate and renal blood flow.
3. Atrial natriuretic peptide.

Causes of salt and water abnormalities

See pages 178–179.

Causes of hypo- and hypernatraemia

See pages 179–180.

POTASSIUM

Factors affecting plasma potassium concentration

ICF K^+ concentration is 30-fold that of the ECF. Potassium enters and leaves the ECF compartment via the intestine, kidney and the various other body cells.

1. *Aldosterone:* via effects on the distal tubule (increases renal excretion).
2. *Acid–base balance:* reciprocal relationship between [K^+] and pH. In acidosis (↑ ECF [H^+]) there is an increase in plasma [K^+], due to reduced entry of K^+ into the cells from the ECF coupled with reduced urinary excretion of the ion. Alkalosis causes a low plasma [K^+] due to a net increase in the entry of potassium into the cells and to an increased urinary loss. K^+ loss from the cells causes an intracellular acidosis, because, there is less available for exchange with Na^+, and some is replaced by H^+.
3. *State of hydration:* K^+ is lost from cells in dehydration and returns into cells when dehydration is corrected.
4. *Insulin* promotes entry of K^+ into cells.
5. In *catabolic states*, e.g. major operations, severe infections, starvation and hyperthyroidism, K^+ is lost from cells. In *anabolic states*, K^+ is taken up by cells.

Causes of hypokalaemia

1. *Increased renal loss*
   Diuretics
   Renal tubular disorders, i.e. diuretic phase of acute renal failure/chronic pyelonephritis
   Diabetic ketoacidosis
   Cushing's syndrome or steroid excess
   Hyperaldosteronism (primary/secondary)
2. *Increased gastrointestinal loss*
   Diarrhoea, vomiting and intestinal fistulae
   Laxative abuse
   Carbenoxolone therapy
   Chronic mucous secreting villous adenomas
3. *Other causes*
   Insulin therapy
   Catabolic states
   Dehydration
   Intravenous therapy with inadequate K^+ supplements
   Insulinoma
   Metabolic or respiratory alkalosis
   Familial periodic paralysis (abnormal redistribution of potassium between ECF and ICF)
   Drugs, e.g. carbenicillin, phenothiazines, amphotericin B and degraded tetracycline

Causes of hyperkalaemia

Acute and advanced chronic renal failure
Potassium-sparing diuretics
Metabolic or respiratory acidosis
Haemolysis (e.g. incompatible blood transfusion), tissue necrosis (e.g. major trauma and burns), severe acute starvation (e.g. anorexia nervosa)
Adrenal insufficiency (Addison's disease)

IRON

Source

- Liver, meat and cereals. Intake 1.5–2 mg/day.

Absorption

- Iron is absorbed by an active process in the upper small intestine (approximately 10%) and passes rapidly into the plasma. It can cross cell membranes only in the ferrous form.
- Factors increasing absorption: vitamin C, alcohol, gastric acid.
- Factors decreasing absorption: tetracycline, phytates, phosphates, gastric achlorhydria.

Storage

- Within the intestinal cell, some of the iron is combined with apoferritin to form ferritin, which is the principal storage form of iron in tissues. Ferritin is lost in the intestinal tract when the cell desquamates.

Transport

- Iron is carried in the plasma in the Fe^{3+} form, attached to a specific binding protein, transferrin, which is normally about one-third saturated with iron. Transferrin-bound iron is stored as ferritin (apoprotein + Fe^{2+}) and haemosiderin (conglomeration of ferritin molecules) in the bone marrow, liver and spleen, but may pass directly to the developing erythrocyte to form haemoglobin.

Loss

- Most of the loss is via the intestinal tract and the skin (approx. 1 mg per day). In women, the mean daily menstrual loss is about 1 mg and during pregnancy 1.5 mg. Negligible amounts appear in the urine.

Distribution of iron in the body (Fig. 6.22)

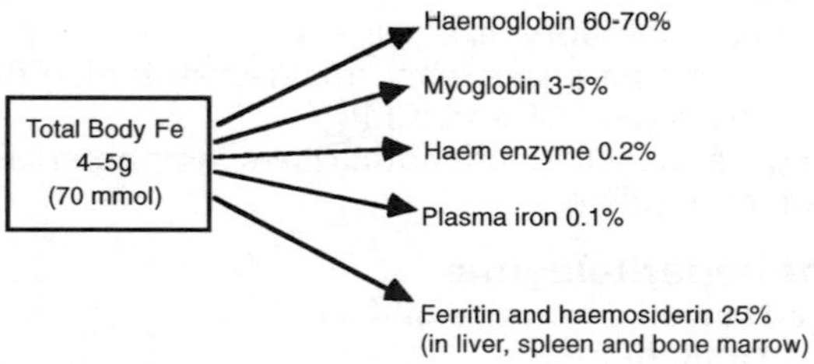

Fig. 6.22

Abnormalities of plasma iron concentration (Fig. 6.16)

Table 6.16

Disorder	*Plasma iron*	*Transferrin or plasma TIBC**	*Plasma ferritin or iron stores*
Fe deficiency	↓	↑	↓
Chronic diseases (e.g. infections, malignancy, inflammatory diseases)	↓	↓ or N	↑ (malignancy)
Haemochromatosis	↑	↓ or N	↑
Pregnancy and oral contraceptives	↑	↑	N
Viral hepatitis	↑	↑ (occ)	↑
β-Thalassaemia (major)	↑ or N	N	↑ or N
Sideroblastic anaemia	↑	N	↑

*TIBC, total iron binding capacity; N, normal. Other causes of ↑ plasma iron include lead poisoning and haemolytic anaemias.

CALCIUM

Functions

1. Calcification of bones and teeth.
2. Regulation of cell metabolism and excitability of nerve and muscle cells.
3. 2nd messenger, e.g. calmodulin (see Note) with ATP.
4. Cardiac conduction.
5. Cofactor in coagulation.

Note: Calmodulin is an intracellular peptide that binds calcium with high affinity. It participates in a variety of different cellular functions requiring calcium, including mitosis, smooth muscle contraction and calcium transport.

Calcium balance

Source

- Present in milk, cheese and eggs.

Distribution in the body

- Most abundant mineral in the body.
- Total body calcium = 32 500 mmol (99% in bone, 1% in teeth as hydroxyapatite, and soft tissues).
- 40–50% of plasma calcium is non-ionized and bound to plasma proteins (mainly albumin).
- 40–50% active and ionized, which is the physiologically important fraction.
- 5–10% complexes with organic anions.

Control of calcium balance

The gastrointestinal tract, kidney and bone control calcium homeostasis through:

1. Vitamin D (1,25-DHCC)
   ↑ Ca^{2+} absorption from the intestine.
   ↑ Ca^{2+} resorption from bone.
2. Parathormone (PTH)
   ↑ production of 1,25-DHCC by kidney.
   ↑ Ca^{2+} resorption from bone.
   ↓ Ca^{2+} excretion in urine, ↑ phosphate excretion.
   ↑ Ca^{2+} absorption by intestine.
3. Calcitonin (minimal clinical significance)
   ↓ Ca^{2+} resorption from bone, ↑ renal excretion of phosphate.
4. Acid–base status
   If ↑ $[H^+]$, less calcium is bound to albumin, e.g. in chronic acidosis, plasma $[Ca^{2+}]$ increases.
   If ↓ $[H^+]$, plasma calcium binds more to albumin and $[Ca^{2+}]$ ↓.

5. Others
   Glucocorticoids, growth hormone and somatomedins, thyroid hormones, oestrogens, insulin, epidermal, fibroblast and platelet-derived growth factor and prostaglandin E_2.

Causes of calcium deficiency

Table 6.17

Disorder	*Plasma phosphate*	*Plasma PTH*	*Plasma alkaline phosphatase*
Chronic renal failure	↑ (or N)	↑	↑ (or N)
Dietary deficiency of vit. D	↓ (or N)	↑ (or N)	↑
Hypoparathyroidism	↑	↓	N
Pseudohypoparathyroidism	↑	↑	N
Renal tubular defects	↓	N	↑ (or N)

N, normal.

Other causes

Hypoproteinaemia, liver disease, acute pancreatitis and drugs, e.g. diuretic therapy, calcitonin, phosphate, diphosphonates, some cytotoxic agents and calcium chelators.

PHOSPHATE

- Major intracellular anion.
- Present in all foods.
- Present with calcium as hydroxyapatite in bones and teeth.

Phosphate balance

- Metabolism follows calcium inversely.
- Acid–base regulation and renal function also affect urinary output of phosphate.

Abnormalities of serum phosphate

Causes of ↑ serum phosphate

Children, haemolysis, renal failure, hypoparathyroidism, acidosis, hypervitaminosis D.

Causes of ↓ serum phosphate

Vitamin D deficiency, hyperparathyroidism, renal tubular disease, malabsorption, chronic alcoholism and excessive use of antacids.

CHLORIDE

Usually parallels the Na^+ concentration

Abnormalities of serum chloride levels

Causes of hyperchloraemia

Hyperventilation
Glomerulonephritis
Eclampsia
Cystic fibrosis (chloride in sweat is ↑ by five times the reference value)

Causes of hypochloraemia

Addison's disease
Diabetes
Intestinal obstruction and vomiting

Causes of hyperchloraemic acidosis and hypochloraemic alkalosis

See page 170.

Causes of hypochlorhydria

1. Pernicious anaemia
2. Gastric carcinoma and ulcer
3. Surgery: vagotomy and subtotal gastrectomy
4. Atrophic gastritis
5. Iron deficiency.

TRACE ELEMENTS

See Table 6.18.
Required intake <100 mg/day; necessary for the function of particular compounds.

Table 6.18 The trace elements.*

Mineral	*Source*	*Function in body*	*Deficiency state and causes*
Iodide	Iodized salt, seafish, milk and eggs	Biosynthesis of thyroid hormones	Cretinism in children Endemic goitre and hypothyroidism in adults
Magnesium (54% found in bone, rest mainly intracellular)	Green vegetables and cereal	Cofactor for many enzymes in metabolism of carbohydrates and fats, e.g. phosphatases and kinases Cofactor in ATP reactions	1. Paraesthesia, tetany 2. Cardiac arrhythmias (usually with hypocalcaemia) Causes: (i) Chronic alcoholism (ii) Malabsorption and fistulae (iii) Diuretic therapy (iv) Chronic dialysis (v) Acute pancreatitis
Copper		Cofactor for some enzymes and for haem synthesis, e.g. *cytochrome* oxidase Transported by albumin and bound to caeruloplasmin	1. Anaemia (hypochromic and microcytic) and neutropaenia 2. Impaired bone mineralization 3. Wilson's disease: deficiency of caeruloplasmin resulting in low plasma copper levels. Excessive copper deposition occurs in the basal ganglia, liver, renal tubules and eye
Zinc	Herrings, beef, liver, eggs and nuts	Cofactor for some enzymes, e.g. carbonic anhydrase, alcohol dehydrogenase and carboxypeptidase	1. Confusion, apathy and depression 2. Acrodermatitis enteropathica, skin ulcers and alopecia 3. Diarrhoea 4. Growth and sexual development retarded

*Other trace elements: manganese, cobalt (cofactor of vitamin B_{12}), fluoride (cofactor of hydroxyapatite), chromium, sulphur (present in methionine and cysteine), molybdenum and selenium (cofactor of glutathione peroxidase).

NUTRITIONAL DEFICIENCIES IN SPECIFIC DISEASES/STATES

DAILY DIETARY REQUIREMENTS (adult male)

- Carbohydrate 400 g (49%)
- Protein 100 g (17%)
- Fat 100 g (34%)
- The ratio of the caloric yield of carbohydrates, protein and fats from biological oxidation is respectively 4:4:9.
- An adult male requires approximately 2500 kcal of energy per day and 6000 kcal for heavy labour.
- These requirements decrease with age, are higher in men than women and are increased by caffeine, thyroxine and catecholamines.

Table 6.19

Disease/state	*Nutritional deficiencies*
Post gastrectomy	Iron, B_{12}
Coeliac disease	Iron, folic acid
Pancreatic disease	Fat-soluble substances: vitamins A, D, E and K
Crohn's disease	Iron, folic acid, potassium and magnesium, B_{12}
Stagnant loop syndrome, alcoholism	Folic acid, thiamine, pyridoxine, protein and calcium
Vegan	B_{12}, iron, occ. calcium and phosphorous
Pregnancy and lactation	↑ in requirements for folate, calcium, phosphorous, magnesium, iron, zinc, iodine, vitamins A and C 15% ↑ in calorie and 50% ↑ in protein requirements

PLASMA PROTEINS

CONSTITUENTS AND FUNCTIONS

These are described in Table 6.20.

USE IN DIAGNOSIS

The patterns of serum proteins on electrophoresis may be used in the diagnosis of disease, e.g.

1. Multiple myeloma: paraprotein band between the α_2 and the γ region; normal or reduced γ-globulin.

Table 6.20 Plasma proteins

Plasma protein	*% of total protein*	*Constituents*	*Function*
Albumin	50–70%		— Maintains plasma volume and distribution of ECF (40% is intravascular) — Acts as a carrier for bilirubin, non-ionized calcium, free fatty acids, hormones (e.g. thyroxine) and drugs (e.g. salicylates) — Minor role as a buffer
α_1-globulins	2–6%	Thyroxine-binding globulins High density lipoproteins (HDL) Orosomucoid Transcortin α_1-anti-trypsin	— Thyroid hormone transport — Lipid transport — Glycoprotein: concentration increases in inflammation — Cortisol-binding globulin — Inhibits proteolytic enzymes (e.g. trypsin and plasmin). High levels in acute illness. Low levels in emphysema and neonatal hepatitis. (Three main phenotypes: normal MM, homozygote ZZ and heterozygote MZ)
α_2-globulins	5–11%	Caeruloplasmin Haptoglobins α_2-macroglobulin Very low density lipoproteins (VLDL)	— Copper transport: low levels in Wilson's disease — Binds to haemoglobin released from damaged red cells and prevents loss of iron in the urine — Inhibits proteolytic enzymes? transport function — Lipid transport
β-globulins	7–16%	Transferrin Low density lipoproteins (LDL) Fibrinogen C3 and C4 complement Plasminogen β_2-microglobulin	— Iron transport — Lipid transport — Fibrinolysis: deficiency states include congenital afibrinogenaemia and disseminated intravascular coagulation — Sensitive indicator of connective tissue disorders: ↑ in glomerulonephritis and infectious diseases; ↓ in disseminated intravascular coagulation, meningococcal meningitis and leukaemia — Fibrinolysis — Used as an index of renal tubular function (GFR)

Table 6.20 *(cont.)*

Plasma protein	*% of total protein*	*Constituents*	*Function*
γ-globulins	11–21%	IgA, IgD, IgE, IgG, IgM Antihaemophilia globulin (AHG) Factor VIII α-Fetoprotein C-reactive protein	— See Table 3.7 pages 89–90 — Deficiency states include haemophilia, Von Willebrand's disease; and disseminated intravascular coagulation — See page 289 — Concentration increases early in acute inflammation. Parallels the ESR but generally positive first: ↑ in chronic infections, cryoglobulinaemia, Hodgkin's disease, macroglobulinaemia, myeloma and rheumatoid arthritis and Crohn's disease; ↓ in lymphomas, nephrotic syndrome, scleroderma and ulcerative colitis

2. Nephrotic syndrome: albumin and sometimes γ-globulin lost in urine; ↑ in α_2 globulin.
3. Liver cirrhosis: ↓ albumin; ↑ production of proteins which migrate in the β–γ region.

Acute phase reactants are plasma proteins whose concentration alters following trauma (e.g. surgery, myocardial infarction), autoimmune disease (e.g. SLE), or infection. Includes fibrinogen, haptoglobins, orosomucoids, C-reactive protein, α_1-antitrypsin, complement and prealbumin. Characterized by an increase in α_1 and α_2 fractions and reduced albumin levels.

CHANGES IN PLASMA PROTEIN CONCENTRATIONS

Causes of raised globulins (mainly α_2-globulins)
Usually secondary to tissue destruction
Malignant disease
Chronic inflammatory conditions
Chronic infections
Nephrotic syndrome

Causes of raised β-globulins
Hepatitis and acute phase reaction

Causes of decreased β-globulins
SLE and autoimmune disorders

Causes of changes in γ-globulins
See pages 101–102.

PLASMA ENZYMES

Table 6.21 Plasma enzymes (see also Table 6.22)

Enzyme	*Causes of raised level*
Alanine amino transferase (ALT or SGPT) Sources: found in the same tissues as AST (see Table 6.22), but ALT present in cytoplasm of hepatocyte only (AST present in cytoplasm and mitochondria of hepatocyte) AST > ALT, if liver cell necrosis severe	Parallels changes in AST, but less affected by trauma or disease of cardiac or skeletal muscle 1. Liver disease, e.g. infectious hepatitis 2. Others: haemolysis, chronic renal failure, dermatomyositis, acute pancreatitis
Alkaline phosphatase (ALP) Sources: bone (heat labile), liver (heat stable), intestine, pancreas and placenta (heat stable)	1. Growing children and pregnancy 2. Bone disease, e.g. metastatic bone disease, Paget's disease, osteomalacia or rickets, hyperparathyroidism

Table 6.21 *(cont.)*

Enzyme	*Causes of raised level*
Alkaline phosphatase – *continued*	3. Liver disease, e.g. obstructive jaundice, cirrhosis, space occupying lesions 4. Malignancy, e.g. bone or liver tumour *Decreased levels in:* Hypophosphatasia or conditions of reduced bone growth, e.g. cretinism
Leucocyte alkaline phosphatase (LAP)	Polycythaemia rubra vera (PRV), secondary polycythaemia and leukaemoid reactions Pregnancy, oestrogens *Decreased levels in:* Chronic myelocytic leukaemia and paroxysmal nocturnal haemoglobinuria
γ-glutamyltransferase (γ-GT) Sources: liver, kidney, pancreas and prostate gland	1. Liver disease, e.g. alcoholic cholestasis 2. Enzyme induction by alcohol, barbiturates and phenytoin 3. Acute pancreatitis (rarely)
Acid phosphatase Sources: prostate, platelets, red cells and Gaucher cells	1. Carcinoma of prostate with metastases 2. After rectal examination or passage of urinary catheter 3. Gaucher's disease 4. Metastatic disease with bony involvement 5. Haemolysis, myeloid leukaemia
Serum amylase Sources: pancreas, salivary glands, ovary, lung and prostate gland	1. Acute pancreatitis, obstruction of pancreatic duct (e.g. carcinoma, stricture or stone) 2. Severe diabetic ketoacidosis. 3. Acute abdominal conditions, e.g. perforated peptic ulcer, ruptured ectopic pregnancy 4. Mumps 5. Tumours, e.g. carcinoma of bronchus, colon and ovary 6. Renal failure 7. Drugs, e.g. morphine and codeine
Angiotensin-converting enzyme (ACE) Source: capillary endothelial cells of lung	1. Active sarcoidosis 2. Liver disease 3. Leprosy 4. Berylliosis, asbestosis and silicosis 5. May also be elevated in TB, carcinoma of the lung, and primary biliary cirrhosis
Pseudocholinesterase Source: liver	*Decreased activity in:* 1. Suxamethonium sensitivity: variants of pseudocholinesterase classified according to dibucaine inhibition number (Normal is 75–80; atypical heterozygote 40–70; and for an atypical homozygote 15–30) 2. Organophosphorous poisoning (anticholinesterases) 3. Liver disease (hepatitis, cirrhosis)

Table 6.22 Enzymes raised after myocardial infarction

Enzyme	*Source*	*First rise (hours)*	*Peak (hours)*	*Duration (days)*	*Other causes of raised levels*
Creatine phosphokinase (CPK)*	Skeletal, cardiac, smooth muscle and brain. Not in liver	6	24–48	3–5	Often non-specific: 1. Crush injuries, surgery, IM injections, severe exercise 2. Muscular dystrophies and in 60% of carriers, polymyositis motor neuron disease, myotonic dystrophy 3. Malignant hyperthermia and delirium tremens 4. Hypothyroidism 5. Diabetic ketoacidosis
Aspartate amino transferase (AST or SGOT)	All tissues including skeletal muscle, liver, heart, pancreas and red cells	6–8	24–48	4–6	1. Liver disease, e.g. cirrhosis (AST > ALT) 2. Haemolytic anaemia 3. Acute systemic infections 4. Skeletal muscle disease, e.g. muscular dystrophies
Lactate dehydrogenase (LDH)†	Widely distributed in skeletal muscle, brain, liver, heart, kidney and red cells	12–24	48–72	7–12	1. Leukaemia, haemolytic anaemia, polycythaemia rubra vera, pernicious anaemia and megaloblastic anaemia 2. Carcinomatosis, Hodgkin's disease 3. Skeletal muscle disease, e.g. muscular dystrophy 4. Cerebral infarction 5. Renal and hepatic disease (hepatitis, obstructive jaundice) 6. Congestive cardiac failure

*CPK has three isoenzymes: MB, myocardium; BB, brain; MM, skeletal muscle

$$\text{Creatine} \xleftrightarrow{\textit{Creatine kinase}} \text{Creatine phosphate} \longrightarrow \text{Creatinine}$$

A constant fraction of the muscle pool creatine phosphate spontaneously cyclizes to creatinine, which is excreted in the urine.

†LDH has five isoenzymes, LD1–5, from different tissues. Hydroxybutrate = isoenzyme 1–2.

TUMOUR PRODUCTS

Carcinoembryonic antigen (CEA)

- Used mainly for detecting recurrent or metastatic disease and for monitoring therapy in carcinoma of the pancreas, liver, colon, rectum, bronchus and breast.
- Also present in individuals with chronic inflammatory bowel disease.

α-Fetoprotein (AFP)

- Normally synthesized by the fetal liver.
- Present in *plasma* in:
  1. Normal fetus
  2. Elevated maternal AFP may indicate fetal neural tube defect, twin pregnancy or fetal distress
  3. Hepatic carcinoma, testicular teratoma and seminoma.
  4. Viral hepatitis, cirrhosis or liver metastases.
- Raised *amniotic fluid* levels present in:
  1. Neural tube defects, e.g. open spina bifida, anencephaly
  2. Congenital nephrotic syndrome
  3. Oesophageal and duodenal atresia.

5-Hydroxyindoleacetic acid (5-HIAA) (Fig. 6.23)

- Increased urinary levels occur in the carcinoid syndrome.
- False positives occur with the ingestion of foods high in serotonin e.g. bananas, avocados.

Metabolism of tryptophan

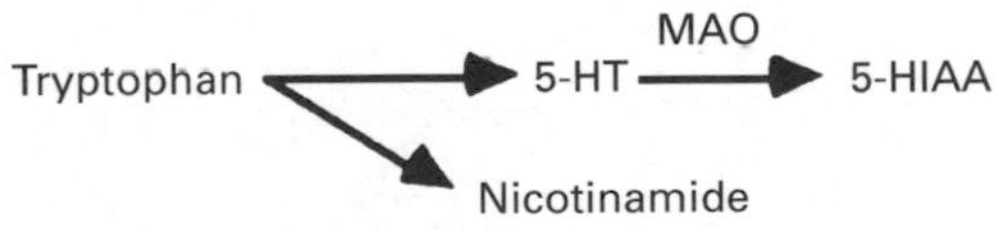

5HT = 5-hydroxytryptamine (serotonin)
5-HIAA = 5-hydroxyindoleacetic acid
MAO = Monoamineoxidase

Fig. 6.23

Vanillyl mandelic acid level (VMA)

A high urinary level present in:

1. Tumours of sympathetic nervous tissue, e.g. phaeochromocytoma, neuroblastoma.
2. Drugs e.g. monoamine oxidase inhibitors (MAOI), phenothiazines, methyl-dopa, tetracyclines and L-dopa.
3. Diet e.g. bananas, vanilla, tea, coffee, ice cream, chocolates.

Gastrin, glucagon and VIP

See page 208.

Multiple endocrine neoplasia (MEN) or pluriglandular syndrome

Two or more endocrine glands secrete excessive amounts of hormones. See Table 6.23.

Table 6.23 Multiple endocrine neoplasia

MEN I	*MEN II*
Parathyroid adenoma	Medullary carcinoma of the thyroid
Pancreatic islets cells (gastrinoma, insulinoma)	Phaechromocytoma
Anterior pituitary gland	Parathyroid carcinoma or adenoma
Adrenal cortex	
Thyroid	

BIOCHEMISTRY OF COAGULATION/FIBRINOLYSIS

THE COAGULATION CASCADE AND FIBRINOLYTIC PATHWAY (Fig. 6.24)

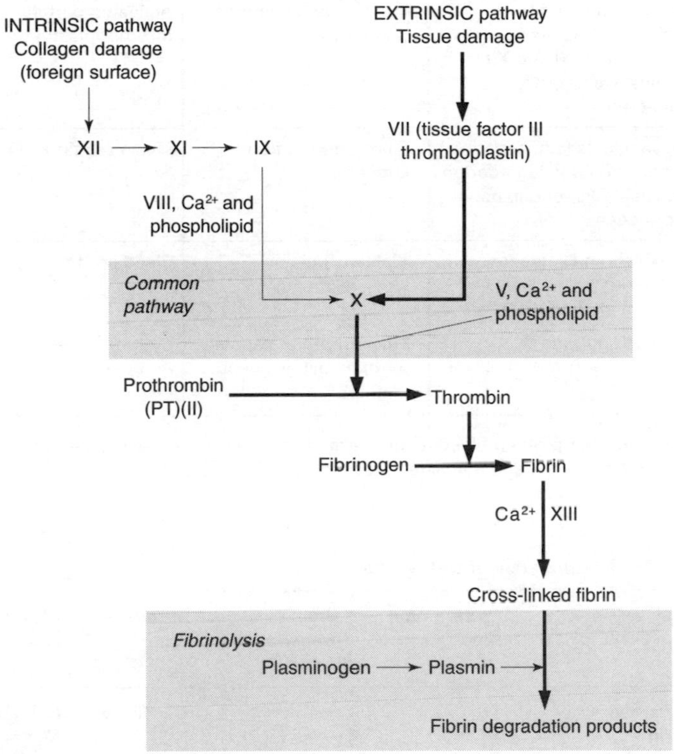

Fig. 6.24

ABNORMALITIES OF COAGULATION

See Tables 6.24 and 6.25

Other causes of abnormal coagulation

Heparin therapy prevents activation of factors II, IX, X, XI and probably VII. Therapy may be monitored using APPT and PTT.

Vitamin K deficiency and *warfarin* treatment affects synthesis of factors II, VII, IX and X.

Disseminated intravascular coagulation (DIC) affects factors I, II, V, VIII and XI.

Liver disease affects factors I, II, V, VII, IX and X.

Table 6.24 Abnormalities of coagulation

Causes of abnormal coagulation	*Function*	*Test*
Deficiency of factors I, II, V, VII, X	Extrinsic and common pathways	Prothrombin time (PT)
Haemophilia A and B Deficiency of factors I, II, V, VIII, IX, X, XI and XII Not sensitive to factor VII deficiency	Intrinsic and common pathways	Activated partial thromboplastin time (APTT)
Anticoagulants (e.g. heparin), presence of fibrin degradation products (FDPs) or depletion of fibrinogen	Fibrinogen to fibrin conversion	Thrombin time (TT)
Von Willebrand's, uraemia and aspirin* Normal in clotting disorders	Platelet function	Bleeding time
Haemophilia A and B	Final common pathway, Intrinsic pathway and platelet function	Clotting time

*Other drugs that prolong bleeding time are phenothiazines, tricyclic antidepressants, dextran, dipyridamole and antihistamines.

Table 6.25 Interpretation of test results

	Prothrombin time	*Partial thromboplastin time*	*Thrombin time*	*Platelet count*
Liver disease	↑	↑	Usually N	N initially
Warfarin	↑	↑	N	N
Factor VII deficiency	↑	N	N	N
Haemophilia	N	↑	N	N
Christmas disease	N	↑	N	N
Heparin	↑	↑	↑	N
Disseminated intravascular coagulation	↑	↑	↑	↓

APPT and PT normal: platelet or vessel defect.
APPT and PT abnormal: defect in common pathway.
APPT normal and PT abnormal: factor VII deficiency.
APPT abnormal and PT normal: defect in intrinsic system.

INTERPRETATION OF LABORATORY FINDINGS

BLOOD

Effects of delayed transport and haemolysis of blood

↑ levels of plasma potassium, phosphate, total acid phosphatase, lactate dehydrogenase and AST.

Prolonged venous stasis during venesection

↑ levels of plasma total Ca^{2+}, total protein, lipids and T4.

Taking blood from 'drip' arm

Electrolyte and glucose concentration approximately equal to composition of infused fluid; dilution of all other concentrations.

Use of wrong bottle

1. EDTA or oxalate: ↓ [Ca^{2+}], ↑ [Na^+] or [K^+]
2. Failure to use a fluoride tube for a blood glucose specimen results in a high glucose reading (fluoride inhibits erythrocyte glycolysis).

Metabolic effects of pregnancy/oral contraceptive therapy

↑ plasma T_4 (due to ↑ thyroxine-binding globulin), ↑ plasma cortisol (due to ↑ cortisol-binding globulin)
↑ TIBC (due to plasma transferrin), ↑ plasma iron
↑ plasma alkaline phosphatase
↑ urinary glucose, and abnormal glucose tolerance tests
↑ serum amylase, ↑ serum cholesterol
Low plasma gonadotrophin, ↑ plasma prolactin.

Drugs that alter thyroid function tests

Lithium carbonate (↓ in protein binding index (PBI), free T4 and ^{131}I uptake)
Phenytoin (↓ in PBI, T4 and T3)
Salicylates (↓ in PBI, T4 and ^{131}I)
Oestrogens and oral contraceptive pill (↑ PBI and T4)
Androgens and anabolic steroids (↓ T4 and ↑ T3 uptake)
Phenylbutazone (↑ PBI, T3 uptake and ↓ ^{131}I)
Propylthiouracil (↓ ^{131}I uptake, T4 and T3).

Laboratory findings in hypothermia (core temperature <35°C)

1. ↑ Hb, haematocrit and plasma viscosity.
2. Thrombocytopaenia and disseminated intravascular coagulation.
3. Hyponatraemia, ↑ blood sugar, creatinine kinase and serum amylase.
4. Thyroid function tests unreliable.

CEREBROSPINAL FLUID (CSF)

COMPOSITION OF CSF

Table 6.26 Composition of cerebrospinal fluid in normal and pathological states

Feature	*Normal values*	*Acute purulent meningitis*	*Aseptic viral meningitis*	*Tuberculous meningitis*
Appearance	Clear	Cloudy	Usually clear	Opalescent
Normal volume	130 ml			
pH	7.3			
Cells/mm³	0–5 lymph.	10–100 000 polymorphs	15–2000 lymph.	250–500 lymph.
Glucose* (mmol/l)	2.8–4.4	low	normal	very low
Protein (g/l)	0.15–0.35	0.5–5.0	0.2–1.25	0.45–5.00
Albumin: globulin ratio	8 : 1			
Chloride	20 mmol/l			
Pressure = 10–18 cmH_2O (lying on side) 30 cmH_2O (standing)				

*Normally 60–70% of plasma level.

CHANGES IN CSF

Causes of low CSF glucose

1. Hypoglycaemia
2. Infection, e.g. bacterial and fungal meningitis, toxoplasmosis
3. Subarachnoid haemorrhage
4. Leukaemia
5. Sarcoidosis.

Causes of raised CSF protein

1. Intracranial haemorrhage
2. Meningitis (tuberculous, bacterial or fungal)
3. Encephalitis
4. Cerebral tumour
5. Carcinomatous neuropathy
6. Neurofibromatosis (especially acoustic barrier neuroma)
7. Guillain–Barré syndrome

} *Inflammatory disease:* Globulin: albumin ratio small due to leakage of albumin via the blood–brain barrier

8. Multiple sclerosis
9. Neurosyphilis
10. SLE
11. Cerebral sarcoidosis

} *Demyelinating disease:* ↑ globulin: albumin ratio because of intrathecal synthesis of immunoglobulin

12. Multiple myeloma
13. Lymphoma
14. Benign paraproteinaemia
15. Diabetic neuropathy

} Monoclonal bands of immunoglobulins

URINE BIOCHEMISTRY

Table 6.27 Values in urine biochemistry

Feature	*Normal values*
Volume	400 ml/day–4 l/day
Specific gravity	1.008–1.030
pH	4.5–7.8
Protein	0–90 mg/day
Urobilinogen	up to 6.7 mmol/day
$[Na^+]$	100–250 mmol/day
$[K^+]$	40–120 mmol/day
Cells	Leucocytes and non-squamous epithelial cells, small number of red cells and some hyaline casts
Osmolality	50–1200 mosmol/kg

Urine casts

1. Hyaline casts (most common) arise from tubules. Do not indicate renal dysfunction.
2. Epithelial/granular casts occur when there is acute inflammation or acute oliguric renal failure.
3. White cell casts occur in medullary inflammation, e.g. pyelonephritis
4. Red cell casts occur in glomerular damage, e.g. SLE and acute glomerulonephritis

Proteinuria (>1.5 g per day)

1. Glomerular proteinuria commonest; due to increased glomerular permeability
2. Tubular proteinuria occurs with renal tubular damage from any cause, especially pyelonephritis (mainly α_2- and β-globulin)
3. Also: Bence–Jones proteinuria, haemoglobinuria and myoglobinuria

Positive Clinitest reaction

Colour change from blue to orange in presence of a reducing agent

Causes

1. Glycosuria e.g. diabetes mellitus, thyrotoxicosis, postgastrectomy, phaeochromocytoma, gross cerebral injury,

severe infection, lag glucose tolerance curve and reduced renal threshold, as in pregnancy.

2. Others
   (i) galactosaemia (galactose)
   (ii) hereditary fructosaemia (fructose)
   (iii) benign fructosuria, pentosuria, and lactosuria
   (iv) alkaptonuria (homogentisic acid)
3. Drugs, e.g. salicylates, isoniazid, L-dopa, vitamin C, tetracyclines

Myoglobinuria

Causes

Crushing injuries
Severe muscle damage due to exercise
Electrical shock
Progressive muscle diseases.

Haemoglobinuria

Causes

Incompatible blood transfusion
Haemolytic anaemias
Burns
Paroxysmal cold haemoglobinuria
Paroxysmal nocturnal haemoglobinuria.

Elevated urinary calcium

Causes

Hyperparathyroidism
Bone tumours
Hypervitaminosis D
Hyperthyroidism
Cushing's syndrome.

Decreased urinary calcium

Causes

Hypoparathyroidism
Vitamin D deficiency
Coeliac disease
Decreased calcium intake

Cystinuria

Causes

Cystinosis
Cystinuria

SYNOVIAL FLUID

- Normal synovial fluid does not clot because it lacks fibrinogen or other clotting factors. Inflammatory processes allow these to enter, so that if the fluid is allowed to stand a clot will form.
- RA cells: 95% of patients with rheumatoid arthritis have RA cells in their synovial fluid.
- LE cells: 30% of patients with rheumatoid arthritis have ANA in their synovial fluid.
- Crystals: monosodium urate crystals are associated with gout.
- Calcium pyrophosphate crystals are associated with chondrocalcinosis.

7. Statistics and epidemiology

CHAPTER CONTENTS

STATISTICS

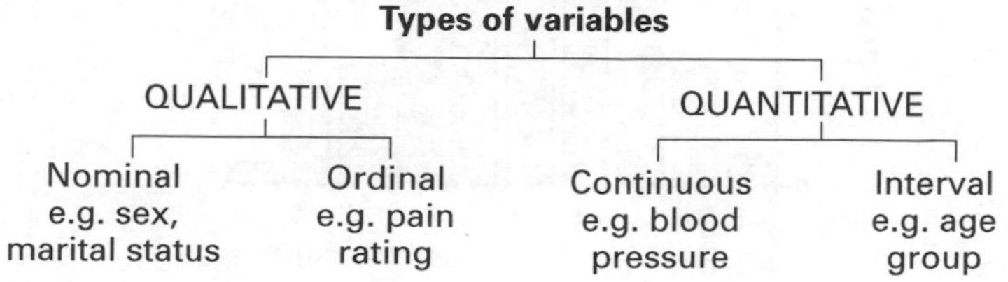

Fig. 7.1

FREQUENCY DISTRIBUTIONS

A frequency distribution shows the values which can be taken by a variable and the frequency with which each value is observed, e.g. pie chart, Venn diagram, bar chart and histogram.

FREQUENCY HISTOGRAM (Fig. 7.1)

- With *non-equal* base lines the *area* of each block is proportional to the frequency.
- With *equal* base lines the *height* of each block is proportional to the frequency.

CUMULATIVE FREQUENCY PLOT (Fig. 7.2)

- The frequency of data in each category represents the sum of the data from that category and from the preceding categories.
- Useful in calculating distributions by percentiles, including the median.

Arithmetic scale: equal distances measure equal absolute distances.
Logarithmic scale: equal distances measure equal proportional differences (i.e. percentage change in a variable).

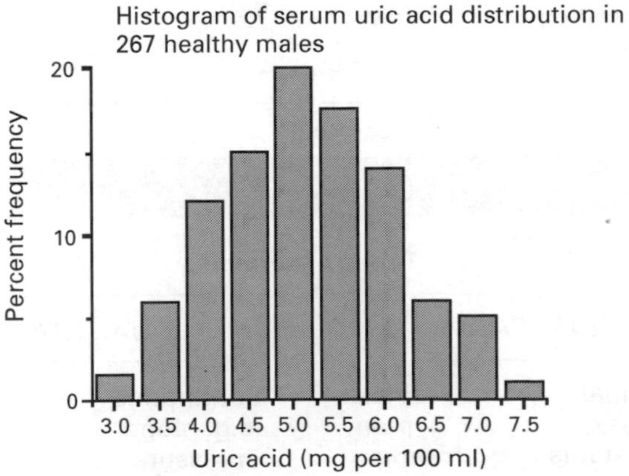

Fig. 7.2

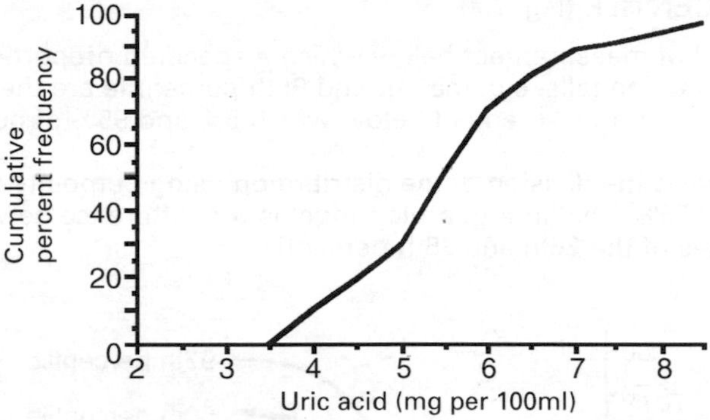

Fig. 7.3

MEASURES OF CENTRAL TENDENCY

$$\textbf{Arithmetic mean} = \frac{\text{Sum of observations}}{\text{Number of observations}}$$

The geometric mean is calculated using first the logarithm of the values, then the arithmetic mean of the logarithm and finally the antilog of the calculated arithmetic mean.

- Used as a substitute for the arithmetic mean when the distribution is skewed, or for describing fractional values, e.g. a series of serum antibody titres. Can only be used for positive values.

The median is the central value of a series of observations arranged in order of magnitude. Unlike the mean, it is not sensitive to extreme values in a series.
The mode is the most frequently observed value in a series of values, i.e. the maximum point in a frequency distribution.

MEASURES OF DISPERSION

(Measures of variation, spread)

1. SAMPLE RANGE

Difference between the highest and lowest values. Disadvantages are that:

1. Range increases as the number of observations increases and extreme values may be unreliable.
2. It provides no information as to the variability of the values between the extremes.

2. PERCENTILE (Fig. 7.4)

The level of measurement below which a specified proportion of the distribution falls, e.g. the 5th and 95th percentile are the values of a particular measurement below which 5% and 95% of people fall.

A *quartile* is the division of the distribution using cutpoints at 25%, 50% and 75%. The 'interquartile range' is the difference between the values of the 25th and 75th percentile.

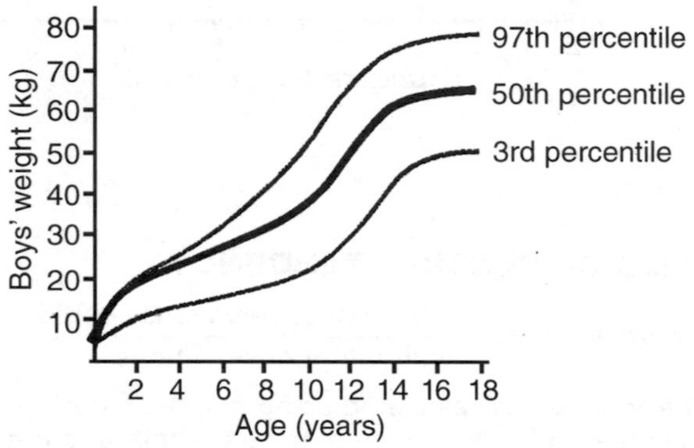

Fig. 7.4

3. VARIANCE AND STANDARD DEVIATION

Measure of spread of observations about the mean.

$$\text{Variance} = \frac{\text{Sum of (individual observations} - \text{mean})^2}{\text{Number of observations}}$$

$$\text{Standard deviation (SD)} = \sqrt{\text{Variance}}$$

4. COEFFICIENT OF VARIATION

- Ratio of the standard deviation of a series of observations to the mean of the observations. It is without units and expressed as a percentage.

$$\text{Coefficient of variation (\%)} = \left(\frac{\text{SD}}{\text{mean}}\right) \times 100$$

- Used to make comparisons of spread when the means are dissimilar, i.e. standard deviation of 10 around a mean of 40 indicates a greater degree of scatter than a standard deviation of 10 around a mean of 400.

PROBABILITY DISTRIBUTIONS

The probability distribution of a random variable is a table, graph or mathematical expression giving the probabilities with which the random variable takes different values.

1. NORMAL OR GAUSSIAN DISTRIBUTION (Fig. 7.5)

- Theoretical, symmetrical bell-shaped distribution.
- Specified by its mean and standard deviation. The mean, median and mode are equal.
- Approximately 68% of the observations fall within one standard deviation of the mean; 95% of observations fall within two standard deviations from the mean and 99% fall within three standard deviations from the mean.

> *Example:* 1000 men have a mean weight of 160 lb with a standard deviation of 10 lb. The population weight is normally distributed. Thus, 680 (68%) of the men have weights of 160 ± 10 lbs (±1SD) or between 150 and 170 lbs, and 997 (99.7%) have weights of 160 ± 30 lbs (±3SD) or between 130 and 190 lbs.

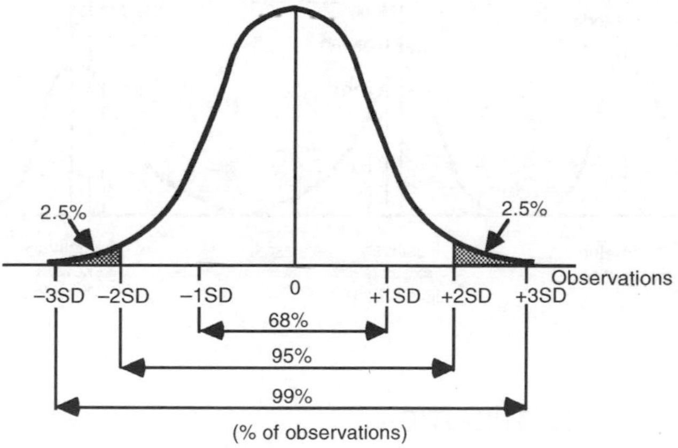

Fig. 7.5

2. SKEWED DISTRIBUTION (Fig. 7.6)

- A distribution that is asymmetric.
- A skewed distribution with a longer tail among the *lower* values is skewed to the *left* or *negatively* skewed.
- A skewed distribution with a longer tail among the *higher* values is skewed to the *right* or *positively* skewed.
- In general, if the curve is skewed, the mean is always towards the long tail, the mode near the short tail, and the median somewhere between the two.

Transformation of data is performed when comparisons are made between two or more samples with unequal variances or when their distributions are non-normal. Logarithmic, square root or square transformations are used most commonly.

3. LOG-NORMAL DISTRIBUTION

This is a skewed distribution when plotted using an arithmetic scale, but is a normal distribution using a logarithmic scale.

4. BINOMIAL DISTRIBUTION

This describes the probability distribution of possible outcomes from a series of data when there are:

1. Only two mutually exclusive outcomes, e.g. success or failure, boy or girl.
2. A known number of independent trials of an event, and the probability of an event or outcome is the same for all trials, e.g. the probability of three male births in a family of six children, where the child's sex is the outcome of the trial.

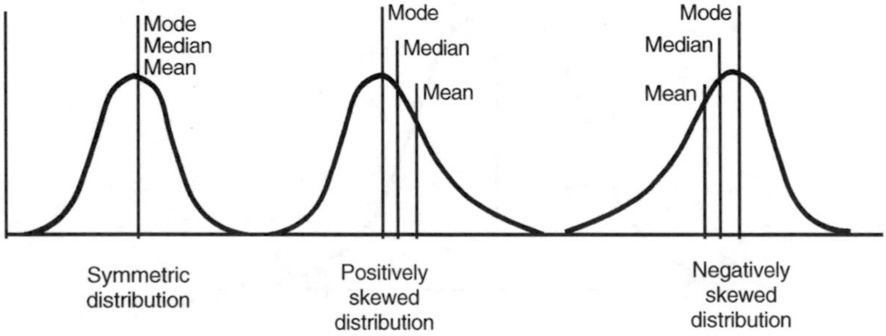

Fig. 7.6

5. POISSON DISTRIBUTION

This describes the probability of occurrence of rare events in a large population. It represents a limiting case of the binomial distribution, e.g. the probability of occurrence of a specific congenital birth defect in a large number of births.

SAMPLING

Used to estimate unknown characteristics of a population, such as:

1. The mean value of some measurement.
2. The proportion of the population with some characteristic.

Statistical inference is the process of inferring features of the population from observation of a sample.
Sampling error may be due to *systematic* or *random errors*.

Systematic errors (biases)

1. *Selection bias* occurs when comparisons are made between groups of patients that differ with respect to determinants of outcome other than those under study. Methods for controlling for selection bias include:
   (i) randomization (see page 317)
   (ii) restricted study eligibility of patients,
   (iii) matching of patients in one study group to those with similar characteristics in the comparison group,
   (iv) stratification (i.e. comparison of rates within groups of individuals who have the same values for the confounding variable),
   (v) adjustment, either using simple methods of standardization or the techniques of multiple linear and logistic regression.
2. *Measurement bias* occurs when the methods of measurement are consistently dissimilar among groups of patients, e.g. recall bias occurs when individuals in one group are more likely to remember past events than individuals in another of the study or control groups. Recall bias is especially likely when the study involves serious disease and the characteristics under study are commonly occurring, subjectively remembered events.
3. *Confounding bias* occurs when two factors 'travel together' and the effect of one is confused or distorted by the other.

Random errors

Such errors are determined by heterogeneity of the population and sample size (see page 309, type I and II errors).

CENTRAL LIMIT THEOREM (Fig. 7.7)

- Means of repeated random samples of a particular size from a population will be normally distributed around the original

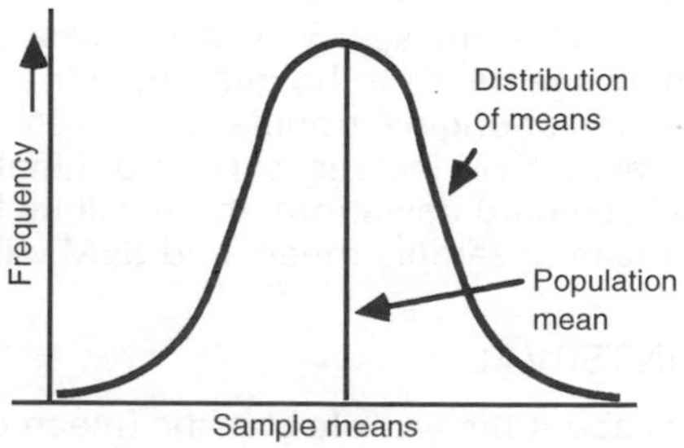

Fig. 7.7

population mean, regardless of the distribution of the observations in the original population, from which the samples were drawn.
- The mean value of the collection of all possible sample means will equal the mean of the original population.

STANDARD ERROR OF THE MEAN (SEM)

- The distribution of the means of these samples has a standard deviation around the population mean. This is called the standard error of the mean and describes the distribution of mean values. It depends on both the standard deviation of the original population and the sample size.

$$\text{Standard error} = \frac{\text{Standard deviation of observations in a sample}}{\sqrt{\text{Sample size}}}$$

- It measures the variability of the sample statistic (mean or proportion) in relation to the true, but unknown, population characteristic, i.e. how accurate is the sample mean as an estimate of the population mean? *(Contrast with the standard deviation which is a measure of the variability of the observations.)*
- Also used when one sample mean is compared to another, and in constructing confidence intervals for a mean or proportion.

> *Example:* Mean systolic blood pressure of 500 randomly selected males from Glasgow was 130 mmHg and the standard deviation was 12.05 mmHg. To determine the precision of this mean, i.e. how closely it gives the true mean blood pressure of males in this district:
>
> $$\text{SEM} = \frac{12.05}{\sqrt{500}} = 0.55 \text{ mmHg}$$

This represents an estimate of the standard deviation of means in the sample of 500.

SEM is affected by two main factors:
1. *Sample size (n):* as n increases, SEM decreases: i.e. to halve SEM, the sample size needs to be quadrupled.
2. *Standard deviation* of original population values: as the standard deviation increases, SEM increases: i.e. if original population is uniform (small standard deviation), there will be little variation from sample mean to sample mean, and SEM will be small.

CONFIDENCE INTERVAL

- It is the interval about the sample statistic (mean or proportion) which contains the unknown true value with a known probability.

- Conventional confidence limits are 90%, 95% and 99%. It is standard practice to use 95% confidence limits.

Sample mean ± 2.56 SE = 99% confidence interval (probability 0.99)

i.e. 99% of *sample means* under normal distribution curve lie within a distance of 2.56 SD from the true population mean, or 99% confident that the interval contains the true population mean. (*Contrast with 99% of observations under any normal distribution curve lie within 2.56 SD from the mean*).

Sample mean ± 1.96 SE = 95% confidence interval (probability 0.95)

Sample mean ± 1.00 SE = 68% confidence interval (probability 0.68)

> *Example:* Metoprolol trial in acute myocardial infarction: n = 698 patients on metoprolol; percent dying within 90 days on metoprolol = 5.7% with a standard error of 0.88%. Therefore, the 95% confidence limits for the true percentage dying on metoprolol = 5.7 ± 1.96 × 0.88 = 4.0% and 7.5% (i.e. 95% confident that if the whole population of eligible patients were given metoprolol, the true percentage dying lies somewhere between 4.0% and 7.5%).

Z SCORE

This is the simplest example of a statistical test. It examines the comparison between a sample mean and a known population mean by calculating the ratio of the difference between means to the standard error.

$$Z = \frac{\text{sample mean} - \text{population mean}}{\text{SEM}}$$

The Z score (or critical ratio) is the number of standard deviations that a value in a normally distributed population lies away from the mean. Thus, in a normally distributed population, 95% of the population lie within 1.96 Z scores of the mean.

HYPOTHESIS TESTING AND STATISTICAL SIGNIFICANCE

NULL HYPOTHESIS

The null hypothesis underlies all statistical tests. It states that there is no difference between the samples or populations being compared, and that any difference observed is simply the result of random variation.

Null hypothesis (H_0): $P_1 - P_2 = 0$ or $P_1 = P_2$

Alternative hypothesis (H_A): $P_1 - P_2 \neq 0$ or $P_1 \neq P_2$

Where P_1 is the probability of a characteristic in sample or population 1, and P_2 is the probability of the same characteristic in the control sample or comparison population 2.

STATISTICAL SIGNIFICANCE

The purpose of significance testing is to assess *how strong is the evidence* for a difference between one group and another, or whether random occurrence could reasonably explain the difference.

Significance level (α)

Conventional significance levels are: 5%, 1% and 0.1%. The smaller the value, the less the likelihood of the difference having occurred by chance. A 5% significance level is most often used for statistical comparisons (i.e. a 5% chance of detecting a difference and rejecting the null hypothesis, when the treatments are actually the same, means that one out of 20 times the result would occur by chance). If chosen at the outset of the study, it expresses the risk the investigator is prepared to accept of a type 1 error (see below) occurring.

Critical level (p value)

The strength of the evidence may also be expressed in terms of probabilities (p values). Conventional p values are 0.05 (5%), 0.01 (1%) and 0.001 (0.1%).

Confidence intervals

These may also be used to provide an indication of the plausible range of the difference between two proportions. The recommendations of the major scientific journals are that confidence limits should be calculated and shown for all results.

One- and two-tailed tests

- *A two-tailed (-sided) test* is concerned with differences between observations in either direction, (i.e. checks both the upper and lower tails of the normal distribution).
  For example, two alternative treatments, A and B are compared, where either A or B may be better.
- *A one-tailed (-sided) test* is only concerned with differences between observations in one direction, (i.e. only one tail of the normal distribution curve), e.g. whether drug A is better than a placebo. The p value for a one-tailed test is generally half that for a two-sided test.

Type I and II errors (Table 7.1)

These concern the incorrect rejection or acceptance of the null hypothesis. There are two types of errors:

1. Type I (α) error: the probability of detecting a significant difference when the parameters, or treatments, are really the same (*significance level* α), i.e. the risk of a false-positive result.
2. Type II (β) error: the probability of not detecting a significant difference when there really is a difference, i.e. the risk of a false-negative result. One minus the type II error ($1 - \beta$) is the *power* of the test to detect a difference.

The power of a test depends on:

1. the significance level
2. the size of the difference you wish to detect
3. the sample size.

Table 7.1 Type I and II errors

Conclusions from observations	*Actual situation*	
	Treatment has an effect	*Treatment has no effect*
Treatment has an effect	True positive $1 - \alpha$	False positive α
Treatment has no effect	False negative β	True negative $1 - \beta$

Determinants of sample size

1. Magnitude of the difference in outcomes between the two treatment groups.
2. Probability of an α (type I) error, i.e. false-positive result. Usually set at 0.05.
3. Probability of a β (type II) error, i.e. false-negative result. Usually set at 0.20.
4. Proportion of patients experiencing the outcome of interest and the variability of observations. An insufficient number of patients may lead to failure to detect the true difference that may exist (type II error).

Clinical versus statistical significance

Statistical significance is not the same as clinical importance. Clinical relevance must be assessed in terms of the magnitude of the difference. A statistically significant difference may not be clinically important and vice versa.

TESTS OF SIGNIFICANCE

- Used for comparisons between estimates (sample means or proportions).

- Two types:
  1. *Parametric*
  2. *Non-parametric*

PARAMETRIC TESTS

Assumptions:
1. The populations from which samples are taken should be normally distributed.
2. The variances of the samples are the same (applies to t test).

Student's t test

- Based on the t distribution and is used for comparing a single small sample with a population or to compare the difference in means between two small samples.
- The t test is inappropriate if more than two means are compared.
- As the sample size increases, the t distribution closely resembles the normal distribution, and at infinite degrees of freedom (see Note), the t and normal distribution are identical.

$$\text{Calculated t value} = \frac{\text{observed difference in means}}{\text{standard error of the difference in means}}$$

- Calculated t value is compared with a critical t value from tables at a predetermined significance level and appropriate degrees of freedom. The larger the value of t (+ or –), the smaller the value of p, and the stronger the evidence that the null hypothesis is untrue.

Note: Degrees of freedom (df) are the number of independently varying quantities, i.e. the number of variables in a series or distribution that can be freely assigned values when the sum of the values is fixed. Used in preference to sample size.

(a) Using paired data

The paired t test compares the means of two small paired observations, either on the same individual or on matched individuals, e.g. comparison of the effects of two drugs on a particular patient, at different points in time.

$$t = \frac{\bar{x}}{\frac{\sqrt{s^2}}{n}}$$

where s = SD.
$\bar{x}$ is the mean difference between the pairs,
and n is the number of pairs.
(df = number of pairs –1.)

(b) Using unpaired data

The unpaired t test compares the means of two small, independent samples e.g. two separate groups of patients.

$$t = \frac{\bar{x}_1 - \bar{x}_2}{s\sqrt{\left(\frac{1}{n_1} + \frac{1}{n_2}\right)}}$$

where s = pooled SD
n_1 and n_2 = number of patients in treatment groups
$\bar{x}_1$ and $\bar{x}_2$ are the means from samples 1 and 2.
(df = $(n_1 - 1) + (n_2 - 1)$)

NON-PARAMETRIC TESTS

- Make no assumptions about the underlying distribution of the sample.
- Used when data is qualitative, i.e. measured by ordinal (rank) scale, or not normally distributed.
- Not as powerful as parametric tests when data is normally distributed.

Examples

1. Chi-square (χ^2) test.
2. Fisher's exact probability test: used to determine the exact probability that an observed distribution is due to chance, when the expected frequencies in any one cell of a contingency table are less than 5.
3. Wilcoxon rank sum test: used for unpaired data.
4. Mann–Whitney U test: gives equivalent results to the Wilcoxon rank sum test.
5. Wilcoxon signed rank test: used for matched or paired data.

Chi-square test

- Used to determine the extent to which an observed series of proportions (or frequencies) differs from an expected series of proportions (or frequencies), or that two or more proportions (or frequencies) differ from one another, based on the chi-square probability distribution.
- Can only be used on count data, and the categories of data used must be mutually exclusive and discrete.

$$\chi^2 = \frac{\text{Sum of (observed} - \text{expected)}^2}{\text{Expected}}$$

- Calculated χ^2 value is compared with a critical value of χ^2 from tables at a predetermined significance level and appropriate degrees of freedom. The larger the value χ^2, the smaller the probability p, and so the stronger the evidence that the null hypothesis is untrue.

Yates' correction factor

The chi-square test is based on a normal approximation of the binomial distribution, and therefore a correction for continuity, called the Yates' correction factor, is often included in the chi-square test equation. The Yates' correction factor is used with small samples, and decreases the chi-square value, so that the null hypothesis is less often rejected.

CORRELATION

Describes the strength of the linear relationship between variables and is denoted by the *correlation coefficient (r)* or *Pearson's product moment correlation coefficient* (Table 7.2).

- Its value can range from –1 to +1.
- A correlation coefficient may be strong but insignificant because of sample size.

Table 7.2 Correlation

Correlation coefficient (r)	*Degree of association*
0.8 to 1.0	Strong
0.5 to 0.8	Moderate
0.2 to 0.5	Weak
0 to 0.2	Negligible

- *Scattergrams* show the relationship between X and Y, e.g. height and weight (Fig. 7.8).
- Spearman's and Kendall's rank correlation coefficients are the non-parametric alternatives to Pearson's correlation coefficient.

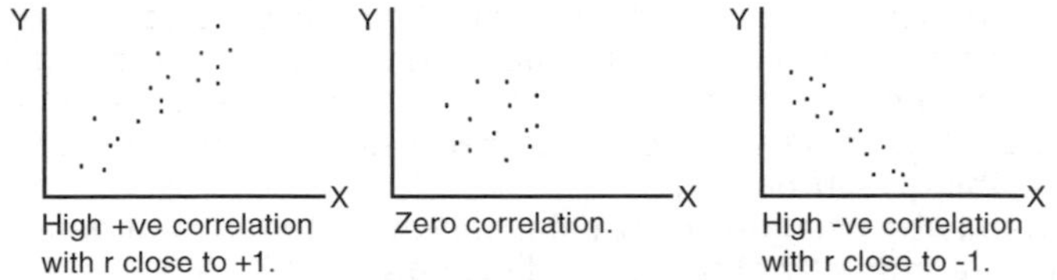

Fig. 7.8

LINEAR REGRESSION

- Mainly used when there is one measured dependent variable and one or more independent variables.
- Used when the main purpose is to develop a predictive model, i.e. to predict Y for a given value of X (Fig. 7.9).

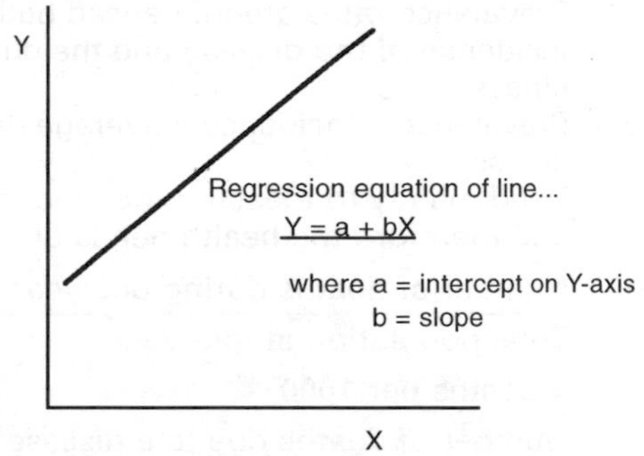

Fig. 7.9

- *Multiple regression* predicts a single dependent variable using a number of independent variables.

EPIDEMIOLOGY

CRUDE RATES

- These are summary rates for a given population, i.e. not standardized for age, sex or other variables, e.g. crude birth and death rate.
- They cannot be used to compare events in different populations because these rates will vary depending on the age–sex composition of the total population.

Incidence rate: $\dfrac{\text{Number of new cases of a disease in a given period}}{\text{Total population at risk during the same period of time}}$

Change in incidence indicates a change in the balance of aetiological factors.

Attack rate: Incidence rate calculated in an epidemic situation, using a particular population observed for a limited period of time.
Normally expressed as a percentage.

Prevalence rate (point): $\dfrac{\text{Total number of cases in a population at one particular time}}{\text{Total population at risk at the time}}$

Point prevalence refers to a particular point in time.
Period prevalence refers to a given time interval.

Prevalence rates are influenced both by the incidence of the disease and the duration of the illness:
Prevalence = Incidence × average duration of illness.
Used mainly to measure the amount of illness and therefore the health needs of a community.

Mortality rate:

$$\frac{\text{Number of deaths during one year}}{\text{Total population at mid-year}} \times 1000$$

= Deaths per 1000

Case fatality rate:

$$\frac{\text{Number of deaths due to a disease in a specified period of time}}{\text{Number of cases of the disease in the same period of time}} \times 100$$

i.e. the risk of dying if the disease is contracted. Normally expressed as a percentage.

Proportionate mortality rate (PMR):

$$\frac{\text{Number of deaths from a given cause in a specified period of time}}{\text{Total number of deaths in the same period of time}} \times 100$$

Used to determine the relative importance of a specific cause of death in relation to all causes of death in a population, e.g. the three leading causes of deaths in the US in 1980 were heart disease (PMR = 38.2%); cancer (PMR = 20.9%) and stroke (PMR = 8.6%).
It is not a rate and therefore does not measure the probability of dying from a particular cause. Usually expressed as a percentage.

ADJUSTED RATES

- These equalize the differences in the populations at risk so that the rates are comparable. Age-adjusted rates are most frequently used.
- The direct and indirect methods of standardization are two statistical methods employed to compute adjusted rates.

Standardized mortality ratio (SMR): Ratio of observed deaths in a particular population to the number that would be expected if a standard mortality rate for that population applied, i.e. age/sex standardized rate. It is calculated using the indirect method of standardization. Usually expressed as a percentage.
If the SMR > 100, then more events are occurring in the population than expected.

SPECIFIC RATES

- These relate only to a specific part of the population, e.g. age, sex, race, occupation, cause-specific death rates, and therefore can be used to compare events in different populations.

Still birth rate:

$$\frac{\text{Number of still births (See Note)}}{\text{Total births (live and still) in the same period of time}} \times 1000$$

Perinatal mortality rate (PMR):

$$\frac{\text{Number of still births and early neonatal deaths (<7 days old) in a period of time}}{\text{Total number of births (live and still) in the same period of time}} \times 1000$$

Infant mortality rate (IMR):

$$\frac{\text{Number of deaths under 1 year of age in a period of time}}{\text{Number of live births in same period}} \times 1000$$

IMR consists of two segments: the neonatal mortality rate (deaths <28 days old) and the postneonatal mortality rate (deaths 28 days to 11 months).

Neonatal and perinatal mortality are generally affected by causes of death related to maternal health, whilst the postneonatal mortality is more closely linked to environmental factors.

Note: Still birth is defined as delivery of a fetus that shows no signs of life after a presumed 28-week gestation.

PRINCIPLES OF STUDY DESIGN

Table 7.3 Simple 2 × 2 table used in cohort and case–control studies

		Disease		*Total*
		Present	*Absent*	
Exposure	Present	a	b	a + b
	Absent	c	d	c + d
Total		a + c	b + d	n

COHORT (PROSPECTIVE OR LONGITUDINAL) STUDIES

Persons exposed (a + b) to the suspected cause and those not exposed (c + d) are followed prospectively over time, to determine the rate of specific diseases or events (Fig. 7.10).

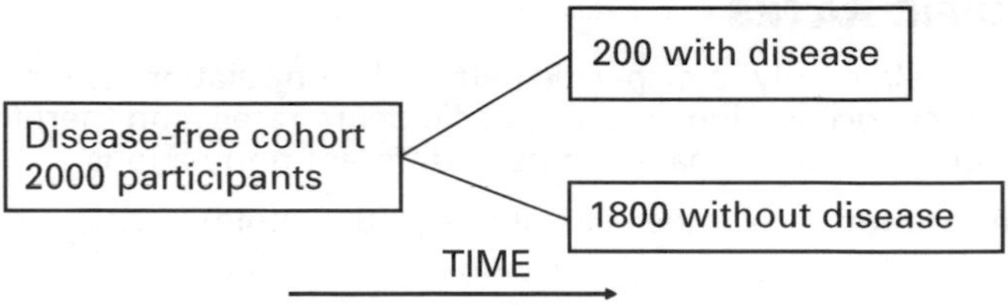

Fig. 7.10

$$\text{Incidence rate in the exposed group} = \frac{a}{a + b}$$

$$\text{Incidence rate in the non-exposed group} = \frac{c}{c + d}$$

Life-table or survival analysis

A method of estimating the survival of a cohort over time, when some individuals are followed for longer periods of time than others. The chance of surviving to any point in time is estimated from the cumulative probability of surviving each of the time intervals that preceded it (syn: Kaplan–Meier life tables).

CASE–CONTROL (RETROSPECTIVE) STUDIES

Persons with a disease (a + c) and those without (b + d) are identified, and then compared regarding specific characteristics to determine their possible association with the disease.

$$\text{Exposure rate among cases} = \frac{a}{a + c}$$

$$\text{Exposure rate among controls} = \frac{b}{b + d}$$

Table 7.4 Comparison of case-control and cohort studies

Case–control	*Cohort*
1. Suitable for rare diseases	1. Suitable for common diseases
2. Short study time	2. Prolonged study time
3. Smaller number of subjects	3. Large number of subjects
4. Bias may occur in the selection of cases and controls and in ascertaining exposure	4. Less selection bias occurs
5. No volunteer subjects needed	5. Subjects usually volunteer
6. Cannot determine incidence	6. Incidence determined

Table 7.5 Methods of controlling for selection bias

Strategy	*Comment*
Randomization	Assigns patients to groups in a way that gives each patient an equal chance of falling into one or the other group
Restriction	Limits the range of characteristics of patients in the study
Matching	For each patient in one group, selects one or more patients with the same characteristics (except for the one under study) for a comparison group
Stratification	Compares rates within subgroups (strata) with otherwise similar probability of the outcome
Adjustment	
Simple	Mathematically adjusts crude rates for one or a few characteristics so that equal weight is given to strata of similar risk
Multiple	Adjusts for differences in a large number of factors related to outcome, using mathematical modelling techniques

CROSS-SECTIONAL STUDIES

Provide information on prevalence, not incidence, i.e. distribution of disease in a population at a particular point in time.

CLINICAL TRIALS

Experimental design used to assess the differences between two or more groups receiving different interventions or treatments.

Effectiveness: The extent to which a treatment produces a beneficial effect when implemented under the *usual* clinical conditions for a particular group of patients.

Efficacy: The extent to which a treatment produces a beneficial effect when assessed under the *ideal* conditions of an investigation.

Randomization: Method of assignment of subjects to either the experimental or control treatments, whereby each patient has an equal chance of appearing in any one treatment group.

- Protects against selection bias in the assignment process.
- Allows the control of other clinical variables which may affect the outcomes under investigation, and so minimizes the effects of systematic error (bias).

Placebo: A pharmacologically inert dummy, identical in appearance to the treatment(s), should normally be used for the control group, when there is no conventional treatment available.

- It dissociates the effects of treatment from the suggestive element imposed by the receipt of treatment.

Double-blinding (masking) technique: Neither the subject nor the investigator knows to which group the subject is assigned.

- Most desirable in trials where the endpoints used are subjective, i.e. improved/unchanged/worse.

Analysis by 'intention to treat': Outcome among all those allocated to treatment after randomization is compared to all those allocated to control, irrespective of whether patients actually received the allocated treatment(s). This avoids introducing bias into the assessment of treatment.

Cross-over or 'within-patient' trial: A comparison of the effects of two or more treatments in the same patient, when the treatments are applied at different points in time in the course of the illness.

- Suitable for the assessment of short-term effects of treatment in relatively stable, chronic conditions.

Meta-analysis: Analysis performed on data from two or more different but similar studies, usually clinical trials, for the purpose of drawing a global conclusion concerning the usefulness of a drug or procedure, the contribution of a risk factor to a disease, or the role of a condition in the aetiology of a disease. The main problems relate to pooling results fron heterogeneous studies.

MEASURES OF EFFECT

Absolute risk: Rate of occurrence of a disease, i.e. incidence.

Relative risk:

$$\frac{\text{Incidence rate among exposed}}{\text{Incidence rate among non-exposed}}$$

$$\frac{a/(a+b)}{c/(c+d)} = \frac{ad}{bc}$$

(When the incidence of disease is *low*, this simplifies to ad/bc.)
Thus, relative risk measures strength of association between a factor and outcome. The

stronger the association between the exposure and the disease, the higher the relative risk.

Attributable risk: Incidence rate among exposed minus the incidence rate among non-exposed
I.e., measures the amount of risk that can be attributed to a particular factor.

Population attributable risk: The excess incidence of disease in a community that is associated with a risk factor. It is a product of the attributable risk and the prevalence of the risk factor in the population.

Population attributable fraction: The fraction of disease in a population that is attributable to exposure to a particular risk factor. It is obtained by dividing the population attributable risk by the total incidence of disease in a population.

Example: Death rate from lung cancer in smokers (i.e. absolute risk) = 0.80/1000/year. Death rate from lung cancer in non-smokers = 0.05/1000/year.
Prevalence of smoking = 50%
Total death rate from lung cancer = 0.50/1000/year
Therefore:

$$\text{Relative risk} = \frac{0.80/1000}{0.05/1000} = 16.0$$

$$\begin{aligned}\text{Attributable risk} &= 0.80/1000/\text{year} - 0.05/1000/\text{year}\\ &= 0.75/1000/\text{year}\end{aligned}$$

$$\begin{aligned}\text{Population attributable risk} &= 0.75/1000/\text{year} \times 0.50\\ &= 0.375/1000/\text{year}\end{aligned}$$

$$\text{Population attributable fraction} = \frac{0.375/1000}{0.50/1000} = 0.75$$

Odds ratio

With a case–control study, it is not possible to obtain a relative risk by dividing the incidence of disease among those exposed by the incidence of disease among those not exposed. An alternative approach uses the odds ratio which is conceptually and mathematically similar to the relative risk.
The odds is itself the ratio of two probabilities:

$$= \frac{\text{Probability of an event}}{1 - \text{probability of an event}}$$

Example:

Odds that a case is exposed $= \frac{a/(a+c)}{c/(a+c)} = \frac{a}{c}$

Odds that a control is exposed $= \frac{b/(b+d)}{d/(b+d)} = \frac{b}{d}$

The ratio of the odds is $\frac{a/c}{b/d} = \frac{ad}{bc}$

Odds ratio and relative risk

The odds ratio is approximately equal to the relative risk only when the incidence of disease is *low*.

ASSOCIATION AND CAUSATION

An association may be artefactual (because of bias in the study), non-causal or causal.

Five criteria adopted as a test of causation

1. Consistency of the association, i.e. dose–response.
2. Strength of the association, i.e. size of relative risk.
3. Specificity of the association, i.e. degree to which one particular exposure produces one particular disease.
4. Temporal relationship of the association, i.e. exposure to factor must precede the development of the disease.
5. Biological plausibility of the association.

Ecological fallacy

The type of error that can occur when the existence of a group association is used to imply the existence of a relationship that does not exist at the individual level.

Cause–effect studies

Types of studies which examine cause–effect relationships and their relative strength of evidence are shown in Table 7.6.

Table 7.6 Study design and strength of evidence

Strong ↑	Clinical trial
	Cohort study
	Case–control study
	Cross-sectional
	Aggregate risk
	Case series
↓ Weak	Case report

SCREENING

Table 7.7 Screening

Test result	*Diagnosis*	
	Disease	*No disease*
Positive	a	b (false + ve)
Negative	c (false – ve)	d

VALIDITY

The ability of a screening test to provide an indication of which individuals have the disease and which do not.
Four components:

1. *Sensitivity* (%) is the test's ability to correctly identify those individuals who truly have the disease.

$$\frac{\text{Persons with the disease detected by the screening test}}{\text{Total number of persons tested with the disease}} \times 100$$

$$= \frac{a}{a + c} \times 100$$

A high sensitivity implies few false negatives (Fig. 7.11) which is important for very rare or lethal diseases, e.g. phenylketonuria.

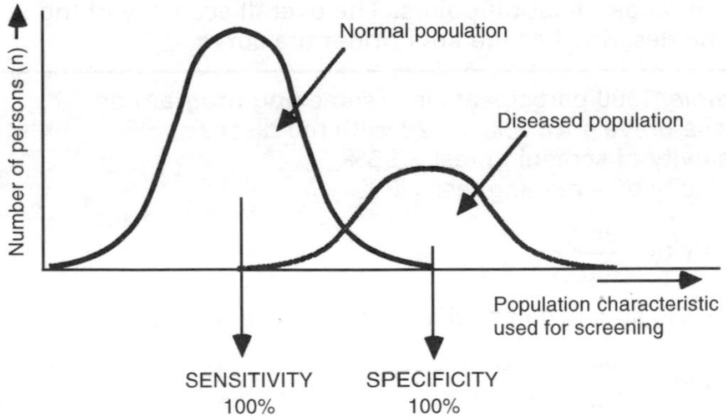

Fig. 7.11

2. *Specificity* (%) is the test's ability to correctly identify those individuals who do not have the disease.

$$\frac{\text{Persons without the disease who are negative to the screening test}}{\text{Total number of persons tested without the disease}} \times 100$$

$$= \frac{d}{b + d} \times 100$$

A high specificity implies few false positives, which is important for common diseases, e.g. diabetes.

3. *Predictive value* (%) is the test's ability to identify those individuals who truly have the disease (true positives) amongst all those individuals whose screening tests are positive.

$$\frac{\text{True positive (a)}}{\text{True positive (a) + false positive (b)}} \times 100$$

The predictive value of a positive test increases with increasing disease prevalence.

- Lowering the screening cut-off level *increases* the sensitivity and number of false positives and *decreases* the specificity and number of false negatives.
- One way to express the relationship between sensitivity and specificity is to construct a receiver operating characteristic (ROC) curve. This may be used to describe the accuracy of a test over a range of cut-off points. The overall accuracy of the test can be described as the area under the curve.

Example: 1000 participants in a screening programme
Disease prevalence 2%, i.e. 20 with the disease
Sensitivity of screening test = 95%
Specificity of screening test = 90%

Sensitivity: $\frac{95}{100} = \frac{a}{a + c}$

a + c = 20; so a (true positive) = 19, c (false negative) = 1

Sensitivity: $\frac{90}{100} = \frac{d}{b + d}$

b + d = 980; so b (false positive) = 98, d (true negative) = 882

Positive predictive value $= \frac{a}{a + b} = \frac{19}{19 + 98} = 16.24\%$

4. *The likelihood ratio* for a particular value of a diagnostic test is defined as: the probability of that test result in the presence of a disease, divided by the probability of the result in people without the disease.
   Likelihood ratios express how many times more (or less) likely a test result is to be found in diseased as compared to non-diseased people.

BASIC REQUIREMENTS OF A SCREENING TEST

1. Test parameters should be high, i.e. high sensitivity and specificity.
2. The test should be applicable to a large number of individuals.
3. The test should be easily and quickly accomplished.
4. The test should not cause harm to the individual being tested.
5. The test should be inexpensive.

8. Clinical pharmacology

CHAPTER CONTENTS

Hyperuricaemia
Hyperkalaemia
Hypokalaemia
Hyponatraemia/inappropriate ADH
Nephrogenic diabetes insipidus
Metabolic acidosis
Osteomalacia
Exacerbation of porphyria

Blood diseases
Aplastic anaemia or neutropaenia
Thrombocytopaenia
Megaloblastic anaemia
Folate deficiency
Haemolytic anaemia
B_{12} deficiency
Methaemoglobinaemia
Lymphadenopathy

Neuropsychiatric
Organic psychoses
Drug withdrawal states
Confusional states
Depression
Extrapyramidal reactions
Peripheral neuropathy
Proximal myopathy
Acute rhabdomyolysis
Exacerbation of myasthenia
Pseudotumour cerebri

Sexual dysfunction
Impotence
Decreased libido
Failure of ejaculation

Otological
Deafness/tinnitus/vertigo

Eye
Corneal opacities
Cataract
Retinopathy
Optic neuritis

Dermatological
Fever
Serum sickness
SLE-like syndrome
Erythema nodosum
Fixed drug eruptions
Erythema multiforme or
Toxic epidermal necrolysis
Pigmentation
Raynaud's syndrome
Photosensitivity
Loss or alteration of taste
Hirsutism/hypertrichosis
Alopecia

GLOSSARY

Pharmacokinetics: Study of the time course of drug absorption, distribution, metabolism and excretion.

Pharmacodynamics: Study of the biochemical and physiological effects of drugs and their mechanisms of action.

Plasma half-life The time taken for drug plasma concentration to fall by 50% (for first-order reactions only). Symbol, $t_{½}$

Steady state: Occurs when the amount of drug administered during the dosage interval equals the amount of drug eliminated during a dosage interval. Dependent on $t_{½}$.
A loading dose or increased frequency of initial doses is used to achieve a steady state more rapidly, e.g. digoxin, phenytoin (Fig. 8.1). The actual steady state

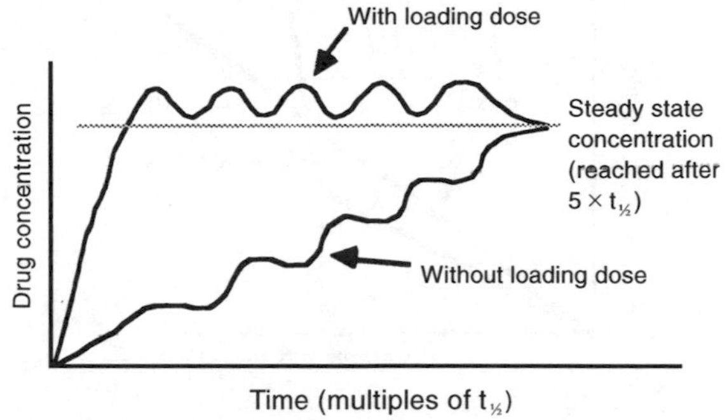

Fig. 8.1

concentration is directly proportional to the size of the dose, and indirectly proportional to the volume of distribution and the eliminator constant.

Clearance: The volume of plasma cleared of drug in unit time. Expressed in ml/min.

Bioavailability: Extent to which a drug is absorbed systemically. It depends on formulation, gut motility, disease states and first-pass effect.

First-pass effect: Metabolic breakdown of certain drugs before entering the systemic circulation on initial passage through either the liver (e.g. propanolol, GTN, lignocaine, pethidine and oestrogens), the intestinal mucosa (e.g. L-dopa, chlorpromazine, ethanol) or lungs (e.g. isoprenaline). This results in some drugs being unavailable if given by certain oral routes.

Volume of distribution (Vd): The theoretical fluid volume which would contain the total body content of a drug at a concentration equal to the plasma concentration. Expressed in m/s/kg. Drugs that are highly lipophilic and extensively tissue-bound have a large volume of distribution, e.g. nortriptyline, chloroquine. Drugs that are poorly lipophilic and highly plasma protein-bound have a low volume or distribution, e.g. warfarin, aspirin gentamicin, theophylline. A knowledge of Vd can be used to determine the size of a loading dose, if an immediate response to treatment is required.

Drug elimination: *First-order (linear) elimination* (Fig. 8.2). Most common type for both drug absorption and elimination. The rate of reaction is directly

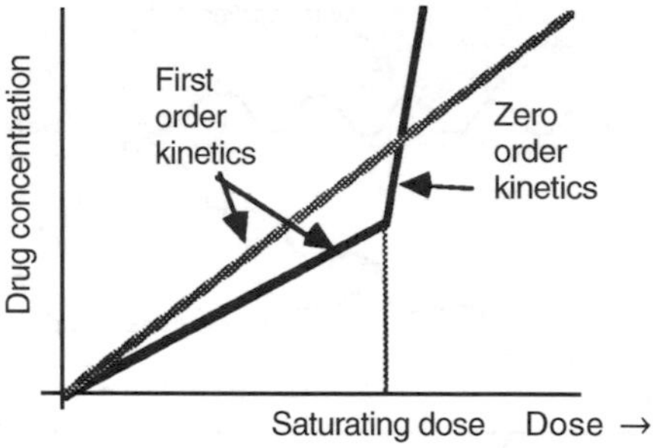

Fig. 8.2

proportional to the amount of drug available, i.e. constant fraction of drug absorbed or eliminated in unit time.

Zero-order elimination (Fig. 8.2). Proceeds at a constant rate and is independent of the amount of drug available. This usually occurs when a high concentration of the drug is present or when the normal elimination mechanism of a drug is saturated, e.g. inhalational anaesthetics or IV infusions. Some first-order reactions may switch to zero-order kinetics when high drug concentrations are present, e.g. hepatic metabolism of phenytoin near the therapeutic level. At this point it is important to adjust the dose in small amounts to avoid toxic effects. Therapeutic monitoring of plasma drug concentrations is used for drugs with a narrow therapeutic range (e.g. lithium), or which show dose-dependent kinetics (e.g. phenytoin).

1. Digoxin
2. Antiarrythmics, e.g. procainamide, quinidine.
3. Anticonvulsants, e.g. phenobarbitone, phenytoin, valproate and carbamazepine.
4. Antibiotics, e.g. aminoglycosides.
5. Others, e.g. theophylline, lithium.

Therapeutic index: Margin of safety of a drug. Ratio of the lethal or toxic dose (LD) and the therapeutically effective dose (ED). In animal experiments, the therapeutic index is often taken as the dose at which 50% of the population respond.

$$\text{Therapeutic index} = \frac{LD_{50}}{ED_{50}}$$

Dose–response curves: Graphs of drug concentration plotted as a function of the response.
Competitive antagonism
In the presence of different concentrations of an antagonist the dose–response curves show parallel displacement but with the same maximal effect, i.e. antagonism can be overcome by raising the concentration of the agonist drug.
Non-competitive antagonism
The maximal effect declines with higher concentrations of the antagonist.

Drug potency: Relative concentrations of two or more drugs that elicit the same effect (Fig. 8.3).

Drug efficacy: Maximal effect that a particular drug may elicit (Fig. 8.3).

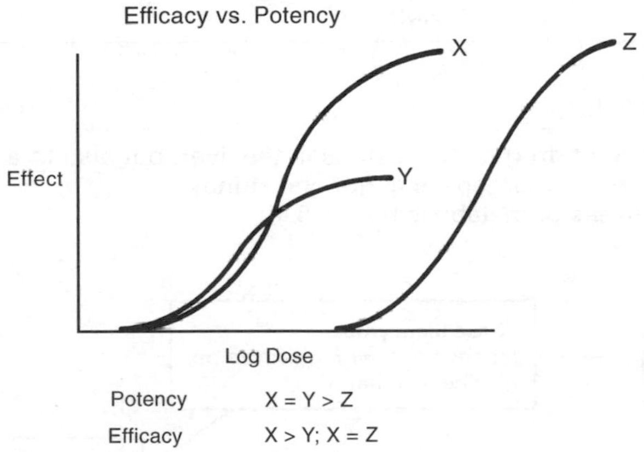

Fig. 8.3

DRUG INTERACTIONS

MAJOR MECHANISMS OF DRUG INTERACTIONS

DRUG ABSORPTION

- Drugs causing decreased absorption, e.g. anticholinergic agents (↓ gastric emptying); cholestyramine (ion exchange resin binder); iron and other chelating agents.
- Drugs causing increased absorption (↑ gastric emptying), e.g. metoclopramide.

PLASMA PROTEIN BINDING (Table 8.1)

- Drug displacement affects drugs that are highly protein-bound, e.g. clofibrate, salicylates, sulphonamides, phenylbutazone, tolbutamide, phenytoin, warfarin.

Table 8.1 Plasma protein binding

Bound drugs	*Displacing drug*	*Effect*
Bilirubin	Sulphonamides Vitamin K Salicylates	Kernicterus
Tolbutamide	Salicylates Phenylbutazone Sulphonamides	Hypoglycaemia
Warfarin	Salicylates Clofibrate Phenylbutazone Phenytoin	Haemorrhage

METABOLISM

- Main site of drug metabolism is in the liver, but also to a lesser extent in other organs, e.g. gut and kidney.
- Two phases of metabolism (Fig. 8.4):

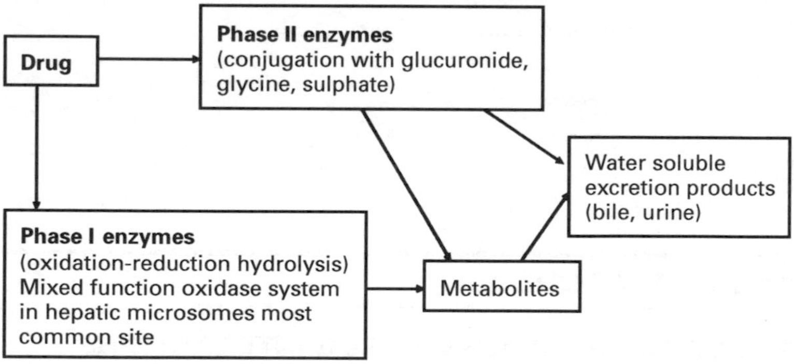

Fig. 8.4

Mixed function oxidase system (MFOS)

Dependent on $NADPH_2$, cytochrome P450 and cytochrome P450 reductase, which catalyse the incorporation of molecular oxygen.

Factors affecting metabolism

1. Enzyme *inducers*, e.g. barbiturates, carbamazepine, griseofulvin, phenytoin and rifampicin.
2. Enzyme *inhibitors*, e.g. allopurinol, cimetidine, ciprofloxacin, erythromycin, isoniazid, chloramphenicol and phenylbutazone.
3. Age, sex and disease states.
4. Genetic constitution: genetic factors influence both *drug response* and *drug metabolism* (see Tables 8.2 and 8.3).

Genetic variation and drug response

Table 8.2 Genetic variation associated with drug sensitivity

Pharmacogenetic trait	*Adverse effects*	*Drugs to avoid*
G6PDH deficiency in erythrocytes (X-linked recessive) Mainly in Africans, some Mediterranean races, Iraqi Jews, Chinese and South-East Asians	Haemolysis (See below and Fig. 8.5)	'Oxidant' drugs **Analgesics:** Aspirin, phenacetin **Antibacterials:** Chloramphenicol, sulphonamides, nitrofurantoin, dapsone, cotrimoxazole **Antimalarials:** Chloroquine, primaquine, quinine, mepacrine **Others:** Quinidine, probenecid
Methaemoglobin-reductase deficiency (autosomal recessive)	Methaemoglobinaemia	As above plus nitrates, nitrites, local anaesthetics
Malignant hyperpyrexia (autosomal recessive)	Hyperpyrexia with muscular rigidity	Suxamethonium
Acute intermittent porphyria (autosomal dominant)*	(See page 264) Pyrexia Abdominal pain Constipation Confusion Peripheral neuropathy Tachycardia ↑BP	**CNS drugs:** Alcohol, barbiturates **Antibacterials:** Rifampicin, sulphonamides, griseofulvin, chloroquine, oral contraceptives **Others:** Phenytoin, sulphonylureas, methyldopa

*Drugs considered safe: *Analgesics*, e.g. salicylates, morphine and related opiates; *antibiotics*, e.g. penicillins, tetracyclines, chloramphenicol; *CNS drugs*, e.g. phenothiazines, diazepam; *antihypertensives*, e.g. propanolol; *others* e.g. digoxin, nitrous oxide, succinylcholine and atropine.

G6PDH deficiency and haemolysis

G6PD maintains low levels of methaemoglobin in red cells. If the methaemoglobin level increases, haemolysis occurs (Fig. 8.5).

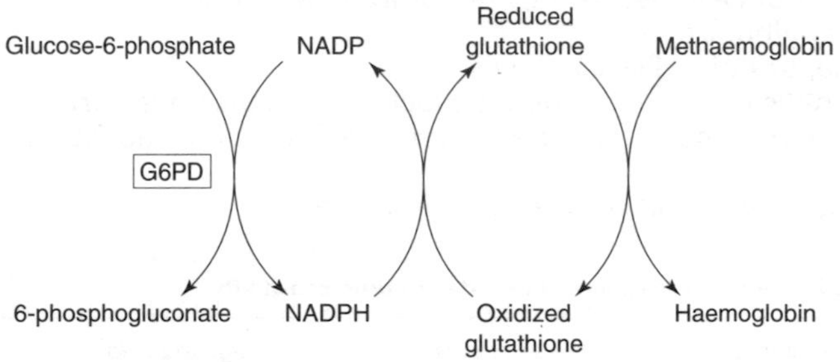

Fig. 8.5

Genetic variation and drug metabolism

Table 8.3 Genetic variation in drug metabolism

Pharmacogenetic trait	*Adverse effects*	*Drugs to avoid or take in reduced dose*
Acetylation (*fast* acetylation = autosomal dominant) (Prevalence of rapid acetylation: Canadian Eskimos, 100%; Japanese 88%; UK, 38%; Egyptians, 18%)	Lupus-like syndrome (see below) or neuropathy in slow acetylators; *fast* acetylators show a diminished response	Hydralazine Isoniazid Procainamide Dapsone Nitrazepam Sulphonamides Sulphasalazine
Suxamethonium sensitivity due to an abnormal plasma pseudocholinesterase (autosomal recessive) (1 in 2500 in UK, but absent in Japanese and Eskimos, rare in Africans)	Prolonged muscle paralysis and apnoea	Suxamethonium
Phenacetin-induced methaemoglobinaemia (autosomal recessive)	Methaemoglobinaemia	Phenacetin

Features of a drug-induced SLE syndrome

1. Equal sex incidence.
2. Most commonly affects persons of HLA type DR4 (i.e. slow acetylators).
3. Dose-related and usually reversible.
4. Renal and CNS disease unlikely.
5. Positive antinuclear antibody.
6. Complement usually unaffected.

EXCRETION

- Changes in urine pH, e.g. alkalinization of urine increases the elimination of phenobarbitone and aspirin in overdose; amphetamine overdose is treated by urine acidification.
- Competition for active renal tubular excretion, e.g. probenecid and penicillin; digoxin and quinidine.
- Drugs which undergo an enterohepatic circulation (EHC) include thyroxine, oestrogens, stilboestrol and rifampicin.
- Dubin–Johnson's syndrome: failure of excretion of bilirubin glucuronide into bile; inherited as autosomal recessive.

PHARMACOLOGIC INTERACTIONS

For example, at drug receptor site (see Tables 8.4–8.27).

ADVERSE EFFECTS AND INTERACTIONS OF DRUGS

Important drug adverse effects and interactions are summarized in Tables 8.4–8.27.

ANTIHYPERTENSIVE DRUGS

Table 8.4 Antihypertensives*

Class/drug	*Adverse effects*	*Interacting drug(s)*	*Interacting effect*
All antihypertensives		Corticosteroids Oral contraceptives NSAIDS	— Antagonism of hypotensive effect (due to fluid retention
Centrally acting	1. Depression and drowsiness 2. Dry mouth 3. Nasal stuffiness 4. Fluid retention		
Methyldopa	*Specific side-effects:* 1. Fever 2. Diarrhoea 3. Failure of ejaculation 4. Positive Coomb's test (20%) 5. Haemolytic anaemia 6. Hepatitis 7. Pancreatitis 8. Gynaecomastia	Tricyclic antidepressants Phenothiazines	— Antagonism of hypotensive effect
Clonidine	*Specific side-effects:* 1. Constipation 2. Rebound hypertension on sudden withdrawal	Tricyclic antidepressants	— Antagonism of hypotensive effect Exacerbates the rebound hypertension in clonidine withdrawal
Moxonidine	1. Similar sedative properties to clonidine but no rebound hypertension	Other antihypertensive agents Benzodiazepines	— Potentiation of antihypertensive effect — Potentiation of sedation

Table 8.4 *(cont.)*

Class/drug	*Adverse effects*	*Interacting drug(s)*	*Interacting effect*
β-**blockers** *Non-selective* Propanolol *Selective* Atenolol Metoprolol Bisoprolol *Intrinsic sympathomimetic activity* Pindolol *Antiarrhythmic properties* Sotalol *Dual antihypertensive action* Labetolol	1. Precipitate cardiac failure 2. Exacerbate Raynaud's and peripheral vascular disease 3. Bradycardia and heart block 4. β-Blockers inhibit hypoglycaemia-related tachycardia 5. Bronchospasm esp. in asthmatics 6. Lethargy, depression, and sleep disturbance 7. Oculocutaneous syndrome (Practolol)	Verapamil (high dose, IV) Disopyramide Oral hypoglycaemics Insulin	— Profound hypotension — Heart failure — Prolonged hypoglycaemic action — Increased hypoglycaemic action of insulin
Vasodilators	1. Headache 2. Flushing 3. Nasal congestion 4. Postural hypotension 5. Tachycardia 6. Fluid retention		
Hydralazine	*Specific side-effects:* 1. SLE syndrome (+ve ANF), esp. with slow acetylators or high dose (> 200 mg/day) 2. Bone marrow depression 3. Peripheral neuropathy		

Table 8.4 *(cont.)*

Class/drug	*Adverse effects*	*Interacting drug(s)*	*Interacting effect*
Prazosin	First-dose dizziness or syncope		
Minoxidil	1. Hypertrichosis 2. Pulmonary hypertension (with long-term treatment)		
Nitrates/nitrites	1. Flushing with severe headache 2. Severe hypotension		
Angiotensin-converting enzyme inhibitors (ACE) *First generation* Captopril Enalapril Lisinopril *Second generation* Fosinopril Perindropril Quinapril Ramipril Trandolapril	1. First-dose hypotension (esp. in renal failure or with diuretics). Hyperkalaemia 2. Rashes. Angio-oedema 3. Proteinuria/haematuria 4. Loss of taste 5. Leucopaenia esp. with pre-existing immune complex disease 6. Persistent dry cough	Potassium-sparing diuretics NSAIDs	— Hyperkalaemia — Antagonism of antihypertensive effect
Angiotensin II antagonists Losartan Valsartan (Angiotensin II binds to the AT_1 receptor which is coupled to a G protein and causes vasoconstriction and aldosterone release. Losartan blocks this effect)	Similar adverse effect profile to ACE inhibitors but without cough, because does not inhibit the breakdown of bradykinin and other lumps. 1. Hypotension, esp. in patients with intravascular volume depletion 2. Hyperkalaemia 3. Angio-oedema		

Table 8.4 *(cont.)*

Class/drug	*Adverse effects*	*Interacting drug(s)*	*Interacting effect*
Calcium antagonists			
Dihydropyridines Nidedipine Nicardipine Amlodipine	1. Vasodilator side-effects (headache and facial flushing, palpitations) 2. Ankle swelling	β-Blockers	↑ Cardiopredepressant effect
Verapamil	1. Bradycardia, AV conduction defects 2. Constipation		
Diltiazem	1. Bradycardia, AV conduction defects 2. Skin rash		
Diuretics			
Thiazides	1. Hypokalaemia 2. Hypomagnesaemia 3. Hyperuricaemia 4. Hyperglycaemia 5. Acute urinary retention 6. Precipitates hepatic encephalopathy 7. Pancreatitis 8. Inhibits Ca^{2+} excretion† 9. Rashes 10. Thrombocytopaenia 11. Impotence (20%)	Digoxin Lithium	— Potentiation of side-effects of thiazides
Loop diuretics	(As above) *Specific side-effects:* 1. Deafness (esp. in renal failure) 2. Thrombocytopaenia 3. ↑ Ca^{2+} excretion 4. ↓ uric acid secretion	Gentamicin Cephalosporins	— ↑ risk of nephrotoxicity and ototoxicity
Potassium-retaining diuretics	1. Hyperkalaemia 2. Gynaecomastia		

**Effect of antihypertensive drugs on serum lipids and lipoproteins*—Thiazide diuretics, ↑ total cholesterol, LDL and triglycerides; β-blockers, ↑ triglycerides and ↓ HDL; prazosin, clonidine and methyldopa, ↓ cholesterol and LDL; angiotension–converting enzyme inhibitors and calcium blockers, no apparent effect on lipid levels.

†Used for treatment of idiopathic hypercalcuria.

ANTIARRHYTHMICS

Table 8.5 Antiarrhythmic drugs: classification of drug actions

Class		*Drugs*
I	Fast sodium channel inhibitors	Ia Quinidine, procainamide, disopyramide Ib Lignocaine, phenytoin, mexiletine, tocainide Ic Flecainide
II	Antisympathetic agents	β-blockers
III	Prolongation of action potential duration	Amiodarone, bretylium, sotalol
IV	Slow calcium channel antagonists	Verapamil, diltiazem
	Not classified	Digoxin, adenine nucleotides

Table 8.6 Antiarrhythmic drugs: adverse effects and interactions

Drug	*Adverse effects*	*Interacting drug(s)*	*Interacting effect*
Digoxin	1. Confusion and insomnia 2. Colour vision defects 3. Xanthopsia 4. Anorexia, nausea and vomiting 5. Arrhythmias esp. (i) Ventricular extrasystoles and bigeminy (ii) Atrial tachycardia with AV block	Hypokalaemia due to potassium-depleting diuretics, corticosteroids, carbenoloxone, and amphotericin B Verapamil β-Blockers Hypercalcaemia Quinidine Amiodarone Also in the elderly, renal failure, hypoxia, severe heart and pulmonary disease	— Digoxin toxicity enhanced
Verapamil	1. Dizziness and constipation 2. Hypotension and AV block 3. Cardiac failure and peripheral oedema	β-Blockers Digoxin	— ↑ AV block — ↑ digoxin levels
Quinidine	1. 'Cinchonism' 2. Cardiac failure, 3. Hypotension, AV block 4. Hypersensitivity	Antihypertensive agents Digoxin Amiodarone Warfarin	— Potentiation of hypotensive effects — ↑ digoxin toxicity — ↑ quinidine levels — ↑ anticoagulant effect
Disopyramide	1. Anticholinergic effects 2. Myocardial depressant	Antihypertensive agents	— Potentiation of hypotensive effects
Procainamide	1. Ventricular arrhythmias 2. SLE syndrome 3. Agranulocytosis 4. Hypersensitivity		

Table 8.6 *(cont.)*

Drug	*Adverse effects*	*Interacting drug(s)*	*Interacting effect*
Lignocaine	1. Hypotension 2. Convulsions 3. Myocardial depression	Phenytoin	— Cardiac depression
Amiodarone	1. Photosensitivity 2. Thyroid dysfunction 3. Fibrosing alveolitis 4. Corneal deposits (do not interfere with sight and reverse on stopping drug) 5. Flattened T wave 6. Tremor, peripheral neuropathy 7. Proarrhythmic effect	Digoxin and warfarin Class I A and C antiarrhythmics β-Blockers, verapamil	— ↑ risk of digoxin and warfarin toxicity — Proarrhythmic effect — ↑ AV block
Adenosine (adenosine receptor agonist used for treatment of supraventricular tachycardias)	1. Short-lived vasodilator effects (flushing, dyspnoea, chest pain, hypotension). Cardiac transplant patients are particularly susceptible 2. Bronchoconstriction in asthmatics 3. Transient heart block	Theophylline Dipyridamole	— ↓ effect of adenosine — ↑ effect of adenosine

ORAL ANTICOAGULANTS AND INTRAVENOUS THROMBOLYTIC AGENTS

Table 8.7 Oral anticoagulants

All produce *increased anticoagulant effect in*: alcoholism, liver disease, renal failure, cardiac failure, thyrotoxicosis, fever and hypoalbuminaemia.

Drug	*Adverse effects*	*Interacting drug(s)*	*Interacting effect*
Warfarin	1. Alopecia 2. Haemmorhagic skin necrosis		↑ **anticoagulant effect**
		NSAIDs Oral hypoglycaemics Metronidazole Cotrimoxazole Ampicillin Cephalosporins Erythromycin Clofibrate Salicylates	— Due to displacement of warfarin from protein binding
		Chloramphenicol Alcohol (acute) Phenylbutazone Cimetidine Amiodarone	— Due to liver enzyme inhibition
		Salicylates (high dose)	— Due to ↓ clotting factor synthesis
		Broad spectrum antibiotics (neomycin)	— Due to ↓ vit. K synthesis
			↓ **anticoagulant effect**
		Barbiturates Phenytoin Rifampicin Carbamazepine Griseofulvin Oral contraceptives	— Due to enzyme induction (sudden ↑ effect when interacting drug is stopped)
		Vitamin K	— Due to increased clotting factor synthesis inhibition
		Cholestyramine	— Due to reduced absorption

Table 8.7 *(cont.)*

Drug	*Adverse effects*	*Interacting drug(s)*	*Interacting effect*
Aspirin	1. GI disturbance and haemorrhage	GI irritants	— ↑ peptic ulceration
	2. 'Salicylism' (deafness, tinnitus and vomiting)	Oral hypoglycaemics	— ↑ hypoglycaemic effect
	3. Hypersensitivity (asthma, urticaria and angio-oedema	Warfarin, NSAIDS	— ↑ anticoagulant effect
	4. Gout (urate retention with low doses (1–2 g/day), uricosuric with high doses)	Steroids	— ↓ aspirin effect
	5. Analgesic nephropathy		
	6. Aggravation of bleeding disorders (hypoprothrombinaemic)		
	7. Reye's syndrome in children		

Intravenous thrombolytic agents

Streptokinase (see Fig. 8.6) Adverse effects: bleeding or allergic reaction. Contraindications include bleeding diathesis, active bleeding (e.g. from a peptic ulcer), recent surgical operation, post cardiac massage, severe uncontrolled hypertension, recent stroke, recent treatment with streptokinase.
Uncontrolled

Anistreplase (anisoylated plasminogen streptokinase activator complex (APSAC)). Same adverse effect profile as streptokinase. Less likely to cause hypertension, but more likely to cause allergy or haemorrhage.

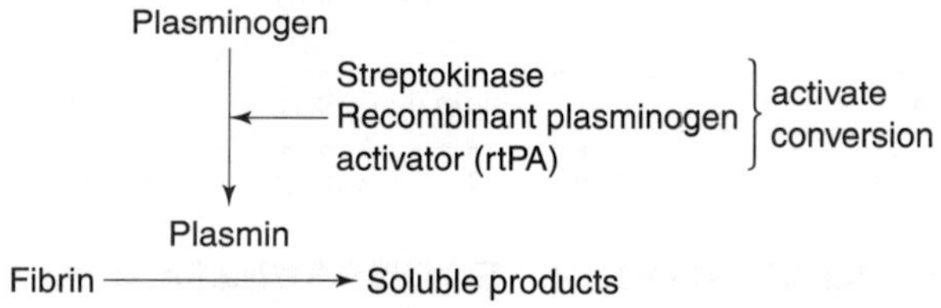

Fig. 8.6

LIPID-LOWERING DRUGS

Table 8.8 Lipid-lowering drugs: Summary of actions

Drug	*LDL*	*HDL*	*Triglycerides*
HMGCoA reductase inhibitors	↓↓	↑	→
Fibrates	↓	↑	↓
Bile acid sequestrant resins	↓	→	→
Others			
Nicotinic acid	↓	↑	↓
Probucol	↓	↓	→

Table 8.9 Lipid-lowering drugs

Drug	*Adverse effects*	*Interacting drug(s)*	*Interacting effect*
HMGCoA reductase	Infrequent		
Simvastatin	1. Skin reactions	Warfarin	— Extensively bound to albumin
Pravastatln	1. Myalgia		
Fluvastatin	1. Headache		
Fibrates			
Bezafibrate	1. GI upsets		
Gemfibrozil	1. Headaches 2. Fatigue 3. Skin reactions		
Resins	1. GI upset	Vitamin K	— Interfere with absorption
	2. Dyspepsia, flatulence	Folic acid Digoxin	

PEPTIC ULCER DISEASE DRUGS

Table 8.10 Drugs used in peptic ulcer disease

Drug	*Adverse effects*	*Interacting drug(s)*	*Interacting effect*
H_2-receptor antagonists Cimetidine Ranitidine Famotidine	1. Confusion 2. Drowsiness 3. Gynaecomastia 4. Galactorrhoea 5. Loss of libido (antiandrogenic effect with cimetidine)	Diazepam Theophylline β-Blockers Phenytoin Quinidine Tricyclic antidepressants Warfarin	— ↑ effect of interacting drugs (cimetidine inhibits cytochrome P450 metabolism)
Proton pump inhibitors			
Omeprazole	1. Mild and infrequent diarrhoea	Diazepam	Omeprazole reduces the clearance and prolongs elimination
Lansoprazole	1. Skin rash 2. Headache	Phenytoin Warfarin	

ANTIDEPRESSANT, ANXIOLYTIC, ANTIPSYCHOTIC AND ANTIMANIC DRUGS

Table 8.11 Antidepressants

Drug	*Adverse effects*	*Interacting drug(s)*	*Interacting effect*
Tricyclic antidepressants *Older tricyclics* e.g. amitryptilene, imipramine, dothiepin *Tetracyclics* e.g. mianserin *5HT-uptake blocks (SSRI)* Mixed e.g. trazodone, lofepramine Selective e.g. fluoxetine *Monoamine oxidase inhibitors* e.g. phenelzine *Thioxanthines* e.g. flupenthixol Newer agents have less cardiotoxic and anticholinergic effects. Selective 5HT inhibitors are not sedating, but can cause nausea, tremor, sexual dysfunction and dizziness	1. Postural hypotension 2. Arrhythmias and conduction defects (quinidine-like), e.g. prolonged PR, QRS, PT intervals, T wave flattening, ST depression 3. Anticholinergic effects 4. Confusion in the elderly 5. Lowering of seizure threshold	Phenothiazines Anticholinergic agents Antihistamines Antiparkinsonian drugs MAOI Ethanol, sedatives	(Phenothiazines, anticholinergic agents, antihistamines, antiparkinsonian drugs) — ↑ anticholinergic effects — (See below) — ↑ CNS effects of interacting drugs
Monoamine oxidase inhibitors (MAOI) *Hydrazine group* e.g. iproniazid, phenelzine *Non-hydrazine groups* e.g. tranylcypromine, pargyline	1. Jaundice 2. Anticholinergic effects	(a) **Tyramine-containing foodstuffs** Mature cheese (cream and cottage cheeses safe), yeast extracts, red wine and beer, chicken liver, broad beans, coffee (b) **Indirect sympathomimetic amines** Tricyclic antidepressants Amphetamines Pethidine Barbiturates L-dopa	(i) Hypertensive crisis (risk of subarachnoid haemorrhage) (ii) CNS excitation, hyperpyrexia (iii) Prolongs actions of interacting drugs

Table 8.12 Anxiolytic drugs

Drug	*Adverse effects*	*Interacting effect*
Benzodiazepines *Longer-acting* Diazepam Chlordiazepoxide Nitrazepam Flurazepam Clonazepam *Shorter-acting* Oxazepam Lorazepam Temazepam *Ultra-short-acting* Midazolam	1. Drowsiness and agitation (esp. in the elderly) 2. Incontinence, nightmares and confusion 3. Excessive salivation 4. Thrombophlebitis with IV injections 5. Respiratory depression, hypotension 6. Withdrawal can be associated with, rebound increased, agitation, hallucinations and seizures	Do not interfere with metabolism of other drugs or with warfarin
Chlormethiazole	1. Nasal, conjuctival and bronchial discomfort 2. Respiratory and CVS depression	

Table 8.13 Antipsychotic and antimanic drugs

Drug	*Adverse effects*	*Interacting drugs*	*Interacting effect*
Lithium carbonate	1. Metallic taste 2. Anorexia and diarrhoea 3. Polyuria and polydypsia 4. Nephrogenic diabetes insipidus 5. Tremor 6. Muscle weakness 7. Goitre and hypothyroidism 8. Leucocytosis 9. ECG and EEG changes *Toxicity:* 10. Slurred speech 11. Coarse tremor 12. Ataxia 13. Confusion and fits	Thiazide diuretics Phenothiazines NSAID Carbamazepine Phenytoin Methyldopa	— ↑ lithium toxicity
Phenothiazines Chlorpromazine Promazine Thioridazine Prochlorperazine Perphenazine Fluphenazine	1. Extrapyramidal effects: (i) Parkinsonism (ii) Dystonic reactions (also with haloperidol) (iii) Akathesia (iv) Tardive dyskinesia 2. Neuroleptic malignant syndrome (potentially fatal hypertension, muscle rigidity and autonomic dysfunction) 3. Glucose intolerance 4. Anticholinergic effects 5. Cardiac arrhythmias and postural hypotension	Alcohol Narcotic analgesics	— ↑ CNS effects of interacting drugs

Table 8.13 *(cont.)*

Drug	*Adverse effects*	*Interacting drugs*	*Interacting effect*
Phenothiazines (*continued*)	6. Gynaecomastia, galactorrhoea 7. Corneal and lens opacities 8. Retinal pigmentation 9. Lowering of seizure threshold 10. Hypothermia in the elderly 11. Hypersensitivity reactions not related to dose —cholestatic jaundice —Skin pigmentation and photosensitivity —Agranulocytosis, leucopaenia and eosinophilia		
Non-phenothiazine neuroleptics Haloperidol (butyropherone) Pimozide (diphenylbutypiperidine) Flupenthixol (thioxanthine) Sulpiride (resubstituted benzamide) Clozapine (dibenzepine)	Less likely to cause sedation or extrapyramidal side effects		

ANTICONVULSANTS

Table 8.14 Anticonvulsants

Drug	*Adverse effects*	*Interacting drug(s)*	*Interacting effect*
All anticonvulsants		Phenothiazines Tricyclic antidepressants	— ↓ anticonvulsant effect (i.e. lowering of convulsive threshold)
Phenytoin	1. Nystagmus, dizziness, ataxia 2. Drowsiness *Long-term effects:* 3. Gum hyperplasia 4. Folate deficiency and megaloblastic anaemia	Disulfuram Warfarin Corticosteroids Carbamazepine	— ↓ effect of phenytoin and Interacting drugs (due to enzyme induction)
		Alcohol	
	5. Hypocalcaemia and osteomalacia 6. Hypersensitivity reactions (idiosyncratic) 7. Rashes, SLE syndrome (idiosyncratic) 8. Lymphadenopathy 9. Slurred speech	Chloramphenicol Isoniazid Warfarin Cimetidine Oestrogens	— ↓ effect of phenytoin (due to drug displacement)
Barbiturates			
Phenobarbitone	1. Tolerance and dependence 2. Sedation 3. ↓ REM sleep 4. Confusion in elderly	Alcohol Narcotic analgesics Antihistamines Antidepressants	— ↑ effect of interacting drugs, i.e. ↑ CNS depression
	5. Precipitates porphyria in susceptible individuals 6. Resp. depression 7. Rashes	Warfarin Corticosteroids Phenothiazines Aminophylline Phenytoin Oral contraceptives	— ↓ effect of interacting drugs (due to liver enzyme induction)

Table 8.14 *(cont.)*

Drug	*Adverse effects*	*Interacting drug(s)*	*Interacting effect*
Sodium valproate	*Concentration-dependent:* 1. Anorexia nervosa and vomiting 2. Tremor 3. Hair loss or curling 4. Peripheral oedema 5. Weight gain *Idiosyncratic:* 6. Hepatoxicity, pancreatitis and thrombocytopaenia (rare) 7. Spina bifida in babies exposed in utero (1%)		— Minor inhibitor of drug metabolism Can ↑ concentrations of other anticonvulsant drugs
Carbamazepine		Erythromycin Lithium Isoniazid	— ↑ Effect of interacting drugs
		Warfarin	— ↓Warfarin effect

ANTIPARKINSONIAN DRUGS

Table 8.15 Antiparkinsonian drugs

Drug	*Adverse effects*	*Interacting drug(s)*	*Interacting effect*
Anticholinergic drugs	1. Confusion	Tricyclic antidepressants	— ↑ anticholinergic effects
Benzhexol	2. Anticholinergic side-effects	Phenothiazines	
Benztropine		Antihistamines	
Orphenadrine			
Procyclidine		MAOI	
L-dopa	1. Nausea and vomiting	Vitamin B_6	— ↓ L-dopa effect
	2. Postural hypotension	Phenothiazines	
	3. Cardiac arrhythmias	Haloperidol	
	4. Dystonic reactions, ('on–off' responses)	Methyldopa	
		Metoclopramide	
		MAOI	
	5. Psychosis, confusion		— ↓ L-dopa effect
	6. Positive Coomb's test		

ALCOHOL

Table 8.16 Alcohol (see also Fig. 8.7)

Adverse effects	*Interacting drugs*	*Interacting effect*
GI		
1. Peptic ulceration; malabsorption 2. Fatty liver 3. Cirrhosis and recurrent pancreatitis	Metronidazole Sulphonylureas (esp. chlorpropamide) Chloramphenicol	— Antabuse reaction. Flushing, abdominal colic, vomiting, dizziness and tachycardia (due to inhibition of aldehyde dehydrogenase)
CVS		
1. Arrhythmia esp. atrial fibrillation 2. Congestive cardiomyopathy	Warfarin Phenytoin Tolbutamide	— ↑ effects of interacting drugs with acute alcohol intoxication (due to enzyme inhibition)
Haematology		
1. Macrocytosis	Phenformin	— ↑ risk of lactic acidosis
Neuropsychiatric		
1. Wernicke's and Korsakoff's syndrome 2. Peripheral neuropathy 3. Cerebellar degeneration 4. Retrobulbar neuropathy 5. Psychoses, hallucinations	Hypnotics Sedatives Narcotic analgesics Antihistamines	— ↑ sedative effects (potentiation of central depression)
Metabolic effects		
1. Hypoglycaemia (↓ gluconeogenesis) 2. Hypertriglyceridaemia and hyperuricaemia 3. ↓ albumin and transferrin synthesis 4. ↑ catecholamine release 5. ↑ lipoprotein synthesis 6. Accumulation of fatty acids, ketoacidosis 7. Diuresis and electrolyte disturbance 8. Haemochromatosis and porphyria cutanea tarda 9. Deficiency of protein, calcium and water-soluble vitamins especially thiamine, folate and pyridoxine		

Metabolism of alcohol (Fig. 8.7)

Ethanol can prevent the lethal effects of the ingestion of ethylene glycol (antifreeze). In the presence of ethanol, ethanol and ethylene glycol compete for alchohol dehydrogenase.

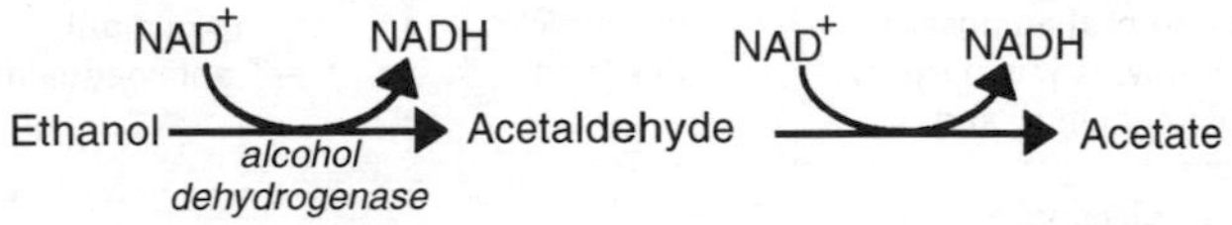

Fig. 8.7

CORTICOSTEROIDS (Tables 8.17 and 8.18)

Table 8.17 Relative properties of various corticosteroids compared to cortisol

Steroid	*Glucocorticoid activity*	*Mineralocorticoid activity*
Cortisol	1.0	1.0
Cortisone	0.7	1.0
Aldosterone	0.3	3000
Fludrocortisone	10	125
Prednisolone	4	1
Dexamethasone	25	0

Table 8.18 Cortisol

Adverse effects	*Interacting drug(s)*	*Interacting effect*
General		
1. Weight gain	Barbiturates Phenytoin Rifampicin	— ↓ corticosteroid effect (due to enzyme induction)
2. Redistribution of body fat (moon face and truncal adiposity)	Warfarin	—↑ anticoagulant effect
3. Skin atrophy, striae, purpura, acne, pigmentation and hirsutism		
4. Cataracts, glaucoma		
CVS/metabolic		
1. Sodium retention and potassium loss		
2. Thirst and polyuria		
3. Hypertension		
4. Hyperglycaemia		
5. Adrenal atrophy and insufficiency (hypotension during anaesthesia and infection)		
Musculoskeletal		
1. Muscle weakness and wasting		
2. Osteoporosis		
3. Growth retardation in children		
4. Aseptic bone necrosis		
GI		
1. Reactivation of peptic ulcer		
Haematological		
1. Polycythaemia		
Immunological		
1. Increased susceptibility to and masking of infection		
2. Reactivation of latent TB		
3. Delayed wound healing		
Psychiatric		
1. Mental disturbances, e.g. euphoria, depression and psychoses		

ORAL CONTRACEPTIVES

Table 8.19 Oral contraceptives
Oestrogens (ethinyloestradiol, norethisterone), progestogens*

Adverse effects	*Interacting drugs*	*Interacting effect*
General		
1. Nausea	Phenytoin	— ↓ contraceptive effect (due to enzyme induction)
2. Headache	Carbamazepine	
3. Fluid retention and weight gain	Phenobarbitone	
4. Hypertension	Rifampicin	
5. Depression	Isoniazid	
6. Loss of libido	Benzodiazepines	
7. Urinary tract infection	Griseofulvin	
8. Genital candidiasis		
9. Jaundice (rare)		
11. Persisting amenorrhoea after stopping pill		
12. Venous thrombosis and embolism		
13. Thrombotic and haemorrhagic stroke		
14. Myocardial infarction		
Metabolic		
1. Precipitate porphyria in susceptible individuals		
2. Impaired glucose tolerance		
3. Increase in cholesterol and triglycerides		
4. Increase in gall bladder disease		
5. ↑ TBG: altered thyroid function tests		
6. Increase in hepatic adenoma (rare) and ? endometrial cancer		

*Adverse effects generally reflect the role of oestrogens. Progestogens may cause irregular menstrual cycles, breakthrough bleeding, amenorrhoea, weight gain and oedema.

Contraindications

Absolute: liver disease, cerebrovascular disease, venous thrombosis, hormone-dependent tumours of the breast, uterus, kidney and malignant melanoma.
Relative: hypertension, gall bladder disease, cardiac failure and nephrogenic oedema.

ORAL HYPOGLYCAEMICS

Table 8.20 Oral hypoglycaemics

Drug	*Adverse effects*	*Interacting drug(s)*	*Interacting effect*
All		Alcohol MAOI β-Blockers* NSAID Aspirin (large doses) Warfarin Chloramphenicol	— ↑ hypoglycaemic effect (due to inhibition of metabolism)
		Corticosteroids Thiazide diuretics Phenothiazines Oral contraceptives Phenytoin Barbiturates Salicylates Lithium Rifampicin As above	— ↓ hypoglycaemic effect (due to enzyme induction)
Sulphonylureas Chlorpropamide Tolbutamide Glibenclamide Glipizide	1. Hypoglycaemia 2. Alcohol intolerance 3. Jaundice (esp. chlorpropamide) 4. Hyponatraemia		
Biguanides Metformin	1. Lactic acidosis 2. Nausea and anorexia 3. Malabsorption of vit. B_{12}	Alcohol	— ↑ risk of lactic acidosis

*Inhibits hypoglycaemia-related tachycardia.

DRUGS USED IN GOUT

Table 8.21 Drugs used in gout*

Drug	*Adverse effects*	*Interacting drug(s)*	*Interacting effect*
Probenecid	1. Rashes 2. Nephrotic syndrome 3. May precipitate acute gout and renal colic	Aspirin (<2 g daily)	— ↓ uricosuric effect
Allopurinol	1. Hypersensitivity reaction 2. May precipitate acute gout	Azathioprine Cyclophosphamide	—↑ toxicity of cytotoxic drugs (due to inhibition of metabolism by xanthine oxidase)
Penicillamine	1. Nausea, loss of taste, rashes 2. Thrombocytopaenia 3. Neutropaenia 4. Proteinuria/nephrotic syndrome		

**Uricosuric drugs:* probenecid (blocks reuptake of uric acid by proximal renal tubule), phenylbutazone, sulphinopyrazone, salicylate in *high* doses (i.e. 5–6 g/day).
Drugs causing gout: thiazide diuretics, loop diuretics, pyrazinamide, ethambutol, salicylate in *low* doses, alcohol, cytotoxic agents, drugs causing haemolysis.
Other drugs: allopurinol (blocks xanthine oxidase), colchicine (binds to microtubular protein and inhibits leucocyte migration).

ANTIBACTERIALS

Table 8.22 Antibacterial drugs (for mechanisms of action see pages 52–53)

Drug	*Adverse effects*	*Interacting drugs*	*Interacting effect*
Penicillins Benzylpenicillin Ampicillin Amoxycillin *Active against β-lactamase-producing bacteria* Flucloxacillin Amoxycillin + clavulanate *Active against Pseudomonas aeroginosa* Carbenicillin Ticarcillin Piperacillin	1. Skin hypersensitivity, fever (including Steven–Johnson syndrome) and anaphylaxis 2. Neurotoxicity, e.g. convulsions (esp. in renal failure and with intrathecal administration) 3. Hyperkalaemia 4. Interstitial nephritis 5. Sodium overload 6. Haemolytic anaemia, thrombocytopaenia		
Tetracyclines	1. Diarrhoea 2. Photosensitivity 3. Candidal infections ↑ urea in patients with impaired renal function 4. Staining of teeth during tooth development	Antacids Oral Fe preparations	— ↓ tetracycline absorption (due to chelation)
Cephalosporins *First generation* Cephradine Cephalexin *Second generation* Cefuroxime* Cephamandole* Cefaclor *Third generation* Cefotaxime Ceftazidime†	1. Hypersensitivity 2. Cross-sensitivity with penicillins (10%) 3. Nephrotoxic (large doses)	Frusemide Alcohol	— ↑ risk of nephrotoxicity — Disulfiram-like reaction

Table 8.22 *(cont.)*

Drug	*Adverse effects*	*Interacting drugs*	*Interacting effect*
Chloramphenicol	1. Dose-related bone marrow depression 2. Non-dose-related aplastic anaemia (rare) 3. Haemolysis in G6PDH deficiency 'Grey baby syndrome'	Warfarin Sulphonylureas Phenytoin Barbiturates	— ↑ effect of interacting drugs (due to liver enzyme inhibition)
Aminoglycosides Gentamicin Amikacin Tobramycin Streptomycin	1. Ototoxicity 2. Nephrotoxicity 3. Malabsorption syndrome (oral neomycin) 4. Aggravation of myasthenia gravis	Frusemide Cephalosporins Amphotericin B }	— ↑ risk of ototoxicity and of nephrotoxicity
Quinolones Ciprofloxacin Ofloxacin	1. GI disturbance 2. Arthritis 3. Lowers seizure threshold	Theophylline	— ↑ side-effects of Theophylline due to ↓ elimination
Nitrofurantoin	1. Nausea and vomiting 2. Rashes and fever 3. Peripheral neuropathy (esp. in renal failure) 4. Hypersensitivity reactions, e.g. pneumonitis 5. Haemolysis in G6PDH deficiency		
Metronidazole	1. GI disturbance 2. Metallic taste 3. Peripheral neuropathy and seizures	Alcohol Warfarin	— 'Antabuse reaction' — ↑ anticoagulant effect (due to enzyme inhibition)

Table 8.22 *(cont.)*

Drug	*Adverse effects*	*Interacting drugs*	*Interacting effect*
Sulphonamides	1. Rashes and photosensitivity 2. Steven–Johnson syndrome 3. Fever 4. Hepatitis 5. Erythema nodosum 6. Kernicterus in the newborn 7. Blood dyscrasias: haemolytic anaemia/ aplastic anaemia 8. Nephrotoxiticity due to crystalluria	Warfarin Phenytoin Sulphonylureas	— ↑ effect of interacting drugs
Glycopeptides			
Vancomycin	1. Thrombophlebitis, 'Red man syndrome'		
Teicoplanin	1. Nausea, anaphylaxis		

*Relatively resistant to β-lactamase.
†Active against *Pseudomonas* infections.

ANTITUBERCULOUS DRUGS

Table 8.23 Antituberculous drugs

Drug	*Adverse effects*	*Interacting drug(s)*	*Interacting effect*
Isoniazid	1. Peripheral neuropathy (corrected by pyridoxine, 50 mg/day) 2. Pellagra-like syndrome 3. Hepatotoxicity and transient rise in aminotransferases +ve ANF and SLE syndrome in slow acetylators 4. Agranulocytosis, haemolytic anaemia	Phenytoin Carbamazepine	— ↑ effects of interacting drugs (due to liver enzyme inhibition)
Ethambutol	1. Retrobulbar neuritis and yellow/green colour vision defects; 2. Transient rise in aminotransferases		
Rifampicin	1. Hepatitis, transient rise in aminotransferases 2. Nephritis 3. Immune thrombocytopaenia 4. Colours urine and sputum pink	Warfarin Oral contraceptives Diazepam Barbiturates β-Blockers Digoxin Oral hypoglycaemics	— ↑ effect of interacting drugs (due to liver enzyme induction)
		Protease inhibitors (indinavit)	— ↑ levels of rifampicin and ↓ levels of indinavir (rifampicin enhances metabolism)
Pyrazinamide	1. Hepatitis; 2. Interstitial nephritis; 3. Hyperuricaemia		
Ansamycin	1. Thrombocytopaenia and leucopaenia 2. GI disturbance	Ketoconazole	— Levels of ansamycin and ketoconazole reduced

ANTIFUNGAL DRUGS

Table 8.24 Antifungal drugs

Drug	*Adverse effects*	*Interacting drug(s)*	*Interacting effect*
Griseofulvin	1. Porphyria in susceptible individuals	Phenobarbitone	— ↑ antifungal effect (due to enzyme induction)
	2. Hepatitis	Warfarin	— ↓ anticoagulant effect (due to enzyme induction)
Amphotericin B	1. Nausea, vomiting and fever 2. Hypersensitivity reactions 3. Nephrotoxicity 4. Normochromic anaemia 5. Hypokalaemia 6. Phlebitis at injection sites	Corticosteroids	— Enhanced potassium loss
Ketoconazole	1. Nausea, vomiting 2. Hepatitis 3. Rashes 4. Gynaecomastia	Warfarin Rifampicin	— ↑ anticoagulant effect — ↓ levels of rifampicin and/or ketoconazole
Fluconazole	GI disturbance	Rifampicin	— ↓ fluconazole levels
Itraconazole	1. Rash 2. Liver damage (fluconazole)	Rifabutin	— ↑ rifabutin levels
Miconazole	1. Reversible liver dysfunction 2. Nausea and vomiting	Warfarin, phenytoin Oral hypoglycaemics	— ↑ effect of interacting drugs (due to protein-binding displacement)
Flucytosine	1. Marrow depression 2. Accumulation in renal failure		

ANTIVIRAL AND ANTIRETROVIRAL AGENTS

Table 8.25 Antiviral drugs

Drug	*Adverse effects*
Amantadine, rimantadine (Influenza A)	1. Renal failure 2. Seizures at high dose
Interferon-alpha (Chronic hepatitis B and C)	1. Influenza-like illness 2. Bone marrow suppression
Foscarnet (CMV retinitis, acyclovir-resistant HSV infections)	1. Nephrotoxicity 2. Hypokalaemia 3. Hypo- and hypercalcaemia
Nucleoside analogues	
Acyclovir (HSV and VZV infections)	1. High therapeutic index 2. Neurotoxicity (<4%) with seizures and hallucinations
Ganciclovir (CMV pneumonia and retinitis)	1. Bone marrow toxicity, Neutropaenia
Cidofovir (CMV infections)	Nephrotoxicity

Table 8.26 Antiretroviral agents

Drug	*Major adverse effects*	*Interacting drug(s)*	*Interacting effect*
Nucleoside reverse transcriptase inhibitors			
Zidovudine (AZT)	1. Anaemia 2. Neutropaenia 3. Myopathy 4. Anorexia 5. Nausea 6. Fatigue 7. Headache 8. Malaise 9. Myalgia 10. Insomnia	Ganciclovir Probenicid	— ↑ risk of haematologic toxicity — ↑ AZT levels
Didanosine (ddI)	1. Pancreatitis (5–9%) 2. Peripheral neuropathy (5–12%) 3. Hyperamylasaemia 4. Diarrhoea 5. Increase in serum urate levels 6. Transaminase elevation	— Avoid drugs that may cause pancreatitis or peripheral neuropathy (e.g. ddC, d4T, isoniazid) — Drugs requiring gastric acidity should be given 2 hours before or after ddI, e.g. tetracyclines, dapsone, ketoconazole and itraconazole	
Dideoxycytidine (ddC)	1. Peripheral neuropathy (17–31%) 2. Pancreatitis 3. Vomiting 4. Rash 5. Stomatitis	Avoid drugs that cause peripheral neuropathy	

Table 8.26 *(cont.)*

Drug	*Major adverse effects*	*Interacting drug(s)*	*Interacting effect*
Stavudine (d4T)	1. Peripheral neuropathy (15–21%) 2. Transaminase elevation 3. Anaemia	Avoid drugs that cause peripheral neuropathy	
Lamivudine (3TC)	1. Headache 2. Nausea 3. Abdominal pain 4. Insomnia		
Protease inhibitors			
Saquinavir	1. Dose-related GI intolerance	Rifampicin	— ↓ saquinavir levels by 80%
		Rifabutin	— ↓ saquinavir levels by 40%
		Phenobarbitone Phenytoin Dexamethasone Carbamazepine	— ↓ saquinavir levels
		Ketoconazole Itraconazole Fluconazole	— ↑ saquinavir levels (inhibition of cytochrome p450)
		Ritonavir	— ↑ saquinavir levels
		Terfenadine Astemizole Cisapride	— saquinavir ↑ drug levels
Indinavir	1. Asymtomatic hyperbilirubinaemia 2. Nephrolithiasis 3. GI intolerance	Ketoconazole	— ↑ indinavir levels
		Rifampicin	— ↓ indinavir levels
		Rifabutin	— ↑ rifampicin and rifabutin levels

Table 8.26 *(cont.)*

Drug	*Major adverse effects*	*Interacting drug(s)*	*Interacting effect*
Protease inhibitors (*continued*)			
Ritonavir	1. GI intolerance 2. Circumoral paraesthesia 3. ↑ cholesterol levels (by 30–40%), and triglyceride levels by 200–300%	Astemizole Amiodarone Cisapride Diazepam Midazolam Piroxicam Rifabutin	Contraindicated because ritonavir is potent inhibitor of p450 system

ANTIMALARIAL DRUGS

Table 8.27 Antimalarial drugs

Drug	*Adverse effects*
Chloroquine (8-aminoquinolines)	1. Retinal and corneal damage 2. Myopathy 3. Photosensitivity 4. Exacerbation of cutaneous porphyria
Primaquine (4-aminoquinolines)	1. Haemolytic anaemia in G6PDH deficiency
Pyrimethamine (diaminopyridamines)	1. Folic acid deficiency 2. Bone marrow depression
Quinine	1. 'Cinchonism' in overdosage
Proguanil (inhibits dihydrofolate, reductase)	1. Apthous mouth ulceration
Mefloquine	1. Neuropsychiatric disturbances Contraindicated in renal and severe hepatic impairment, past psychiatric history, epilepsy, cardiac condition defects, lactation and pregnancy

IMMUNOSUPPRESSANT DRUGS

CYTOTOXIC DRUGS (Fig. 8.8)

Adverse effects

- Antiproliferative effects e.g. marrow suppression, ulceration of GI tract, and, especially with cyclophosphamide, infertility, hair loss, cystitis.
- Steroid effects, e.g. cushingoid appearance, hypertension, diabetes, peptic ulceration, stunted growth, osteoporosis, avascular bone necrosis, cataracts, myopathy.
- Infection: viral, e.g. CMV, HSV, VZV; fungal, e.g. aspergillus, candida, pneumocystitis; bacterial, e.g. tuberculosis, listeria, nocardia.
- Malignancy, e.g. lymphomas, skin tumours.
- Teratogenesis.

OTHER ANTICANCER DRUGS (NON-CYTOTOXIC)

Cyclosporin A

- Main immunosuppressant action is against T-cells. Blocks IL-2.
- *Adverse effects*: hepatotoxicity, nephrotoxicity, hypertension, hypertrichosis gingival hyperplasia and tremor. Increased incidence of lymphoma. Marked absence of bone marrow problems.

Cell cycle and phase specificity of cytotoxic agents

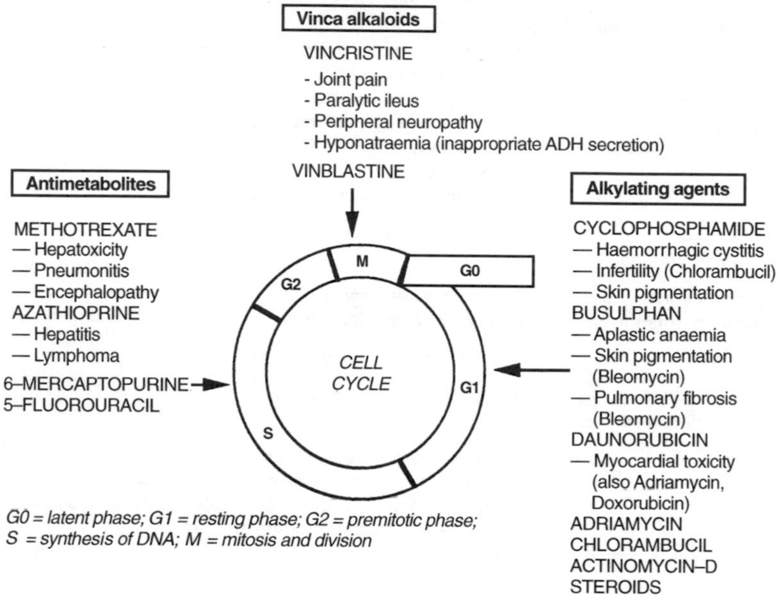

Fig. 8.8

Tamoxifen

- Treatment of oestrogen-dependent cancer.
- *Adverse effects*: hot flushes, nausea and vomiting, hypercalcaemia and ocular changes, i.e. retinopathy and ↓ visual acuity.

Antilymphocyte globulin

- *Adverse effects*: serum sickness, fever.

Colony-stimulating factors (CSF)

E.g. granulocyte-CSF (G-CSF), granulocyte macrophage-colony-stimulating factor (GM-CSF).

- Stimulate haematopoiesis. Produced by recombinant DNA technology.
- *Adverse reactions*: bone pain and liver dysfunction with G-CSF, and rashes, fever and myalgia with GM-CSF. Vasculitis, deep vein thrombosis and pulmonary embolus have been reported with high-dose GM-CSF.

ADVERSE EFFECTS IN SPECIAL RISK GROUPS

DRUGS IN PREGNANCY

Adverse effects may occur at any time but especially during the first trimester.

1st trimester (Table 8.28)

Period of greatest risk is considered to be 3rd–11th week of pregnancy ('teratogenesis').

Table 8.28 Drugs in pregnancy: 1st trimester

Teratogenic drugs	*Adverse effects*
Cytotoxic drugs e.g. methotrexate, cyclophosphamide	Fetal malformations
Thalidomide	Phocomelia, congenital heart disease and stenosis
Androgens Danazol	Virilization and other congenital defects
Diethylstilboestrol	Adenocarcinoma of vagina
Warfarin	Fetal warfarin syndrome*
Alcohol	Fetal alcohol syndrome†
Radioactive iodine	Fetal thyroid damage
Others: live vaccines, oral contraceptives, lithium, and amphetamines	

*Hypoplastic nose, upper airway difficulties, optic atrophy, mental handicap.
†Mental handicap, microcephaly, congenital heart disease, renal anomaly, growth retardation, cleft palate, characteristic facies.

2nd and 3rd trimester (Table 8.29)

Drugs with important adverse effects on fetal growth and development.

Table 8.29 Drugs in pregnancy: 2nd and 3rd trimester

Drug	*Adverse effects*
Aminoglycosides	Ototoxicity
Tetracyclines	Impaired fetal bone growth, teeth discoloration
Chloramphenicol	Peripheral vascular collapse ('grey baby syndrome')
Sulphonamides	Kernicterus, methaemoglobinaemia
Quinine, chloroquine	Retinopathy, congenital deafness, corneal opacities
Antithyroid drugs	Neonatal hypothyroidism and goitre
Aspirin*	Haemorrhagic disease of the newborn
NSAIDs†	Kernicterus, premature closure of ductus arteriosus
Thiazide diuretics, β-blockers	Neonatal thrombocytopaenia Fetal bradycardia
High concentrations of O_2 (> 35%)	Retrolental fibroplasia and blindness
Opiates, barbiturates, diazepam	Respiratory depression, drowsiness
Lithium	Congenital heart disease (Ebstein's complex)
Sodium valproate	Neural tube defect (1–2%), hypospadias, microstomia, developmental delay
Corticosteroids	Growth inhibition
Cytotoxic drugs	Inhibition of intellectual development

*Heparin is the drug of choice for anticoagulation at any time during pregnancy, since it does not cross the placenta.
†Prostaglandin-synthetase inhibitors.

DRUGS EXCRETED IN BREAST MILK

Drugs to be avoided when breast feeding

1. Antibiotics, e.g. aminoglycosides, sulphonamides, tetracycline, metronidazole, chloramphenicol.
2. Anti-TB drugs, e.g. isoniazid.
3. CNS drugs, e.g. narcotic analgesics, benzodiazepines, chlorpromazine.
4. Antithyroid drugs, e.g. carbimazole, radioactive iodine.
5. Anticonvulsant drugs, e.g. phenytoin, phenobarbitone
6. Anticoagulant drugs, e.g. phenindiones (warfarin and heparin are acceptable). Aspirin is associated with a theoretical risk of Reye's syndrome.
7. Cytotoxic drugs and high dose corticosteroids.

Lactation is suppressed by: frusemide, bromocriptine, oestrogens.

Drugs safe in breast feeding

1. Penicillins, cephalosporins.
2. Theophylline, salbutamol by inhaler, prednisolone.
3. Sodium valproate, carbamazepine, phenytoin.
4. Beta-blockers, methyldopa, hydralazine.
5. Warfarin, heparin.
6. Haloperidol, chlorpromazine.
7. Tricyclic antidepressants.

DRUGS IN THE ELDERLY (Table 8.30)

Table 8.30 Drugs in the elderly

Drugs to be used with caution	*Adverse effects*
Benzodiazepines (especially if long $t_{1/2}$)	— Prolonged CNS depression
Barbiturates	— Confusional states, hypothermia
Phenothiazines	— Hypotension, parkinsonism, extrapyramidal reactions, hypothermia
Antiparkinsonian drugs, (e.g. benzhexol, L-dopa) Anticholinergic drugs and Tricyclic antidepressants	— ↑ anticholinergic effects, hallucinations and disorientation
Antihypertensive agents	— More prone to postural hypotension
Diuretics	— Hypokalaemia, hypomagnesaemia, incontinence
Digoxin	— Toxic effects more common
Anticoagulants	— ↑ risk of haemorrhage

DRUGS IN LIVER DISEASE (Table 8.31)

Table 8.31 Drugs in liver disease

Drugs to be used with caution	*Adverse effects*
Drugs whose main route of metabolism is via the liver, e.g. phenytoin, warfarin, narcotic analgesics, theophylline, corticosteroids, barbiturates, phenothiazines and antimicrobials (clindamycin, rifampicin, isoniazid, ethambutol, erythromycin)	— ↑ risk of toxic effects
Drugs causing fluid retention, e.g. NSAIDS, corticosteroids	— Exacerbate fluid retention
Sedative drugs	— May precipitate hepatic encephalopathy
Hepatotoxic drugs	— Dose-dependent and hypersensitivity reactions more likely
Diuretics (especially non-potassium sparing)	— May precipitate hepatic encephalopathy

DRUGS IN RENAL DISEASE

Drugs accumulate in renal failure if excreted mainly or entirely by the kidney.

Drugs to be avoided

1. Antimicrobials, e.g. tetracyclines, nitrofurantoin, amphotericin B.
2. Cardiovascular drugs, e.g. potassium-sparing diuretics, potassium supplements.
3. Narcotic analgesics, e.g. meperidine.
4. Aspirin and NSAIDs.
5. Psychotropic drugs, e.g. lithium.

Drugs requiring dose adjustment in renal failure

1. Antimicrobials, e.g. penicillin G, ampicillin, aminoglycosides, cephalosporins, sulphonamides, vancomycin, metronidazole.
2. Cardiovascular drugs, e.g. methyldopa, digoxin, procainamide, disopyramide and ACE inhibitors, flecainide.
3. Others, e.g. chlorpropamide, insulin, H_2-antagonists.

Drugs which can be used in normal dose

1. Antimicrobials, e.g. cloxacillin, oxacillin, clindamycin, chloramphenicol, doxycycline, erythromycin, pyrimethamine, rifampicin and isoniazid.
2. Cardiovascular drugs, e.g. clonidine, calcium antagonists, hydralazine and prazosin, thiazide and loop diuretics.
3. Narcotic analgesics, e.g. codeine, morphine, naloxone, pentazocine and propoxyphene.

4. Psychotropic drugs, e.g. barbiturates, tricyclic antidepressants, haloperidol.
5. Oral anticoagulants, e.g. warfarin and phenindione.
6. Others, e.g. steroids, tolbutamide and theophylline.

ANTIDOTES USED IN OVERDOSE

Table 8.32 Antidotes used in overdose

Drug	*Antidote*
Digoxin	Fab antibody fragments to digoxin
Iron	Desferioxamine (chelating agent)
Lead	Penicillamine or calcium sodium edetate
Heavy metals (arsenic, mercury or gold)	Dimercaprol or D-penicillamine
Anticholinesterases	Pralidoxime (cholinesterase reactivator) and atropine (competitive antagonist at acetylcholine receptor)
Cyanide*	Sodium thiosulphate or cobalt edetate
Paracetamol (acetaminophen)	N-acetyl cysteine† or methionine
Methanol	IV ethanol (competes with alcohol dehydrogenase)
Carbon monoxide	Oxygen
Opiates	Naloxone/naltrexone (competitive antagonist at opiate receptor)
Benzodiazepines	Flumazenil
Warfarin	Vitamin K
Monoamine oxidase inhibitors	Hypertensive crisis: α-blocker, chlorpromazine and β-blocker

*Inhibits cytochrome oxidase by complexing copper in the carrier. This prevents the reduction of molecular oxygen and causes the complete reduction of all electron transport carriers.

†After an overdose of paracetamol, the predominant pathways of elimination by conjugation to sulphate and glucuronic acid become saturated. An increasing amount of the drug is activated by the cytochrome p450 system and conjugated with the sulphahydryl group of glutathione. When the stores of glutathione are depleted, the reactive intermediates of paracetamol bind covalently to liver macromolecules, causing liver necrosis. Early administration of N-acetyl cysteine replenishes glutathione stores which protect against paracetamol toxicity.

Drugs for which dialysis in overdosage may be indicated

Salicylates
Methanol
Barbiturates
Lithium carbonate
Procainamide
Disopyramide
Aminoglycosides
Cephalosporins
Sulphonamides

Drugs not significantly removed by dialysis

Dextropropoxiphene
Benzodiazepines
Phenytoin
Phenothiazines
Tricyclic antidepressants
Oral hypoglycaemics
β-Blockers
Digoxin
Hydralazine
Rifampicin
Tetracycline
Benzylpenicillin
Flucloxacillin
Amphotericin
Erythromycin

High concentrations of antimicrobial drugs in CSF, bile and urine (Table 8.33)

Table 8.33 Antimicrobial drugs achieving high concentrations in CSF, bile and urine

CSF	*Bile*	*Urine*
Chloramphenicol	Penicillins	Penicillins
Erythromycin	Cephalosporins	Cephalosporins
Isoniazid	Erythromycin	Aminoglycosides
Pyrazinamide		Sulphonamides
Rifampicin		Nitrofurantoin
Flucytosine		Nalidixic acid
		Ethambutol
		Flucytosine

SUMMARY OF DRUG-INDUCED DISEASE

CARDIOVASCULAR SYSTEM

HYPERTENSION

Corticosteroids, ACTH
Oral contraceptives
Non-steroidal anti-inflammatory drugs (NSAIDs)
MAOI with sympathomimetic agents
Clonidine and methyldopa withdrawal

CONGESTIVE CARDIAC FAILURE/FLUID RETENTION

As above plus —
Arterial vasodilators, e.g. minoxidil and hydralazine
β-Blockers
Verapamil

EXACERBATION OF ANGINA

Vasopressin, oxytocin
β-Blocker withdrawal
Excessive thyroxine
α-Blockers
Hydralazine

DIRECT MYOCARDIAL TOXICITY

Cytotoxic agents, e.g. doxorubicin, daunorubicin, vincristine
Anaesthetic agents, e.g. halothane
Alcohol

RESPIRATORY SYSTEM

BRONCHOSPASM

β-Blockers
Aspirin, NSAIDs
Cholinergic drugs, e.g. pilocarpine
Cholinesterase inhibitors, e.g. pyridostigmine
Prostaglandin $F_2\alpha$
Any drug causing anaphylaxis

PULMONARY FIBROSIS

Cytotoxic agents, e.g. busulphan, bleomycin and methotrexate
Nitrofurantoin
Sulphasalazine
Prolonged high dose oxygen
Practolol
Amiodarone

PLEURAL REACTION

Practolol
Drug-induced lupus syndrome, e.g. procainamide, hydralazine
Bromocriptine
Methotrexate

ACUTE PULMONARY OEDEMA

Salicylates
β-Blockers
Narcotics, e.g. methadone and diamorphine
Contrast media

RENAL SYSTEM

DIRECT NEPHROTOXICITY: ACUTE TUBULAR NECROSIS

Antibiotics, e.g. aminoglycosides, tetracyclines and amphotericin B
Cytotoxic agents (due to uric acid deposition)
Solvents, e.g. CCl_4, ethylene glycol
Paracetamol overdose
Heavy metals, e.g. mercury, bismuth
Radio-iodinated contrast media
Drug combinations:
1. Cephaloridine and frusemide
2. Gentamicin and frusemide

ACUTE INTERSTITIAL NEPHRITIS

Antibiotics, e.g. penicillins, sulphonamides, tetracycline
Anti-TB drugs, e.g. rifampicin, streptomycin
Frusemide, thiazide diuretics
NSAIDs, analgesic abuse
Radiation nephritis
Phenytoin

RENAL TUBULAR ACIDOSIS

Degraded tetracycline
Amphotericin B
Acetozolamide

NEPHROTIC SYNDROME (accounts for 2% cases)

Penicillamine
Gold salts and other heavy metals
Mercurials
NSAIDs
Probenecid
Angiotensin-converting enzyme inhibitors, e.g. high dose captopril

URINARY RETENTION

Diuretics with prostate enlargement
MAOI
Anticholinergic agents, e.g. tricyclic antidepressants, disopyramide

GASTROINTESTINAL SYSTEM

OESOPHAGEAL ULCERATION

Tetracycline
Ferrous salts
Doxycycline
Disodium etidronate (bisphosphonate used in treatment of osteoporosis)

NAUSEA AND VOMITING

Digoxin
Opiates
Oestrogens
L-dopa
Theophylline
Bromocryptine
Tetracycline
Quinidine

PANCREATITIS

Azathioprine
Sulphonamides
Methyldopa

DIARRHOEA

Antibacterial drugs
Digoxin
Magnesium salts
Laxative abuse

CONSTIPATION

Opiates
Anticholinergic drugs
Phenothiazines
Aluminium hydroxide
Ferrous salts

HEPATITIS (2–3 weeks after exposure)

Halothane (repeated administration)
MAOI
Anticonvulsants
Methyldopa
Anti-TB, e.g. rifampicin, isoniazid, pyrizinamide

INTRAHEPATIC CHOLESTASIS ± HEPATITIS

(Hypersensitivity 3–6 weeks after exposure)
Phenothiazines
Tricyclic antidepressants
NSAIDs
Sulphonylureas
Anti-TB drugs, e.g. rifampicin, isoniazid
Antibiotics, e.g. erythromycin, carbenicillin, sulphonamides

CHOLESTASIS ALONE

Anabolic steroids
Oral contraceptives

HEPATOXINS

Tetracycline
CCL_4
Paracetamol
Methotrexate
Aflatoxin

ENDOCRINE SYSTEM

GALACTORRHOEA

Methyldopa
Phenothiazines, haloperidol
L-dopa
Metoclopramide
Cimetidine
Benzodiazepines
Oestrogens
Tricyclic antidepressants

GYNAECOMASTIA

Antiandrogens:
Spironolactone (without galactorrhoea)
Cimetidine (without galactorrhoea)
Methyldopa
Phenothiazines
Tricyclic antidepressants
Cytotoxic agents
Digoxin (without galactorrhoea)
Oestrogens

HYPOTHYROIDISM

Iodides
Antithyroid drugs, e.g. carbimazole, thiouracil
Lithium
Amiodarone

VAGINAL CARCINOMA

Diethylstilboestrol (administered to mother)

METABOLIC

HYPERGLYCAEMIA

Corticosteroids
Oral contraceptives
Diuretics (loop and thiazide)

HYPOGLYCAEMIA

Alcohol
Salicylates and NSAIDs
β-Blockers

HYPERCALCAEMIA

Antacids (Ca^{2+} salts)
Vitamin D
Thiazide diuretics
Oestrogen therapy in cancer

HYPERURICAEMIA

See page 268.

HYPERKALAEMIA

Potassium-sparing diuretics
Cytotoxic agents
Steroid withdrawal
ACEI, e.g. captopril, enalapril

HYPOKALAEMIA

(See also page 180.)
Diuretics
Laxative abuse
Corticosteroids
Amphotericin B
Insulin

HYPONATRAEMIA/INAPPROPRIATE ADH

See page 180.

NEPHROGENIC DIABETES INSIPIDUS

Lithium
Demethylchlortetracycline

METABOLIC ACIDOSIS

See page 169.

OSTEOMALACIA

Anticonvulsants (long-term), e.g. phenytoin, barbiturates

EXACERBATION OF PORPHYRIA

See page 331.

BLOOD DISEASES

APLASTIC ANAEMIA OR NEUTROPAENIA

1. Cytotoxic agents
2. Antibiotics, e.g. chloramphenicol, sulphonamides, methicillin, ampicillin, cotrimoxazole
3. Anti-TB, e.g. rifampicin
4. Antimalarials, e.g. pyrimethamine, chloroquine
5. Antirheumatic agents, e.g. gold salts, penicillamine, NSAID (phenylbutazone)
6. Dapsone
7. Antithyroid, e.g. carbimazole
8. Oral hypoglycaemics, e.g. sulphonylureas
9. Anticonvulsants, e.g. carbamazepine, phenytoin
10. Tricyclic antidepressants
11. Anticoagulants, e.g. phenindione
12. Diuretics, e.g. thiazides, frusemide
13. Psychotropic drugs, e.g. phenothiazines, clozapine (agranulocytosis, 1:300)
14. Antiarrhythmics, e.g. quinidine, procainamide

THROMBOCYTOPAENIA

As above, but especially:
Diuretics (thiazide and loop)
Antirheumatic agents, e.g. aspirin, NSAIDs
Antibiotics, e.g. rifampicin, carbenicillin, cotrimoxazole, quinine, quinidine
Methyldopa
Anticonvulsants, e.g. phenytoin, carbamazepine
Heparin

MEGALOBLASTIC ANAEMIA (Fig. 8.9)

FOLATE DEFICIENCY

Dihydrofolate reductase inhibitors, e.g. methotrexate, pyrimethamine, trimethoprim

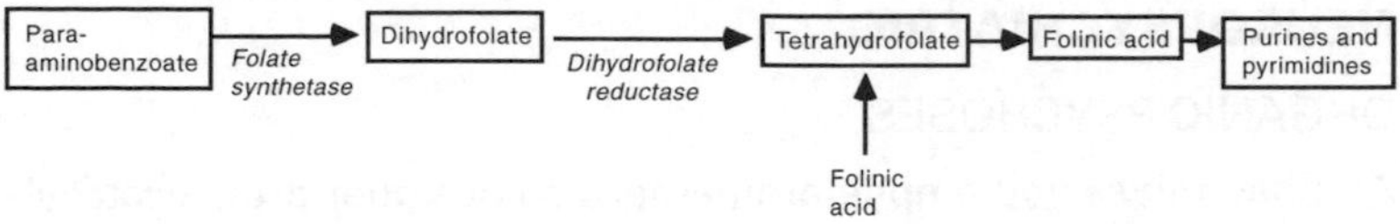

Fig. 8.9

Sulphonamides
Impaired absorption, e.g. cholestyramine, sulphasalazine
Uncertain mechanisms, e.g. anticonvulsants, ethanol and oral contraceptives

HAEMOLYTIC ANAEMIA

- Mainly in G6PDH deficiency (see page 331).
- Immune haemolysis

  Type I: Antibodies directed against the drug, e.g. penicillin, quinidine, methyldopa, dapsone

  Type II: Drug combines with an antibody and immune complex absorbed onto cells, e.g.
  Isoniazid
  Phenacetin
  Quinine, quinidlne
  Sulphonamides
  Sulphonylureas

  Type III: Autoimmune (autoimmune haemolytic anaemia)
  Methyldopa (+ve Coomb's test)
  L-dopa
  Mefenamic acid
  Cephalosporins (+ve Coomb's test)
  Rifampicin.
- Drugs with direct toxicity, e.g. phenacetin abuse.

B_{12} DEFICIENCY

Colchicine
Neomycin
Metformin

METHAEMOGLOBINAEMIA

See page 265.

LYMPHADENOPATHY

Phenytoin
Phenybutazone
Dapsone

NEUROPSYCHIATRIC

ORGANIC PSYCHOSES

Amphetamines and amphetamine-derived designer drug 'ecstasy'
Anticholinergic drugs, e.g. atropine, benzhexol, L-dopa, and dopamine agonists, e.g. bromocriptine
Steroids
Phencyclidine, e.g. PCP: 'angel dust'
Cannabis

DRUG WITHDRAWAL STATES

Benzodiazepines
Clonidine
Barbiturates
Opiates
Alcohol

CONFUSIONAL STATES

Alcohol
Sedatives and hypnotics, e.g. barbiturates, benzodiazepines
Tricyclic antidepressants
Phenothiazines
Anticholinergic drugs
Antiparkinsonian drugs, e.g. benzhexol, L-dopa
Opiates
Digoxin
Isoniazid

DEPRESSION

Corticosteroids
Centrally acting antihypertensives e.g. methyldopa, clonidine
β-Blockers
Oral contraceptives (4–6% of cases)
Phenothiazines
Opiates, benzodiazepines,
Alcohol
L-dopa

EXTRAPYRAMIDAL REACTIONS

Parkinsonism
Phenothiazines e.g. chlorpromazine
Butyrophenones e.g. haloperidol
Metoclopramide
Carbon monoxide

Dystonic reactions
Tricyclic antidepressants
L-dopa, bromocriptine
Methyldopa
Oral contraceptives (chorea)

PERIPHERAL NEUROPATHY

Cytotoxic agents, e.g. vincristine, vinblastine
Antibiotics, e.g. nitrofurantoin, streptomycin, metronidazole nalidixic acid, chloramphenicol
Oral hypoglycaemics, e.g. sulphonylureas
Anti-TB, e.g. isoniazid, ethambutol
MAOI, e.g. phenelzine
Tricyclic antidepressants
Amiodarone

PROXIMAL MYOPATHY

Corticosteroids
Chloroquine
Amiodarone
Oral contraceptives
Amphotericin B

ACUTE RHABDOMYOLYSIS

Diamorphine
Barbiturates
Diazepam
Isoniazid
Amphotericin B

EXACERBATIONS OF MYASTHENIA

Aminoglycosides
Polymixins
Opiates

PSEUDOTUMOUR CEREBRI (papilloedema)

Corticosteroids
Oral contraceptives
Tetracyclines
Hypervitaminosis A

SEXUAL DYSFUNCTION

IMPOTENCE

Antihypertensives, e.g. methyldopa, clonidine
β-Blockers
Antidepressants, e.g. tricyclics
Antiandrogens, e.g. cimetidine, cyproterone acetate

DECREASED LIBIDO AND ERECTILE IMPOTENCE

Antihypertensives, e.g. clonidine, methyldopa, β-blockers and thiazide diuretics
Sedatives, e.g. opiates, ethanol
Cytotoxic drugs
Lithium

FAILURE OF EJACULATION

Antihypertensives, e.g. methyldopa
Psychotropic agents
Tricyclic antidepressants

OTOLOGICAL

DEAFNESS/TINNITUS/VERTIGO

Aminoglycosides
Quinine and quinidine ('cinchonism')
Salicylates
Frusemide

EYE

CORNEAL OPACITIES

Phenothiazines, esp. chlorpromazine
Chloroquine
Amiodarone
Indomethacin
Corticosteroids
Vitamin D

CATARACT

Corticosteroids
Phenothiazines, esp. chlorpromazine
Cytotoxic agents, e.g. busulphan, chlorambucil

RETINOPATHY

Chloroquine, quinine
Phenothiazines, esp. high dose thioridazine
Penicillamine
Indomethacin

OPTIC NEURITIS

Anti-TB, e.g. ethambutol, streptomycin, isoniazid
Digoxin
Alcohol
Chloramphenicol

DERMATOLOGICAL

FEVER (± other features of hypersensitivity)

Antihistamines
Hydralazine, methyldopa
Isoniazid, nitrofurantoin
Penicillin
Salicylates
Quinidine, procainamide
Phenytoin
Chlorambucil, 6-mercaptopurine

SERUM SICKNESS

Aspirin
Penicillins
Streptomycin
Sulphonamides

SLE-LIKE SYNDROME

Antibiotics, e.g. griseofulvin, penicillin, streptomycin, tetracyclines, sulphonamides
Anti-TB drugs, e.g. isoniazid
Anticonvulsants, e.g. carbamazepine, phenytoin
Antihypertensives, e.g. hydralazine, methyldopa
Antiarrhythmics, e.g. practolol, procainamide
Antirheumatics, e.g. gold, phenylbutazone

ERYTHEMA NODOSUM

Antibiotics, e.g. penicillin, sulphonamides
Dapsone
Salicylates, phenylbutazone
Sulphonylureas, e.g. chlorpropamide
Oral contraceptives
Gold salts

FIXED DRUG ERUPTIONS

Antibiotics, e.g. penicillins, sulphonamides, tetracyclines
Phenytoin
Salicylates, phenylbutazone
Barbiturates
Antihistamines
Quinine
Captopril
Dapsone

ERYTHEMA MULTIFORME OR STEVEN–JOHNSON SYNDROME

Barbiturates
Salicylates, phenylbutazone
Antibiotics, e.g. tetracycline, sulphonamide
Phenytoin, carbamazepine
Thiazide diuretics
Chlorpropamide

TOXIC EPIDERMAL NECROLYSIS

Barbiturates
Phenytoin
Penicillin

PIGMENTATION

ACTH
Phenothiazines
Amiodarone
Antimalarials, e.g. chloroquine, androgens
Cytotoxic agents, e.g. bulsulphan, cyclophosphamide
Phenytoin
Heavy metals, e.g. gold salts, mercury, arsenic
Corticosteroids,
Hypervitaminosis A
Oral contraceptives

RAYNAUD'S SYNDROME

Ergotamine
β-Blockers
Clonidine

PHOTOSENSITIVITY

Antibiotics, e.g. sulphonamides, tetracyclines, griseofulvin, nalidixic acid
Sulphonylureas
Thiazide diuretics
Phenothiazines
Oestrogens and progesterones

LOSS OR ALTERATION OF TASTE

Penicillamine
Griseofulvin
Lithium
Metronidazole
Gold salts
ACE inhibitors

HIRSUTISM/HYPERTRICHOSIS

Diazoxide
Minoxidil
Corticosteroids

ALOPECIA

Cytotoxic agents
Anticoagulants, e.g. heparin
Withdrawal of oral contraceptives
Antithyroid agents
L-dopa
Gold salts

Index